Concepts and Practice of Humanitarian Medicine

Concepts and Practice
of Humanitarian Medicine

Edited by

S. William A. Gunn, MD, FRCSC, FRCSI(Hon), DSc(Hon), Dr h c
President, International Association for Humanitarian Medicine
Formerly Head, Emergency Humanitarian Operations, World Health
Organization

Michele Masellis, MD
Director, International Association for Humanitarian Medicine
President, Mediterranean Council for Burns and Fire Disasters

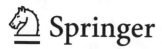 Springer

S. William A. Gunn
International Association
for Humanitarian Medicine
Bogis-Bossey
Switzerland

Michele Masellis
Mediterranean Council
for Burns and Fire Disasters
Palermo
Italy

ISBN: 978-1-4419-2471-1   e-ISBN: 978-0-387-72264-1

This book is dedicated to

the vision of Dr George Brock Chisholm, O.C.
and to

the action of the World Health Organization,
1948–2008

Preface

Parallel with their spectacular and life-saving advances in biotechnology, the health sciences have been increasingly strengthening their responsibility and humanitarian action. Current inequalities, conflicts, and stresses, however, continue to disadvantage the health and well being of an unacceptably large proportion of the world's population, whether in developing countries, in industrially insalubrious environments, in disaster situations, in chronic poverty, or in sick opulence. Several intergovernmental and non-governmental institutions, in particular the World Health Organization and the medical profession, address these issues boldly, yet the problem continues and in many aspects is becoming worse. In the face of this situation, a group of concerned professionals from many disciplines established the International Association for Humanitarian Medicine Brock Chisholm, based on the principles of the United Nations, the Red Cross, the World Health Organization, the WHO Collaborating Centre, and WHO's founding father, Dr G. Brock Chisholm.

The beginnings of the Association go back to 1984, to the Brock Chisholm Memorial Trust, now incorporated as the International Association for Humanitarian Medicine Brock Chisholm (IAHM), with an expanded mission.

This is not a question of repeating a Red Cross, or Médecins Sans Frontières, or Save the Children, nor, of course, of duplicating any of the specialized functions of the World Health Organization or of Amnesty International. It is not a question of rushing to an epidemic focus, disaster site, refugee camp, or torture prison. Many, many are doing these, and are doing them well. Certainly basic, essential care must be made available, and there are those who make them available. Yet Health for All remains far from being within the reach of all. We would like to be in a position of helping that dream come true. It is every human being's right to have access to such essential care, the human right to health.

Besides such basic health care, many working in developing countries and disaster situations have noted with dismay that any patient needing a slightly advanced, let alone specialized, treatment usually falls by the wayside. Without in any way encroaching upon programmes of primary health care or disaster relief, IAHM would like to and can fill this niche, can respond to these situations and provide the kind of specialized health care that is not available in poor country x or disaster site y, all within a humanitarian philosophy. To this end, IAHM has an open-ended network of hospitals on the one hand, and of health providers and specialists on the other, who, in many countries, have formally agreed to look after such patients, without charge, on an entirely humanitarian basis. It has been christened World Open Hospital (WOH), and any hospital or any physician can join it any time. Therefore:

In conceptual yet tangible ways IAHM aims at:

- promoting the precept of health as a human right;
- strengthening the contribution of health as a bridge to peace;
- advancing humanitarian principles in the practice of medicine;
- facilitating the availability of Health for All.

In practical terms the Association will additionally:

- provide specialized medical and surgical treatment, free of charge, in or from countries where such treatment is not possible;
- mobilize hospitals in developed countries to receive, and doctors to treat, such patients entirely on a humanitarian basis;
- provide similar services in disaster situations;
- collaborate with institutions pursuing similar objectives.

Our definition of humanitarian medicine should facilitate understanding the spirit and mission of the International Association for Humanitarian Medicine Brock Chisholm:

> While all medical intervention to reduce a person's sickness and suffering is in essence humanitarian, Humanitarian Medicine goes beyond the usual therapeutic act and promotes, provides, teaches, supports, and delivers people's health as a human right, in conformity with the ethics of Hippocratic teaching, the principles of the World Health Organization, the Charter of the United Nations, the Universal Declaration of Human Rights, the Red Cross Conventions and other covenants and practices that ensure the most humane and best possible level of care, without any discrimination or consideration of material gain.

In 2005, the International Association for humanitarian Medicine published the first book entirely dedicated to humanitarian medicine. This is a sequel to that volume, expanding the basic concepts and adding 14 chapters. Like its predecessor, this new edition is respectfully offered to the global and humanitarian health community.

S.W.A. Gunn
M. Masellis

Acknowledgments

This publication and its predecessor *Humanitarian Medicine* have been made possible through the continuous collaboration of the Brock Chisholm Memorial Trust, the International Association for Humanitarian Medicine, and with the generous financial assistance of the Sicilian Regional Parliament. These expressions of support are gratefully acknowledged.

Special thanks are also due to the Regents, authors, participating experts, and humanitarian health organizations for their valuable scientific, medical, and moral contributions to the mission and growth of humanitarian medicine.

The sources of articles reproduced by gracious permission have been duly acknowledged in the respective chapters. Bill Tucker and Khristine Queja of Springer Science are to be thanked for valuable editorial assistance.

Contents

Part IV   Disasters and Conflicts

Part V   Science, Research and Perspectives

Part VI   Society, Health and Equity

The Contributors

Kofi Annan
Former Secretary General
of the United Nations
Nobel Peace Prize, 2001

Jean Philippe Assal
Formerly Professor
of Therapeutic Education
University of Geneva
Member International Committee
of the Red Cross
Regent of the International Association
for Humanitarian Medicine

Yves Beigbeder
Formerly of the United Nations
and the World
Health Organization
Regent of the International Association
for Humanitarian Medicine

Rosalie Bertell
President-Emerita
International Institute
of Concern for Public Health
Regent, International Association
for Humanitarian Medicine

Boutros Boutros-Ghali
Former Secretary General
of the United Nations

Manuel Carballo
Doctor of Medicine
Executive Director of the
International Organization
for Migration

Jan T. Christenson
Secretary General
Global Forum for Humanitarian
Medicine in Cardiology
and Cardiac Surgery

Paddy Dewan
Professor of Paediatric Urology
University of Melbourne
Director Kind Cuts for Kids programme
Regent of the International Association
for Humanitarian Medicine

Xavier Emmanuelli
Director
SAMU Social
Paris
Co-founder of Médecins sans Frontières
Nobel Peace Laureate 1999
Regent, International Association for
Humanitarian Medicine

Fernando Fabò
Reverend, Pontifical Council
for Health Pastorate
The Vatican

Jean Marie Fonrouge†
Late Director of Humanitarian Action
International Carrefour Foundation
Paris
Regent, International Association
for Humanitarian Medicine

G. Gargano
Department of Obstetrics
and Gynaecology
Modena

William C. Gibson
Chancellor Emeritus
University of Victoria
Canada
Regent, International Association
for Humanitarian Medicine

S.William A. Gunn
President
International Association
for Humanitarian Medicine
President Emeritus
World Association for Disaster
and Emergency Medicine

C. Rollins Hanlon
Past President
Executive Consultant
American College of Surgeons
Regent, International Association
for Humanitarian Medicine

Kendall Ho
Professor
Knowledge Transmission
University of British Columbia
Health Advisor
Government of B.C. Regent
International Association
for Humanitarian Medicine

Sir Robert Jackson†
Former Under-Secretary General
Special Advisor to the Secretary
General
United Nations

Radana Königová
Professor of Burns Surgery
Charles University
Prague
Regent, International Association
for Humanitarian Medicine

Jong-Wook Lee†
Late Director-General
of the World Health Organization

Gudjón Magnússon
Dean, Nordic School of Public Health
Regent, International Association
for Humanitarian Medicine

Halfdan Mahler
Director-General Emeritus
World Health Organization
Regent, International Association
for Humanitarian Medicine

Giuseppe Masellis
Director
Department of Obstetrics
and Gynaecology
Modena

Michele Masellis
Director
International Association
for Humanitarian Medicine
President, Mediterranean Council
for Burns and Fire Disasters

Hanifa Mezoui
Chief of NGO Section
Department of Economic
and Social Affairs
United Nations

Helena Nygren-Krug
Health and Human Rights Strategy Unit
World Health Organization

Anthony Piel
Former Legal Counsel
and Director of Cabinet
World Health Organization

Joseph Rotblat†
Professor Emeritus
of Physics
University of London
President Emeritus
Pugwash Conferences
Nobel Peace Prize 1995
Regent, International Association
for Humanitarian Medicine

Shashi Tharoor
Former Under-Secretary General
for Communications
and Public Information
United Nations

D. Vezzani
Department of Obstetrics
and Gynaecology
Modena

Jaap A. Walkate†
Late Ambassador
Former Chairman of the
Board of Trustees
United Nations Fund
for Victims of Torture
and Regent, International
Association for Humanitarian Medicine

Ivan Wilhelm
Professor of Physics
Rector of Charles
University
Prague

Preamble

As an overall introduction, a brief mission statement and the definition of Humanitarian Medicine are given here to express the concepts and practices outlined in this book.

The International Association for Humanitarian Medicine Brock Chisholm*

A professional, non-profit, non-governmental organization that promotes and delivers health care on the principles of humanitarian medicine, named after Dr Brock Chisholm, first director-general of the World Health Organization. In particular, it provides medical, surgical, nursing, and rehabilitation care to patients in or from developing countries deficient in the necessary specialized expertise; brings relief to victims of disasters where health aid is lacking; mobilizes hospitals and health specialists in developed countries to receive and treat such patients free of charge; promotes the concept of health as a human right and bridge to peace; and advocates humanitarian law and humanitarian principles in the practice of medicine.

Humanitarian Medicine

While all medical intervention to reduce a person's sickness and suffering is in essence humanitarian, Humanitarian Medicine goes beyond the usual therapeutic act and promotes, provides, teaches, supports, and delivers peoples' health as a human right, in conformity with the ethics of Hippocratic teaching, the principles of the World Health Organization, the Charter of the United Nations, the Universal Declaration of Human Rights, the Red Cross Conventions and other covenants and practices that ensure the most humane and best possible level of care, without any discrimination or consideration of material gain.

---

* Founded in 1984 at the World Health Organization, Geneva, by Mrs Grace Brock Chisholm and Dr S. William A. Gunn, as The Brock Chisholm Memorial Trust, and registered in Italy in 2000 as the International Association for Humanitarian Medicine Brock Chisholm. http://www.iahm.org

Part I
The Fundamentals:
Human Rights and Health

Chapter 1
The Right to Health

S. W. A. Gunn, MD, FRCSC, DSc(Hon), Dr h c

Until barely a few decades ago, health had mostly been regarded as a personal matter, implying a reciprocal relationship between patient and physician, as codified by the Hippocratic Oath. Today, however, health is considered a human right, with not only medical but also complex philosophical, ethical, socioeconomic, political, and legal implications. Additionally, children, the handicapped, the wounded, and the disaster-stricken have their particular fundamental rights, such that the problem of health becomes a concrete issue within international and humanitarian law.

I am a physician. Moreover, I am an international health worker with ties to the World Health Organization, the European Centre for Disaster Medicine, and the International Association for Humanitarian Medicine. I shall therefore approach my theme as a citizen, physician, disaster relief provider, and international doctor. I shall address the issue of "The Right to Health".

I propose to construct my statement on six basic instruments: the Universal Declaration of Human Rights, the Constitution of WHO, the United Nations Declaration of the Rights of the Child, the Red Cross Conventions, the UN Convention on Economic, Social and Cultural Rights, and the mission statement of the International Association for Humanitarian Medicine Brock Chisholm.

The establishment of the United Nations in 1945 was a momentous event not only in global geopolitics but also in international health. The San Francisco Conference, where the UN Charter was signed, considered it wise that a universal health organization be set up. The ensuing International Health Conference approved the establishment of a new body, which began life on 7 April 1948 under the name of the World Health Organization and under the directorship of Dr Brock Chisholm. The basic principle behind the constitution of WHO was the then totally new—not to say controversial—concept of man's right to health, which implies the right to access to health.

1.1 The Instruments

I Although, chronologically, the *Universal Declaration of Human Rights* was in fact signed after the ratification of the WHO Constitution, I shall take it up first as it covers a wider field. Of the 30 articles (Rights) that the Declaration contains, Article 25 is particularly concerned with the right to health. It states the following:

1. Everyone has the right to a standard of living adequate for the health and well-being of himself and of his family, including food, clothing, housing and medical care and necessary services.
   It further establishes that
2. Motherhood and childhood are entitled to special care and assistance.

II Eight months before this Declaration was signed, the *WHO Constitution* had already injected new dimensions of social thinking, let alone new concepts of health. Its preamble states that "the enjoyment of the highest attainable standard of health is one of the fundamental rights of every human being ... and that Governments are responsible for the health of their peoples."
It further enounces the principle that health is a matter of international politics, since "the health of all peoples is fundamental to the attainment of peace and security."
Article 1 clearly points out the objective of WHO. This "... shall be the attainment by all people of the highest possible level of health." And boldly— indeed for its times iconoclastically—WHO defines health as a state of complete physical, mental, and social well-being, and not merely the absence of disease or infirmity.
One can easily grasp the vastness and depth of the interpretation and its implications on the provision of and access to health services everywhere.

III Health rights begin early in life. The *UN Declaration of the Rights of the Child*, signed in November 1959, proclaims the following Principles:

1. The child shall enjoy the benefits of social security. He shall be entitled to grow and develop in health: to this end special care and protection shall be provided both to him and to his mother, including adequate pre-natal and post-natal care. The child shall have the right to adequate nutrition, housing, recreation, and medical services.
2. The child who is physically, mentally, or socially handicapped shall be given the special care required.

As in many other instruments, the child is also protected in the Universal Declaration on the Eradication of Hunger and Malnutrition. Endorsed in December 1974, it proclaims that "Every child has the inalienable right to be free from hunger and malnutrition." The sunken eyes of starving children seen daily on our screens, and the constant breach of all the solemn declarations mentioned above, constitute a flagrant breach of human rights, a breach perpetrated not uncommonly by kleptocratic leaders who rob and starve the very populations they are supposed to govern and protect.

IV *The International Red Cross* has specific principles for the protection of health.

1. The Geneva Conventions of 12 August 1949 clearly protect the health and integrity of civilian populations and noncombatants as of right, and

2. The Additional Protocols of 1977 ensure that, even in war and combat conditions, medical personnel are protected without discrimination, so that they can perform their duties to uphold health.

V *UN International Convention on Economic, Social and Cultural Rights* of 2000 establishes "The right to the highest attainable standard of health. Its Article 12 provides the most comprehensive statement on the right to health in international human rights law.

Article 12.1: States parties recognize the right of everyone to the enjoyment of the highest attainable standard of physical and mental health.

Article 12:2 enumerates a number of obligations and steps to be taken by the States . . . to achieve the full realization of this right.

It is important to note that this right is not confined to the right of health care alone. Indeed, the Convention acknowledges that the right to health embraces a wide range of social and economic factors that promote conditions in which people can lead a healthy life and extends to the underlying determinants of health, such as food, water, sanitation, housing, schools, poverty, conflicts, and the environment.

VI *The International Association for Humanitarian Medicine Brock Chisholm* continues the spirit of the Dr Brock Chisholm Memorial Trust, founded in 1984 to perpetuate the ideals, legacy, and action of the first director-general of WHO. Let me define Humanitarian Medicine. On first thought, all medicine, it may be argued, is humanitarian, but:

> While all medical intervention to reduce a person's sickness and suffering is in essence humanitarian, Humanitarian Medicine goes beyond the usual therapeutic act and promotes, provides, teaches, supports, and delivers peoples' health as a human right, in conformity with the ethics of Hippocratic teaching, the principles of the World Health Organization, the Charter of the United Nations, the Universal Declaration of Human Rights, the Red Cross Conventions, and other covenants and practices that ensure the most humane and best possible level of care, without any discrimination or consideration of material gain.

The right to health is not to be understood as *ipso facto*, a right to be healthy. The right confers both freedoms and obligations designed to promote health. Naturally these rights must be guaranteed and provided in practice, and at present, the universally accepted strategy to ensure health for all is through the national and international efforts in support of essential primary health care available to all.

1.2 Health for All

"Health for All" is in fact the name of the long-term thrust pioneered by WHO and supported by all countries as a realizable social goal and human right. If health is a human right, and human rights are for all humans—as indeed they are—then health too must be for all. And that is just what the WHO vision is about. In fact, in 1977, the World Health Assembly, drawing attention to the vast health inequalities that exist throughout the world and to the inequitable distribution of resources to deal with this human tragedy, decided that the main social target of WHO for the coming decades would be the attainment, by all citizens of the world, of a level of health that would permit them to lead a socially productive life. That is the pragmatic and at once humanitarian concept of "Health for All," based on the strategy of Primary Health Care.

The fundamental principle on which the program and the strategy is based is that a country shall develop its own health policies in the light of its own particular health problems, its social situation, political mechanisms, and economic possibilities, within a structured program of sustainable development. The United Nations and the World Bank have espoused the cause, and countries actively promote it. There is no question, however, of creating a pseudo nirvana where all disease will have been abolished. Yet several things are clearly attainable: preventable illness should and can be prevented; there should and can be early diagnosis, treatment, and rehabilitation for treatable conditions; there should and can be better continuing management for nontreatable diseases; and increasing regard must be paid not only to the length of life but also to the quality of life. The fundamental right of man demands this.

1.3 The Cost

Studies show that tremendous improvements in children's and peoples' health can be achieved for as little as 0.5% of the yearly gross national product per capita. This is by any standard a reasonable cost, around a hundredth of what is spent on health by people in most of the affluent countries. Indeed, as William Gibson points out, the terrible cost of not doing health research, the main cost of providing health for all would be in not doing anything, or going on in our old ways. For then the burden would be more disease, less health, less development, less social justice, more pauperization, more misery, and a somber horizon for freedom and peace. No, the price and the effort are worthwhile, and the International Association for Humanitarian Medicine, named after the first director-general of the Organization that has spearheaded this social revolution, is entirely committed to it.

1.4 Full Circle

Health is a human right. And as early as 1948, WHO proclaimed that "the health of all peoples is fundamental to the attainment of peace and security." Conversely, a later World Health Assembly declared that "Peace is the most significant factor for the attainment of Health for All."

What a beautiful circle: health > human right > security > peace > health > human right.

Bibliography

Berner P., Fonrouge J.M., Gunn S.W.A.: Legal, diplomatic and geopolitical concepts for physicians on international humanitarian missions. Prehosp. Disaster Med., 14: S. 87, 1999.

Butros-Ghali B.: From peace keeping to peace building. Lecture by the Secretary General, UN doc. PR/SG/SM/1330, May 1992.

Gunn S.W.A.: Health research in an interdependent world. Canad. J. Public Health, 72: 245, 1981.

Gunn S.W.A.: The implementation of the right to health through international cooperation. Colloquy on Health Protection, International Institute of Humanitarian Law, 1983.

Gunn S.W.A.: Le droit de l'enfant à la santé. Symposium Croix Rouge/Croissante Rouge, Inst. Internat. de Droit Humanitaire, San Remo, 1985.

Gunn S.W.A.: Disaster Medicine and emergencies. The international community's response. J. Irish Coll. Phys Surg., 17: 14, 1988.

Gunn S.W.A.: The right to health. Cemec Monography no. 2, Cemec, San Marino, 1989a.

Gunn S.W.A.: Il diritto alla salute. Medicina a Morale, 5: 895, 1989b.

Gunn S.W.A.: Multilingual Dictionary of Disaster Medicine and International Relief. Kluwer Academic Publishers, Dordrecht, Boston, London, 1990.

Gunn S.W.A.: Il presupposto umanitario nel soccorso. Oplitai, 6 (5): 7, 1993a.

Gunn S.W.A.: The role of the military in non-military disasters. Proceedings of the International Military Medical Symposium. Saudi Arabia, 1993b.

Gunn S.W.A., Masellis M.: The WHO Collaborating Centre for Prevention and Treatment of Burns and Fire Disasters. Ann. Burns Fire Disasters, 11: 3–6, 1998.

Gunn S.W.A.: Disaster Medicine, humanitarian medicine. Prehosp. Disaster Med., 15: S. 53, 2000a.

Gunn S.W.A.: Disasters and conflicts. Encyclopedia of Life Support Systems, UNESCO, Paris, 2000b.

Gunn S.W.A.: The Right to health. Doctoral address. J. Humanitarian Med., 1: 1–3, 2000c.

Mahler M.: Social justice. The underpinning for leadership in local and global health. Brock Chisholm oration, WHO, 1998.

United Nations: The right to the highest attainable standard of health. Convention on Economic, Social, and Cultural Rights, Document E/C.12/2004/4, 11, UN, Aug. 2000.

Whitehead M.: Equity and ethics in health. World Health Organization Regional Committee for Europe, Dec. EUR/R44/Tech. Disc./1 Rev. 1, 1994.

World Health Organization: Principles of the rights of patients in Europe, including a model for a declaration on the rights of patients. Copenhagen, WHO Europe, 1994.

World Health Organization: Basic Documents, WHO, Geneva, 2005.

Chapter 2
Health and Human Rights—A Public Health Perspective

Gudjón Magnússon, MD, PhD

Health and Human Rights may at first sight look like two separate issues. Both valued highly but distributed very unevenly. Both desirable but hard to sustain. At a closer look, we will find that Health and Human Rights are not only closely linked but interrelated and highly synergetic.

Health and Human Rights is a relatively new topic in public health training in Europe, but has a longer history in the USA. The first course in Health and Human Rights at the Nordic School of Public Health took place in 1995 and was organized jointly with the Harvard School of Public Health in Boston, USA. This was a great success and inspired two summer courses and is now part of the standard courses offered at the Nordic School.

The reasons for the increased interest in Health and Human Rights are many and varied. First, it has to do with global trends:

– the demographic revolution;
– human rights initiatives;
– market economy;
– regional integrations;
– increased role for non-governmental organizations (NGOS);
– globalization.

According to one source, one of the 20th century's hallmark achievements is its progress in human rights. In the year 1900, more than half the world's people lived under colonial rules, and no country gave all its citizens the right to vote. Today, some three-quarters of the world live under democratic regimes. Over 25 years (1974–1999), multi-party electoral systems were introduced in 113 countries. Europe is making human rights a key priority, as is clearly shown in the work of the Council of Europe and from the impact of the European Court of Human Rights.

Market economy can be seen both as a threat to human rights and health and also as a promoter of freedom and human development. It has been interesting to observe how human rights records of different applicant countries to the World Trade Organization have figured in the debate as to whether or not they should be allowed to become members.

The increased importance of non-governmental organizations is well recognized. During only one decade (1991–1999), the number of NGOs worldwide increased from 23,600 to 44,000 in 1999. The roles of the NGOs vary widely, but include being a watchdog for social injustice and initiating new measures to assist and care for those most in need.

Finally, the effects of globalization can be similar to market economy, either seen as a real threat to health and human rights or as increased opportunity to promote health and human rights.

In the Human Development Report 2000, it is noted that

> The mark of all civilizations is the respect they accord to human dignity and freedom. All religious and cultural traditions celebrate these ideals. Yet, throughout history, they have been violated. Every society has known racism, sexism, authoritarianism, xenophobia— depriving men and women of their dignity and freedom. And in all regions and cultures the struggle against oppression, injustice and discrimination has been common. That struggle continues today in all countries, rich and poor.

2.1 Health and Human Rights—How Linked?

The first relationship, Health $\rightarrow$ Human Rights, concerns the potential impact of health policies, programmes, and practices on human rights. The challenge is to negotiate the optimal balance between promoting and protecting public health and promoting and protecting human rights. A good example is the optimal balance between individual freedom of movement and the societal needs to isolate an individual or groups of individuals to reduce the risk of spreading a communicable disease.

The second relationship, Health $\rightarrow$ Human Rights, expresses that violations or lack of implementation of any or all human rights have negative effects on physical, mental, and social well-being (health). This is particularly true in times of war, conflict, and political repressionand also in peacetime. A good example is torture of human beings.

The third relationship, Health $\longleftrightarrow$ Human Rights, underlines that the best possible results are obtained when health and human rights act in synergy.

2.2 What Do We Mean by Health?

WHO has defined health as "a state of complete physical, mental and social well-being and not merely the absence of disease or infirmity." This definition, which dates back to 1948 when WHO was founded, has been criticized for being more political than operational. A goal that is impossible to reach! Several attempts to revise the definition have been made like the one presented here:

Health is a condition of well-being free of disease or infirmity and a basic and universal human right. R. Saracci, BMJ, 1997

The focus is put on health being a basic and universal human right. Even WHO is using more than one definition depending on what purpose the definition is being used for. If we look at Health21—The Target Document for Health Development in the 21st Century in the European Region—we see this definition:

Health is the reduction in mortality, morbidity and disability due to detectable disease or disorder, and an increase in the perceived level of health.

What is new here is the emphasis on "reduction due to *detectable* diseases and disorders, and an *increase* in the perceived level of health."

At the Fourth International Conference on Health Promotion, we see yet another development in the definition:

Health is a resource for everyday life, not the object of living. It is a positive concept emphasizing social and personal resources as well as physical capabilities.

Here the emphasis is on seeing health as a resource and not as the object of living.
When it comes to Health Impact Assessment, we find this definition:

Health is the highest attainable level of physical, mental and social well-being. It includes capacity to cope with physical, psychological and social stress. A more easy to measure but also more restricted aspect of health is the absence of indications of somatic or psychic illness.

The first part of the definition derives from the WHO Constitution, but the emphasis is on coping with long-term illnesses, disorders and stress.

Finally, we have the "Health Poem" by the Danish poet Piet Hein that he wrote to celebrate WHO's 40th Anniversary.

Health is not bought with a chemist's pills
Nor saved by the surgeon's knife
Health is not only the absence of ills
But the fight for the fullness of life.

Before proceeding, it is important to make clear that modern concepts of health derive from two different disciplines, medicine and public health. While medicine focuses on the health of the individual, public health emphasizes the health of populations. At the Nordic School of Public Health, we favour this definition of public health:

Public Health can be said to be: the science and art of preventing disease, prolonging life and promoting health through organized efforts of society.

The Acheson Report, 1988

2.3 Health and Human Rights in Professional Training

The Nordic School and the Council of Europe arranged jointly the First European Conference on Health and Human Rights in Strasbourg, 15–16 March 1999. More than 300 participants met to share and gain knowledge. The main conclusions were the need to

– Ratify and respect all international treaties relating to health and human rights;
– Recognize that equitable access to health care, good quality services, and high professional standards are an integral part of human rights and that their absence may constitute violations of human rights;
– Take measures to ensure health services of a high quality, paying special attention to vulnerable groups and to the rights of patients;
– Pay due attention to the opportunities as well as the serious ethical and medical risks in the context of the development of new technologies in the biological and medical fields;
– Focus attention on preventive care and promotion of health as important measures for individual and public health, thus adding quality of life;
– Support humanitarian work in areas of tension and conflict and safeguard security and human rights for the benefit of the assisted populations and the humanitarian aid workers;
– Acknowledge the link between health and social cohesion.

Furthermore, educational authorities and universities were invited to

– Introduce health and human rights education programmes in the curricula of universities and schools, in particular schools of Public Health.

At the Nordic School we have taken on that challenge to integrate teaching in Health and Human Rights in one curriculum and are offering training courses in all the topics related to Health and Human Rights. We sincerely believe that Health and Human rights is an indispensable tool in promoting health, preventing disease, ensuring basic rights, and reducing suffering worldwide.

Bibliography

Health and Human Rights: A reader. Mann J.M., Gruskin S., Grodin M.A., Annas E.J., (eds). Routledge Publ.: 1999a.
Health and Human Rights. Report from the European Conference held in Strasbourg March 1999. Stefan Winter (ed.). NHV-Report 2: 1999b.
Health Impact Assessment: From theory to practice. Report on the Leo Kaprio Workshop, Nordic School of Public Health, October 1999. NHV-Report 9: 2000.
Health21: An introduction to the Health for All policy framework for the WHO European region. Copenhagen, WHO, European Health For All series 5: 1998.
Human Rights and Human Development. Human Development Report 2000. UNDP, 2000.

Public health in England: The report of the Committee of Inquiry into the Future Development
    of the Public Health Function. Presented to Parliament by the Secretary of State for Social
    Services by command of Her Majesty, January 1988.
Saracci R.: The World Health Organization needs to reconsider its definition of health. Br. Med. J.,
    10, 314: 1409–20, 1997.

Chapter 3
Health for All or Hell for All?
The Role of Leadership in Health Equity

Halfdan Mahler, MD

Let me start by giving you a very brief account of my first and last encounter with Dr Brock Chisholm, in New Delhi 52 years ago. As the only director-general in WHO's history, Dr Chisholm insisted on having individual briefing by all field staff when he visited countries. After having listened to my ecstatic account of the National Tuberculosis Program, he looked at me intently and said, "Dr Mahler, you have far too much sympathy and far too little empathy for poor Indians." Had Dr Chisholm been here today, I hope he might agree that I have learnt my lesson. I believe that Milan Kundera had it right when he wrote in one of his books: "The struggle against human oppression is the struggle between memory and forgetfulness." For instance, I believe that the many who over and over again ridicule WHO's definition of health in its Constitution have forgotten this Constitution and its Health definition. So let me remind all of the intrinsic beauty and pertinence of this definition: "Health is a state of complete physical, mental, and social well-being, and not merely the absence of disease or infirmity." Let me also remind the forgetful about the link between the inspirational and the practical in that this Constitution has only one article defining "The Objective of the World Health Organization shall be the Attainment by All Peoples of the Highest Possible Level of Health." For my personal enlightenment, one of the architects of this WHO definition, a partisan during the Second World War, explained it to me in the following way:

> I have experienced this complete physical, mental, and social well-being many times as a partisan when I decided to risk my life for something I thought was vitally important, namely freedom from occupation. Complete physical well-being, in that I as an individual could make a difference against a huge army of occupation.
> Complete mental well-being, in that I fully realized my existential freedom by deciding to risk my life for something vitally important. Complete social well-being, in that I knew that should I not come back alive somebody from my partisan group would take care of my family.

And so, in facing death, this partisan maintained that he had experienced the innate and transcendental meaning of WHO's Health definition.

I am convinced that health is politics and that politics is health as if all people truly mattered. I am, therefore, also convinced that political action for health—locally and globally—requires moral and intellectual stimulation. I am, furthermore, morally and intellectually convinced that the Health for All Vision and the Primary Health Care Strategy provide significant starting forces and added impetus for health development all over the world. Such development is based on the principle that those who have little in health and wealth will generate much more for themselves, and those that have much will have no less, but will have it with a better social conscience.

I see startling patterns of inequities in the health scores throughout our miserable world. I'm not talking about a first, or second, or third, or fourth world—I'm talking about one world—the only one we have got to share and care for. And I continue to support the resolve to provide levels of health that will allow all people of this ONE WORLD to lead socially and economically satisfying and productive lives.

I have always maintained that people's own creativity and ingenuity are the keys to their and the world's progress. People's apathy can turn development dreams into stagnating nightmares. The transformation of social apathy into social and economic productivity is the point of embarkation of all sustainable and cumulatively growing human development. And an adequate level of health is a basic ingredient that fuels this transformation. What the billions of people throughout the developing world need and want is what everyone, everywhere, needs and wants: the well-being of those they love; a better future for their children; an end to gross injustice; and a beginning of hope. So development is about the creation and expansion of opportunities for human beings to realize what they consider to be their positive destiny. It is a complex, often messy process involving the interplay of physical, social, economic, and political variables. And we are not talking about dealing with physical sciences and controlled environments where quantifiable elements can be introduced and results predicted. We are talking about human institutions and cultures, ways in which people organize themselves to effect change in their social environments. We are talking about human expectations, perceived rights, preference values, and people's emotions and attitudes about those rights and values.

Equity, especially in ensuring essential health and socioeconomic care, and particularly as it relates to vulnerable groups such as the poor, children, women, the elderly, the disabled, remains for me a primordial objective of all development. Indeed, I consider equity a moral imperative to which all social and economic activities must be subsumed. I do believe that a greater degree of equity, to assure a more just and reasonable equality of health opportunity, is an absolute necessity for the preservation of a sane local and global humanity. Let us not forget that there are still thousands of millions of humans caught in the absolute poverty trap—a condition of life so characterized by malnutrition, illiteracy, and ill health as to be beneath any definition of human decency.

How then, in today's largely amoral, if not immoral, world, is "social conscience" on the part of leaders generated? Rarely in human history has this kind of leadership been so essential—so vital; leadership to propagate new values in society, particularly values that are concerned with social progress; leadership of involvement, of responsibility, of objectivity and of compassion.

It has been said that leaders have a significant role in creating the state of mind, that is, the society. They can express the values that hold the society together. They can bring to consciousness the society's sense of its own needs, values, and purposes. Only by doing this will it, in my opinion, become possible for all of us on board Spaceship Earth to steer it away from our present course towards Hell for

All, towards the course of Health for All! And let us not forget that visionaries have always been the true realists of humankind's history.

It is my firm personal conviction that leadership is nothing if it is not linked to the collective purposes of the society. The effectiveness of the leaders must be gauged, not by their charisma, or their visibility, or the so-called power they hold, but by the actual social change they create, measured by the satisfaction of human needs and expectations. I do speak of moral leadership, where values have a decisive place, where leaders assume consummate responsibility for their commitments, and thereby produce social change that is truly relevant to the needs, aspirations, and values of the society.

And the vision of a commitment to remove social inequities cannot be introduced as a one-shot piece of magic. It must be introduced time after time. It must be incorporated in the political system and supported through the strategic and decision-making processes. It must be reinforced continuously through the diligent pursuit of facts and the fearless exposure of the facts that cry out for social justice.

A question often raised is, "Can health truly form a leading edge for social justice, especially when we are dealing with situations where the basic issue is survival; where people are trapped in the vicious circle of extreme poverty, ignorance and apathy?"

I can best answer this question by referring to the events that led to the creation of the Health for All movement and to this movement, in my opinion, becoming a leading edge in the promotion of equity and social justice.

The World Health Assembly decided in 1977 that the main social target of Governments and WHO in the coming decades should be the attainment of what is known locally and globally as "Health for All." And the World Health Assembly described that as a level of health that will permit all the people of the world to lead socially and economically satisfying and productive lives. Please note that the World Health Assembly did not consider health as an end in itself, but rather as a means to an end. That end is human development as characterized by social and economic productivity and well-being. You will also note that the social aspect preceded the economic aspect. That is also as it should be. When people are mere pawns in an economic growth and profit game, that game is so often lost for the poor. But when people themselves can contribute actively and voluntarily to the social development of the society in which they live, whether in such fields as shaping public policies, providing social support to others, undertaking voluntary action for the health and education of society, or through all kinds of cultural activities, in other words when people are socially productive, there is much hope for economic productivity too.

This morally binding contract of Health for All was the basis of The Primary Health Care Strategy, which implied a commitment not only to a reorientation of the conventional health care system—which rather should be called "medical repair systems"—but to a shift towards people's own control over their health and well-being to the extent that they would be willing to handle in fact profound social reforms in health. This implies a continuous empowerment process whereby people acquire the skill and will to become the social carriers of their own health and well-being.

Therefore, I do believe that the fundamental values of social justice and equity are firmly embedded in the vision of Health for All and the strategy of Primary Health Care. And this vision and strategy can indeed be a strong force and leading edge for achieving social justice and equity. Health may not be everything, but without health there is very little to well-being.

The question is often asked: "Can we afford the cost of social justice and equity?" I would propose a counterquestion: "Can we afford the cost of social and economic destabilization inherent in today's pursuit of profit-maximization?" The costs generated through the creation of a just and equitable health care system may indeed cause some economic turbulence. But equitable cost containment can be introduced, and resources can be reallocated. Justice and fiscal responsibility do not have to be incompatible. They will be so only if there is a breakdown of political nerve. While there has been solid progress in a few countries towards Health for All, progress towards social justice and health equity remains strictly limited. A major reason—in my opinion—for this limited progress in the application of the Health for All vision through the Primary Health Care Strategy has been the lack of politically sensitive ammunition generated through clinical, epidemiological, sociological, and operations research. Therefore, much more leadership must be generated as a collective force from all levels of the local and global society towards accelerating the abatement of today's gross health inequities.

I believe it is obvious, if present inequity trends continue undimished, that our world will become more crowded, more polluted, less stable ecologically, and much more vulnerable to socioeconomic and political devastation. I believe the most turbulent transition will be that associated with the establishment of equity between all earth citizens.

Health for All leadership—locally and globally—is moved by a vision which cannot tolerate the unacceptable inequities of life, and which has faith in the potential of people, in their inherent ability to develop, and to take responsibility for their own destiny.

I do believe that the leaders are there who are willing to take up these challenges. They are those in leading political positions who can emphasize social values and be politically sensitive to them, who feel strongly about equity issues, and who can find ways to motivate and mobilize others. They are the leaders in the communities—able to take up the cause of justice and equity more strongly, prepared to adjust their own traditional values and approaches and willing to take risks. They are the leaders of thousands of civil society organizations, such as IAHM, at local and global level already fighting for equity in health. They are the leaders in educational and scientific institutions—able to visualize the scope for improving human conditions and thus willing to focus their intellectual energies accordingly—and also willing to motivate future generations towards social values promoting equity. Last but not least, they are potentially among the leaders of all the world's religions, willing to add the spiritual dimension in the fight for justice and equity.

Those who are fighting for social justice and equity must be even more than ready to look, to listen, to probe, and to learn, and be brave enough to fearlessly evaluate progress or lack of progress in abating inequities. Only by highlighting inequities is it possible to redress them. This struggle for equity can often be frustrating, since development knows no limits. The more you move along its road the more you want to move. You cannot blame people if they strive to join up with those who are further along the road than they are. That is only human nature. Injustices, however, have to be seen through the eyes of those who are farthest behind on that road. But we must not let the injustices take over. Indeed we must not!

Chapter 4
The Declaration of Alma-Ata on Primary Health Care

International Conference on Primary Health Care

On 12 September 1978, gathered in Alma-Ata, then in the USSR, the World Health Organization and its Member States solemnly signed the Declaration of Alma-Ata on Primary Health Care. This was to become the global spearhead for peoples' health and the foundation of the concept of Health for All. To celebrate that momentous humanitarian event, we give here the full text of the Declaration of Alma-Ata.

The International Conference on Primary Health Care, meeting in Alma-Ata this twelfth day of September in the year nineteen hundred and seventy-eight, expressing the need for urgent action by all governments, all health and development workers, and the world community to protect and promote the health of all the people of the world, hereby makes the following Declaration:

I   The Conference strongly reaffirms that health, which is a state of complete physical, mental and social well-being, and not merely the absence of disease or infirmity, is a fundamental human right and that the attainment of the highest possible level of health is a most important world-wide social goal whose realization requires the action of many other and social economic sectors in addition to the health sector.

II The existing gross inequality in the health status of the people particularly between developed and developing countries as well as within countries is politically, socially and economically unacceptable and is, therefore, of common concern to all countries.

III Economic and social development, based on a New International Economic Order, is of basic importance to the fullest attainment of health for all and to the reduction of the gap between the health status of the developing and developed countries. The promotion and protection of the health of the people is essential to sustained economic and social development and contributes to a better quality of life and to world peace.

IV The people have the right and duty to participate individually and collectively in the planning and implementation of their health care.

V   Governments have a responsibility for the health of their people which can be fulfilled only by the provision of adequate health and social measures. A main social target of governments, international organizations and the whole world community in the coming decades should be the attainment by all peoples of the world by the year 2000 of a level of health that will permit them to lead a socially and economically productive life. Primary health care is the key to attaining this target as part of development in the spirit of social justice.

VI Primary health care is essential health care based on practical, scientifically sound and socially acceptable methods and technology made universally accessible to individuals and families in the community through their full participation and at a cost that the community and country can afford to maintain at every stage of their development in the spirit of self-reliance and self-determination. It forms an integral part both of the country's health systems, of which it is the central function and main focus, and of the overall social and economic development of the community. It is the first level of contact of individuals, the family and community with the national health system bringing health care as close as possible to where people live and work, and constitutes the first element of a continuing health care process.

VII   Primary health care:

- reflects and evolves from the economic conditions and sociocultural and political characteristics of the country and its communities and is based on the application of the relevant results of social, biomedical and health services research and public health experience;
- addresses the main health problems in the community, providing promotive, preventive, curative and rehabilitative services accordingly;
- includes at least: education concerning prevailing health problems and the methods of preventing and controlling them; promotion of food supply and proper nutrition; an adequate supply of safe water and basic sanitation; maternal and child health care, including family planning; immunization against the major infectious diseases; prevention and control of locally endemic diseases; appropriate treatment of common diseases and injuries; and provision of essential drugs;
- involves, in addition to the health sectors, all related sectors and aspects of national and community development, in particular agriculture, animal husbandry, food, industry, education, housing, public works, communications and other sectors; and demands the coordinated efforts of all those sectors;
- requires and promotes maximum community and individual self-reliance and participation in the planning, organization, operation and control of primary health care, making fullest use of local, national and other available resources; and to this end develops through appropriate education the ability of communities to participate;
- should be sustained by integrated, functional and mutually supportive referral systems, leading to the progressive improvement of comprehensive health care for all, and giving priority to those most in need;
- relies, at local and referral levels, on health workers, including physicians, nurses, midwives, auxiliaries and community workers as applicable, as well as traditional practitioners as needed, suitably trained socially and technically to work as a health team and to respond to the expressed health needs of the community.

VIII   All governments should formulate national policies, strategies and plans of action to launch and sustain primary health care as part of a comprehensive national health system and in coordination with other sectors. To this end, it will be necessary to exercise political will, to mobilize the country's resources and to use available external resources rationally.

IX   All countries should cooperate in a spirit of partnership and service to ensure primary health care for all people since the attainment of health by people in any one country directly concerns and benefits every other country. In this context the joint WHO/UNICEF report on primary health care constitutes a solid basis for the further development and operation of primary health care throughout the world.

X   An acceptable level of health for all the people of the world by the year 2000 can be attained through a fuller and better use of the world's resources, a considerable part of which is now spent on armaments and military conflicts. A genuine policy of independence, peace, détente and disarmament could and should release additional resources that could well be devoted to peaceful aims and in particular to the acceleration of social and economic development of which primary health care, as an essential part, should be allotted its proper share.

The International Conference on Primary Health Care calls for urgent and effective national and international action to develop and implement primary health care throughout the world and particularly in developing countries in a spirit of technical cooperation and in keeping with a New International Economic Order. It urges governments, WHO and UNICEF, and other international organizations, as well as multilateral and bilateral agencies, non-governmental organizations, funding agencies, all health workers and the whole world community to support national and international commitment to primary health care and to channel increased technical and financial support to it, particularly in developing countries. The Conference calls on all the aforementioned to collaborate in introducing, developing and maintaining primary health care in accordance with the spirit and content of this Declaration.

Chapter 5
Health and Human Rights:
In 25 Questions and Answers

Helena Nygren-Krug

5.1 Health and Human Rights Norms and Standards

5.1.1 Q.1 What Are Human Rights?

Human rights are legally guaranteed by human rights law, protecting individuals and groups against actions that interfere with fundamental freedoms and human dignity. They encompass what are known as civil, cultural, economic, political and social rights. Human rights are principally concerned with the relationship between the individual and the state. Governmental obligations with regard to human rights broadly fall under the principles of *respect, protect and fulfil.*

> All human rights are universal, indivisible and interdependent and interrelated. The international community must treat human rights globally in a fair and equal manner, on the same footing, and with the same emphasis. While the significance of national and regional particularities and various historical, cultural and religious backgrounds must be borne in mind, it is the duty of States, regardless of their political, economic and cultural systems, to promote and protect all human rights and fundamental freedoms.
>
> Vienna Declaration and Programme

5.1.2 Q.2 How Are Human Rights Enshrined in International Law?

In the aftermath of Second World War, the international community adopted the Universal Declaration of Human Rights (UDHR, 1948). However, by the time that States were prepared to turn the provisions of the Declaration into binding law, the Cold War had overshadowed and polarized human rights into two separate categories. The West argued that civil and political rights had priority and that economic and social rights were mere aspirations. The Eastern bloc argued to the contrary that rights to food, health and education were paramount and civil and political rights secondary. Hence two separate treaties were created in 1996—the International Covenant on Economic, Social and Cultural Rights (ICESCR) and the International

Covenant on Civil and Political Rights (ICCPR). Since then, numerous treaties, declarations and other legal instruments have been adopted, and it is these instruments that encapsulate human rights.

5.1.3 Q.3 What Is the Link Between Health and Human Rights?

There are complex linkages between health and human rights:

- Violations or lack of attention to human rights can have serious health consequences;
- Health policies and programmes can promote or violate human rights in the ways they are designed or implemented;
- Vulnerability and the impact of ill health can be reduced by taking steps to respect, protect and fulfil human rights.

The normative content of each right is fully articulated in human rights instruments. In relation to the right to health and freedom from discrimination, the normative content is outlined in Questions 4 and 5, respectively. Examples of the language used in human rights instruments to articulate the normative content of some of the other key human rights relevant to health follow:

- *Torture*: "No one shall be subjected to torture or to cruel, inhuman or degrading treatment or punishment. In particular, no one shall be subjected without his free consent to medical or scientific experimentation."
- *Violence against children*: "All appropriate legislative, administrative, social and educational measures to protect the child from all forms of physical or mental violence, injury or abuse, neglect or negligent treatment, maltreatment or exploitation, including sexual abuse . . ." shall be taken.
- *Harmful traditional practices*: "Effective and appropriate measures with a view to abolishing traditional practices prejudicial to the health of children" shall be taken.
- *Participation*: The right to ". . . active, free and meaningful participation."
- *Information*: "Freedom to seek, receive and impart information and ideas of all kinds."
- *Privacy*: "No one shall be subjected to arbitrary or unlawful interference with his privacy . . ."
- *Scientific progress*: The right of everyone to enjoy the benefits of scientific progress and its applications.
- *Education*: The right to education, including access to education in support of basic knowledge of child health and nutrition, the advantages of breast-feeding, hygiene and environmental sanitation and the prevention of accidents.
- *Food and nutrition*: "The right of everyone to adequate food and the fundamental right of everyone to be free from hunger . . ."

- *Standard of living*: Everyone has the right to an adequate standard of living, including adequate food, clothing, housing and medical care and necessary social services.
- *Right to social security*: The right of everyone to social security, including social insurance.

5.1.4 Q.4 What Is Meant by "The Right to Health"?

> The right to health does not mean the right to be healthy, nor does it mean that poor governments must put in place expensive health services for which they have no resources. But it does require governments and public authorities to put in place policies and action plans which will lead to available and accessible health care for all in the shortest possible time. To ensure that this happens is the challenge facing both the human rights community and public health professionals.
>
> United Nations High Commissioner for Human Rights, Mary Robinson

The right to the highest attainable standard of health (referred to as "the right to health") was first reflected in the WHO Constitution (1946) and then reiterated in the 1978 Declaration of Alma-Ata and in the World Health Declaration adopted by the World Health Assembly in 1998. It has been firmly endorsed in a wide range of international and regional human rights instruments (Figure 5.1).

The right to the highest attainable standard of health in international human rights law is a claim to a set of social arrangements—norms, institutions, laws, an

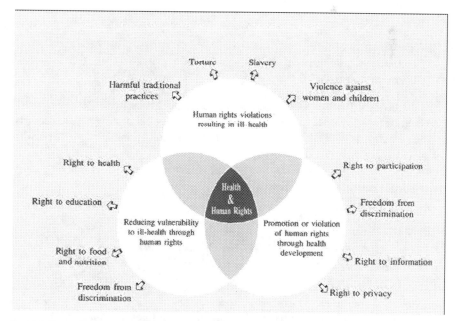

Fig. 5.1 Examples of the links between *Health* and *Human Rights*

enabling environment—that can best secure the enjoyment of this right. The most authoritative interpretation of the right to health is outlined in Article 12 of the ICE-SCR, which has been ratified by 145 countries (as of May 2002). In May 2000, the Committee on Economic, Social and Cultural Rights, which monitors the Covenant, adopted a General Comment on the right to health. General Comments serve to clarify the nature and content of individual rights and States Parties' (those states that have ratified) obligations. The General Comment recognized that the right to health is closely related to and dependent upon the realization of other human rights, including the right to food, housing, work, education, participation, the enjoyment of the benefits of scientific progress and its applications, life, non-discrimination, equality, the prohibition against torture, privacy, access to information and the freedoms of association, assembly and movement.

Furthermore, the Committee interpreted the right to health as an inclusive right extending not only to timely and appropriate health care but also to the underlying determinants of health, such as access to safe and potable water and adequate sanitation, an adequate supply of safe food, nutrition and housing, healthy occupational and environmental conditions, and access to health-related education and information, including sexual and reproductive health.

The General Comment sets out four criteria by which to evaluate the right to health.

a *Availability*. Functioning public health and health care facilities, goods and services, as well as programmes, have to be available in sufficient quantity.
b *Accessibility*. Health facilities, goods and services have to be accessible to everyone without discrimination, within the jurisdiction of the State party. Accessibility has four overlapping dimensions:

   – Non-discrimination;
   – Physical accessibility;
   – Economic accessibility (affordability);
   – Information accessibility.

c *Acceptability*. All health facilities, goods and services must be respectful of medical ethics and culturally appropriate, sensitive to gender and life cycle requirements, as well as being designed to respect confidentiality and improve the health status of those concerned.
d *Quality*. Health facilities, goods and services must be scientifically and medically appropriate and of good quality.

5.1.5 Q.5 How Does the Principle of Freedom from Discrimination Relate to Health?

Vulnerable and marginalized groups in societies tend to bear an undue proportion of health problems. Overt or implicit discrimination violates a fundamental human rights principle and often lies at the root of poor health status. In practice, discrimination can manifest itself in inadequately targeted health programmes and restricted access to health services.

Discrimination manifests itself in a complex variety of ways, which may, directly or indirectly, impact upon health. For example, the Declaration on the Elimination of Violence against Women recognizes the link between violence against women and the historically unequal power relations between men and women.

The prohibition of discrimination does not mean that differences should not be acknowledged, only that different treatment—and the failure to treat equal cases equally—must be based on objective and reasonable criteria intended to rectify imbalances within a society.

In relation to health and health care, the grounds for non-discrimination have evolved and can now be summarized as proscribing

> any discrimination in access to health care and the underlying determinants of health, as well as to means and entitlements for their procurement, on the grounds of race, colour, sex, language, religion, political or other opinion, national or social origin, property, birth, physical or mental disability, health status (including HIV/AIDS), sexual orientation, civil, political, social or other status, which has the intention or effect of nullifying or impairing the equal enjoyment or exercise of the right to health.

5.1.6 Q.6 What International Human Rights Instruments Set Out Governmental Commitments?

Governments decide freely whether or not to become parties to a human rights treaty. Once this decision is made, however, there is a commitment to act in accordance with the provisions of the treaty concerned. The key international human rights treaties, the International Covenant on Economic, Social and Cultural Rights (ICESCR, 1996) and the International Covenant on Civil and Political Rights (ICCPR, 1966), further elaborate the content of the rights set out in the Universal Declaration of Human Rights (UDHR, 1948), and contain legally binding obligations for the governments that become parties to them. Together, these documents are often called the "International Bill of Human Rights."

Building upon these core documents, other international human rights treaties have focused on either specific groups or categories of populations, such as racial minorities, women and children, or on specific issues, such as torture. In considering a normative framework of human rights applicable to health, human rights provisions must be considered in their totality.

The Declarations and Programmes of Action from UN world conferences, such as the World Conference on Human Rights (Vienna, 1993), the International Conference on Population and Development (Cairo, 1994), the World Summit for Social Development (Copenhagen, 1995), the Fourth World Conference on Women (Beijing, 1995) and the World Conference Against Racism, Racial Discrimination, Xenophobia and Related Intolerance (Durban, 2001), provide guidance on some of the policy implications of meeting governments' human rights obligations.

5.1.7 Q.7 What International Monitoring Mechanisms Exist for Human Rights?

The implementation of the core human rights treaties is monitored by committees of independent experts known as treaty monitoring bodies, created under the auspices of and serviced by the United Nations. Each of the six major human rights treaties has its own monitoring body which meets regularly to review State Party reports and to engage in a "constructive dialogue" with governments on how to live up to their human rights obligations. Based on the principle of transparency, States are required to submit their progress reports to the treaty bodies, and to make them widely available to their own populations. Thus reports can play an important catalytic role, contributing to the promotion of national debate on human rights issues, encouraging the engagement and participation of civil society, and generally fostering a process of public scrutiny of governmental policies. At the end of the session, the treaty body makes concluding observations which include recommendations on how the government can improve its human rights record. Specialized agencies such as WHO can play an important role in providing relevant health information to facilitate the dialogue between the State Party and the treaty monitoring body.

Other mechanisms for monitoring human rights in the United Nations system include the Human Rights Council and the Sub-Commission on the Promotion and Protection of Human Rights. These bodies appoint special rapporteurs and other independent experts and working groups to monitor and report on thematic human rights issues (such as violence against women, sale of children, harmful traditional practices and torture) or on specific countries. In addition, the post of High Commissioner for Human Rights was created in 1994 to head the United Nations human rights system. The High Commissioner's mandate extends to every aspect of the United Nations human rights activities: monitoring, promotion, protection and coordination.

Regional arrangements have been established within existing regional intergovernmental organizations. The African regional human rights instrument is the African Charter on Human and People's Rights, which is located within the African Union. The regional human rights mechanism for the Americas is located within the Organization of American States and is based upon the American Convention of Human Rights. In Europe, a human rights system forms a part of the Council of Europe. Key human rights instruments are the European Convention on the Protection of Human Rights and Fundamental Freedoms and the European Social Charter. The 27-member state organization—the European Union—has detailed rules concerning human rights issues and has integrated human rights into its common foreign policy. In addition, the Organization for Security and Cooperation in Europe (OSCE), a 55-member state organization, has separate mechanisms and agreements. In the Asia-Pacific region, extensive consultations among Governments are underway concerning the possible establishment of regional human rights arrangements.

5.1.8 Q.8 How Can Poor Countries with Resource Limitations Be Held to the Same Human Rights Standards as Rich Countries?

Steps towards the full realization of rights must be deliberate, concrete and targeted as clearly as possible towards meeting a government's human rights obligations. All appropriate means, including the adoption of legislative measures and the provision of judicial remedies as well as administrative, financial, educational and social measures, must be used in this regard. This neither requires nor precludes any particular form of government or economic system being used as the vehicle for the steps in question.

The principle of progressive realization of human rights imposes an obligation to move as expeditiously and effectively as possible towards that goal. It is therefore relevant to both poorer and wealthier countries, as it acknowledges the constraints due to the limits of available resources, but requires all countries to show constant progress in moving towards full realization of rights. Any deliberately retrogressive measures require the most careful consideration and need to be fully justified by reference to the totality of the rights provided for in the human rights treaty concerned and in the context of the full use of the maximum available resources. In this context, it is important to distinguish the inability from the unwillingness of a State Party to comply with its obligations. During the reporting process, the State Party and the Committee identify indicators and national benchmarks to provide realistic targets to be achieved during the next reporting period.

5.1.9 Q.9 Is There, Under Human Rights Law, an Obligation of International Cooperation?

Malaria, HIV/AIDS and tuberculosis are examples of diseases which disproportionately affect the world's poorest populations, placing a tremendous burden on the economies of developing countries. In this regard, it should be noted that although the human rights paradigm concerns obligations of States with respect to individuals and groups within their own jurisdictions, where the human rights instruments refer to the State's resources, they include international assistance and cooperation.

In accordance with Articles 55 and 56 of the Charter of the United Nations, international cooperation for development and the realization of human rights is an obligation of all States. Similarly, the Declaration on the Right to Development emphasizes an active programme of international assistance and cooperation based on sovereign equality, interdependence and mutual interest.

In addition, the ICESCR requires each State that is party to the Covenant to "take steps, individually and through international assistance and cooperation, especially economic and technical, to the maximum of its available resources, with a view to achieving progressively the full realization of the rights recognized [herein]."

In this spirit, "the framework of international cooperation" is referred to, which acknowledges, for instance, that the needs of developing countries should be taken into consideration in the area of health. The role of specialized agencies is recognized in human rights treaties in this context. For example, the ICESCR stresses that "international action for the achievement of the rights . . . includes such methods as . . . furnishing of technical assistance and the holding of regional meetings and technical meetings for the purpose of consultation and study organized in conjunction with the Governments concerned."

5.1.10 *Q.10 What Are a Government's Human Rights Obligations in Relation to Other Actors in Society?*

As government roles and responsibilities include increased reliance on non-state actors (health insurance companies, etc.), governmental health systems must ensure the existence of social safety nets and other mechanisms to ensure that vulnerable population groups have access to the services and structures they need.

The obligation of the State to protect human rights means that governments are responsible for ensuring that non-state actors act in conformity with human rights law within their jurisdiction. Governments are obliged to ensure that third parties conform with human rights standards by adopting legislation, policies and other measures to assure adequate access to health care, quality information and so on, and an accessible means of redress if individuals are denied access to these goods and services. An example of this is the obligation of governments to ensure the regulation of the tobacco industry in order to protect its population against infringements of the right to health, the right to information and other relevant human rights provisions.

In the corporate and NGO contexts, there is a proliferation of voluntary codes which reflect international human rights norms and standards. Increasing attention to the human rights implication of work in the private sector has resulted in human rights being placed higher on the business agenda, with several businesses beginning to incorporate concern for human rights into their daily operations.

5.2 Integrating Human Rights in Health

5.2.1 *Q.11 What Is Meant by a Rights-Based Approach to Health?*

A rights-based approach to health refers to the processes of:

- Using human rights as a framework for health development.
- Accessing and addressing the human rights implications of any health policy, programme or legislation.

- Making human rights an integral dimension of the design, implementation, monitoring and evaluation of health-related policies and programmes in all spheres, including political, economic and social.

Substantive elements to apply, within these processes, could be as follows:

- Safeguarding *human dignity.*
- Paying attention to those population groups considered most vulnerable in society. In other words, recognizing and acting upon the characteristics of those affected by health policies, programmes and strategies—children (girls and boys), adolescents, women and men; indigenous and tribal populations; national, ethnic, religious and linguistic minorities; internally displaced persons; refugees; immigrants and migrants; the elderly; persons with disabilities; prisoners; economically disadvantaged or otherwise marginalized and/or *vulnerable groups.*
- Ensuring health systems are made *accessible* to all, especially the most vulnerable or marginalized sections of the population, in law and in fact, without discrimination on any of the prohibited grounds.
- Using a *gender* perspective, recognizing that both biological and socio-cultural factors play a significant role in influencing the health of men and women, and that policies and programmes must consciously set out to address these differences.
- Ensuring *equality and freedom from discrimination*, advertent or inadvertent, in the way health programmes are designed or implemented.
- *Disaggregating* health data to detect underlying discrimination.
- Ensuring free, meaningful and effective *participation* of beneficiaries of health development policies or programmes in decision-making processes which affect them.
- Promoting and protecting *the right to education* and the right to seek, receive and impart *information* and ideas concerning health issues. However, the right to information should not impair the right to *privacy*, which means that personal health data should be treated confidentially.
- Only limiting the exercise or enjoyment of a right by a health policy or programme as a last resort, and only considering this legitimate if each of provisions reflected in *the Siracusa principles* is met (see Question 13).
- Juxtaposing the human rights implications of any health legislation, policy or programme with the desired public health objectives and ensuring the *optimal balance* between good public health outcomes and the promotion and protection of human rights.
- Making *explicit linkages to international human rights norms and standards* to highlight how human rights apply and relate to a health policy, programme or legislation.
- Making the attainment of the right to *the highest attainable standard of health* the explicit ultimate aim of activities, which have as their objective the enhancement of health.
- Articulating the concrete government *obligations* to respect, protect and fulfil human rights.

- Identifying *benchmarks and indicators* to ensure monitoring of the progressive realization of rights in the field of health.
- Increasing *transparency* in and *accountability* for health as a key consideration at all stages of programme development.
- Incorporating *safeguards* to protect against majoritarian threats upon minorities, migrants and other domestically "unpopular" groups, in order to address power imbalances. For example, by incorporating redress mechanisms in case of impingements on health-related rights.

5.2.2 Q.12 What Is the Value-Added of Human Rights in Public Health?

Overall, human rights may benefit work in the area of public health by providing the following:

- Explicit recognition of the highest attainable standard of health as a "human right" (as opposed to a good or commodity with a charitable construct);
- A tool to enhance health outcomes by using a human right approach to designing, implementing and evaluating health policies and programmes;
- An "empowering" strategy for health which includes vulnerable and marginalized groups engaged as meaningful and active participants;
- A useful framework, vocabulary and form of guidance to identify, analyse and respond to the underlying determinants of health;
- A standard against which to assess the performance of governments in health;
- Enhanced governmental accountability for health;
- A powerful authoritative basis for advocacy and cooperation with governments, international organizations, international financial institutions and in the building of partnerships with relevant actors of civil society;
- Existing international mechanisms to monitor the realization of health as a human right;
- Accepted international norms and standards (e.g. definitions of concepts and population groups);
- Consistent guidance to States as human rights crosscut all UN activities;
- Increased scope of analysis and range of partners in countries.

5.2.3 Q.13 What Happens if the Protection of Public Health Necessitates the Restriction of Certain Human Rights?

There are a number of human rights that cannot be restricted in any circumstance, such as freedom from torture and slavery, and freedom of thought, conscience and religion. Limitation and derogation clauses in the international human rights instruments recognize the need to limit human rights at certain times.

Public health is sometimes used by States as a ground for limiting the exercise of human rights.

A key factor in determining if the necessary protections exist when rights are restricted is that each one of the five criteria of the Siracusa Principles must be met. Even in circumstances where limitations on grounds of protecting public health are basically permitted, they should be of limited duration and subject to review.

Interference with freedom of movement when instituting quarantine and isolation for a serious communicable disease—for example, Ebola fever, syphilis, typhoid or untreated tuberculosis—are examples of restrictions on rights that may, under certain circumstances, be necessary for the public good, and therefore could be considered legitimate under international human rights law. By contrast, a state which restricts the movements of, or incarcerates, persons with HIV/AIDS, refuses to allow doctors to treat persons believed to be opposed to a government or fails to provide immunization against the community's major infectious diseases, on grounds such as national security or the preservation of public order, has the burden of justifying such serious measures.

5.2.4 Q.14 What Implications Could Human Rights Have for Evidence-Based Health Information?

The process that gives birth to an internationally recognized human right is generated from the pressing reality on the ground. For example, the development of a declaration on the rights of indigenous populations stems from the recognition that this is a vulnerable and marginalized population group lacking full enjoyment of a wide range of human rights, including rights to political participation, health and education. In other words, the establishment of human rights norms and standards is itself evidence of a serious problem and governmental recognition of the importance of addressing it. The existence of human rights norms and standards should therefore stimulate the collection of evidence, indicating the data needed to tackle complex health challenges. For example, disaggregating data beyond traditional markers could detect discrimination on the basis of ethnicity against indigenous and tribal peoples, which is considered an underlying determinant of their overall poor health status. However, the political sensitivities which underpin human rights in exposing how different population groups are treated, and why, hamper the extent to which human rights are welcomed as a driving force for data collection.

More widely accepted is the notion that human rights are relevant to the way in which health data should be collected. This includes the choice of the methods of data collection which must include considerations on how to ensure respect for human rights, such as privacy, participation and non-discrimination. Secondly, international instruments can be helpful in defining various population groups. For example, the ILO Convention Concerning Indigenous and Tribal Peoples provides an authoritative basis for identifying and differentiating indigenous and tribal peoples from other population groups.

5.2.5 *Q.15 How Can Human Rights Support Work to Strengthen Health Systems?*

Human rights provide a standard against which to evaluate existing health policies and programmes, including highlighting the differential treatment of individual groups of people in, for example, manifestations, frequency and severity of disease and governmental responses to it. Human rights norms and standards also form a strong basis for health systems to prioritize the health needs of vulnerable and marginalized population groups. Human rights moves beyond averages and focuses attention on those population groups in society which are considered most vulnerable (e.g. indigenous and tribal populations; refugees and migrants, ethnic, religious, national and racial minorities), as well as putting forward specific human rights which may help guide health policy, programming and health system processes (e.g. the right of those potentially affected by health policies, strategies and standards to participate in the process in which decisions affecting their health are made).

5.2.6 *Q.16 What Is the Relationship Between Health Legislation and Human Rights Law?*

Health legislation can be an important vehicle towards ensuring the promotion and protection of the right to health. In the design and review of health legislation, human rights provide a useful tool to determine its effectiveness and appropriateness in line with both human rights and public health goals. In this context, HIV/AIDS has caused many countries to revisit their public health laws, including in relation to quarantine and isolation.

Restrictive laws and policies that deliberately focus on certain population groups without sufficient data, epidemiological and otherwise, to support their approach may raise a host of human rights concerns. Two examples in this regard are health policies concerning the involuntary sterilization of women from certain population groups that are justified as necessary for their health and well-being and sodomy statutes criminalizing same-sex sexual behaviour that are justified as necessary to prevent the spread of HIV/AIDS.

Government capacity to develop national health policy and legislation that conforms to human rights obligations needs to be strengthened. This includes developing the tools to review health-related laws and policies to determine whether, on their face or application, they violate human rights, and providing the means to rectify any violation which exists.

5.2.7 Q.17 How Do Human Rights Apply to Situational Analyses of Health in Countries?

Increased attention to human rights may, firstly, broaden the scope of situational health analyses in countries, and secondly, as a result, allow new partners to be identified. New areas of attention include consideration of the health components of national human rights action plans and, conversely, the inclusion of human rights in national health strategies and action plans. Given that human rights obligations relevant to health rest with the government as a whole, health and human rights goals need to figure in policies and plans which may be generated outside the health sector per se but which have a strong bearing on health, such as national food and nutrition policies and plans. The focus on vulnerable population groups draws attention to how national legislation and development policies impact upon the status of such groups, which institutions work to protect their best interests, and how civil society movements represent them. Finally, the reports to and comments from the United Nations human rights treaty monitoring bodies and the views of civil society organizations are another issue for consideration.

Practical implications may be to engage at the national level with a greater range of Ministries other than Health Ministries, for example, Justice Ministries and those with responsibility for human rights (including independent human rights institutions), women's affairs, children's affairs, education, social affairs, finance and so on. UN agencies and other intergovernmental organizations working on human rights, international and national human rights NOGs, national human rights institutions, ombudspersons, national human rights commissions, human rights think-tanks and research institutes also constitute fruitful partners for advancing the global health agenda.

5.3 Health and Human Rights in a Broader Context

5.3.1 Q.18 How Do Ethics Relate to Human Rights?

Ethics are norms of conduct for individuals and for societies. These norms derive from many sources, including religion, cultural tradition and reflection, which accounts in part for the complexity within each ethical outlook. Ethics as a system of norms employs many component concepts, including obligations and duties, virtues of character, standards of value and goodness in outcomes and consequences of action, standards of fairness and justice in allocation of resources and in reward and punishment.

Human rights refer to an internationally agreed upon set of principles and norms embodied in international legal instruments. These international human rights principles and norms are the result of deep and long-standing negotiations among Member States on a range of fundamental issues. In other words, human rights are generated by governments through a consensus-building process.

Work in ethics needs to take into account human rights norms and standards, not only in substance but also in relation to the processes of ethical discourse and reasoning. For example, where issues concern a specific population group, individuals representing this group should be participants in any determination of the ethical implications of the issues affecting them. Ethics is particularly useful in areas of practice where human rights do not provide a definite answer, for example, in new and emerging areas where human rights law has not been applied or codified, such as human cloning.

5.3.2 *Q.19 How Do Human Rights Principles Relate to Equity?*

Equity means that people's needs, rather than their social privileges, guide the distribution of opportunities for well-being. This means eliminating disparities in health and in health's major determinants that are systematically associated with underlying social disadvantage within a society. Within the human rights discourse, the principle of equity is increasingly serving as an important non-legal generic policy term aimed at ensuring fairness. It has been used to embrace policy-related issues, such as the accessibility, affordability and acceptability of available health care services. The focused attention on vulnerable and disadvantaged groups in society in international human rights instruments reinforces the principle of equity. Also, at the international level, human rights instruments address equity by encouraging international cooperation to realize rights as well as addressing intrastate relations, most notably in the United Nations Declaration on the Right to Development.

5.3.3 *Q.20 How Do Health and Human Rights Principles Apply to Poverty Reduction?*

The right to a standard of living adequate for health and well-being, including necessary social services, and the right to security in the event of sickness, disability, old age or other lack of livelihood are enshrined in the Universal Declaration of Human Rights. The Committee on Economic, Social and Cultural Rights has defined poverty as "a human condition characterized by sustained or chronic deprivation of the resources, capabilities, choices, security and power necessary for the enjoyment of an adequate standard of living and other civil, cultural economic, political and social rights."

Human rights empower individuals and communities by granting them entitlements that give rise to legal obligations on others. Human rights can help to equalize the distribution and exercise of power both within and between societies, mitigating the powerlessness of the poor. As economic and social rights, such as the right to health, are increasingly gaining weight through increased normative clarity and application, they will provide an important tool for poverty reduction.

A human rights approach also requires the active and informed participation of the poor in the formulation, implementation and monitoring of strategies which may affect them.

Accountability, transparency, democracy and good governance are essential ingredients to addressing poverty and ill health. Legal rights and obligations, at the domestic and international level, demand accountability: effective legal remedies, administrative and political accountability mechanism at the domestic level, as well as human rights monitoring at the international level. Overall, human rights provide a holistic framework to poverty reduction, demanding consideration of a spectrum of approaches, including legislation, polices and programmes.

5.3.4 Q.21 How Does Globalization Affect the Promotion and Protection of Human Rights?

Globalization is a term used to cover many different phenomena, most of which concern increasing flows of money, goods, services, people and ideas across national borders. This process has brought benefits to many peoples and countries, lifting many people from poverty and bringing greater awareness of people's entitlement to basic human rights. In many cases, however, the globalization process has contributed to greater marginalization of people and countries that have been denied access to markets, information and essential goods such as new life saving drugs.

Within the human rights community, certain trends associated with globalization have raised concern with respect to their effect on states' capacity to ensure the protection of human rights, especially for the most vulnerable members of society. Located primarily in the economic–political realm of globalization, these trends include an increasing reliance upon the free market; a significant growth in the influence of international financial markets and institutions in determining national policies; cutbacks in public sector spending; the privation of functions previously considered to be the exclusive domain of the state; and the deregulation of a range of activities with a view to facilitating investment and rewarding entrepreneurial initiative. These trends serve to reduce the role of the state in economic affairs, and at the same time increase the role and responsibilities of private (non-state) actors, especially those in corporate business, and also those in civil society. Human rights analysts are concerned that such trends limit the ability of the state to protect the vulnerable from adverse effects of globalization, and enforce human rights.

In this context, the United Nations Committee on Economic, Social and Cultural Rights has emphasized the strong and continuous responsibility of international organizations, as well as the governments that have created and manage them, to take whatever measures they can in the context of globalization to assist governments to act in ways which are compatible with their human rights obligations and to seek to devise policies and programmes which promote respect for those rights.

5.3.5 Q.22 How Does International Human Rights Law Influence International Trade Law?

Recently, the United Nations human rights system has begun addressing trade laws and practices in relation to human rights law, and, in turn, the World Trade Organization (WTO) and other organizations dealing with trade have begun to consider the human rights implications of their work.

For example, the question of access to drugs has been increasingly addressed in the context of human rights. In an unprecedented move, the Commission on Human Rights in 2001 adopted a resolution on access to medication in the context of pandemics, such as HIV/AIDS which reaffirms that access to medication in this context is a fundamental element for the progressive realization of the right to health. States are called upon to pursue policies which would promote the availability, accessibility and affordability for all without discrimination of scientifically appropriate and good quality pharmaceuticals and medical technologies used to treat pandemics, such as HIV/AIDS. They are also asked to adopt legislation or other measures to safeguard access to such pharmaceuticals and medical technologies from any limitations by third parties.

Also in relation to the question of access to drugs, the relationship between the Agreement on the Trade Related Aspects of Intellectual Property Rights (TRIPS) and human rights was considered in a report to the Sub-Commission on Human Rights in 2001 by the High Commissioner for Human Rights. This report notes that of the 141 Members of the WTO, 111 have ratified the ICESCR. Members should therefore implement the minimum standards of the TRIPS Agreement bearing in mind both their human rights obligations as well as the flexibility inherent in the TRIPS Agreement, and recognizing that "human rights are the first responsibility of Governments."

Article 15 of the International Covenant on Economic, Social and Cultural Rights recognizes "the right of everyone to enjoy the benefits of scientific progress and its applications." This right places obligations on governments to take the steps necessary to conserve, develop and diffuse science and scientific research, as well as ensure freedom of scientific enquiry. The implications of this right for health issues have only recently begun to be explored, for example, with respect to access to drugs for developing countries.

5.3.6 Q.23 What Is Meant by a Rights-Based Approach to Development?

There is increasing recognition, within the UN system and beyond, that development itself is not only a human right as recognized in the United Nations Declaration on the Right to Development (1986) but that the development process must, in itself, be consistent with human rights. In this regard, the Office of the High Commissioner of Human Rights (OHCHR) has advocated a rights-based approach to development as a conceptual framework for the process of human development that is normatively based on international human rights. This approach integrates the norms, standards and principles of the international human rights system into the plans, policies and processes of development.

The norms and standards are those contained in the wealth of international treaties and declarations. The principles include those of participation, account-ability, non-discrimination and attention to vulnerability, empowerment and express linkage to international human rights instruments.

> A rights-based approach to development describes situations not simply in terms of human needs, or of developmental requirements, but in terms of society's obligations to respond to the inalienable rights of individuals, empowers people to demand justice as a right, not as charity, and gives communities a moral basis from which to claim international assistance when needed.
>
> United Nations Secretary-General, Kofi Annan

5.3.7 Q.24 How Do Human Rights Law, Refugee Law and Humanitarian Law Interact with the Provision of Health Assistance?

The large number and changing nature of emergencies and conflicts, including the explosion of religious and ethnic turmoil around the world, has prompted the need for new thinking and approaches within the UN system and beyond. Fresh attention is being drawn to the international legal framework for dealing with these emergen-cies, in particular the relationship between humanitarian law, human rights law and refugee law and their applicability in a changing crisis environment.

Refugee law acts to protect refugees by spelling out specific legal provisions protecting the human rights of refugees, most notably through the United Nations Convention Relating to the Status of Refugees (1950) and its protocol (1966).

Human rights, humanitarian law and refugee law are distinct yet closely related branches of the international legal system. Human rights and refugee law were developed within the UN framework and thus have similar underpinnings. Humani-tarian law, however, has profoundly different origins and uses different mechanisms for its implementation. All branches of law have, however, a fundamental common objective: the respect for human dignity without any discrimination whatsoever as to race, colour, religion, sex, birth or wealth, or any similar criteria. In addition, they share a great number of detailed objectives and conceptual similarities.

Humanitarian law is the law of armed conflict or the law of wars: a body of rules which in wartime protect persons who are not or no longer participating in the hostilities and which limit methods and means of warfare. The central instruments of humanitarian law are the four 1949 Geneva Conventions and their two Additional Protocols of 1977.

Efforts are underway to ensure that international human rights and humanitarian law principles provide the standard and reference for humanitarian action by the United Nations and its agencies as well as other actors. Health practices in preparing for, assessing, implementing and evaluating the impact of health assistance in the context of an armed conflict need to be grounded within a framework of international law.

The sick and wounded, health workers, medical equipment, hospitals and various medical units (including medical transportation) are all protected under humanitarian law principles. Moreover, denying access to medical care in some circumstances could constitute a war crime.

Overall, humanitarian action in the field of health represents action towards the fulfilment of the right to health in situations where the threats to health are greatest. Moreover, in the provision of health care in emergency situations, consideration of the human rights dimensions can help ensure that strategies pay particular attention to vulnerable groups.

The particular vulnerability of refugees, internally displaced and migrants requires a special emphasis on human rights. Within these groups, women as single heads of households, unaccompanied minors, persons with disabilities and the elderly are in need of special attention. Specific human rights principles exists that provide guidance in ensuring protection in emergencies against exposure of vulnerable groups to risk factors of diseases and ill health.

5.3.8 Q.25 How Do Human Rights Relate to Health Development Work in Countries?

Human rights are upheld as a cross-cutting issue in the United Nations' development work at country level. The Common Country Assessment (CCA) and the United Nations Development Assistance Framework (UNDAF) provide the major principles upon which a human rights-based approach to development is founded. The CCA and UNDAF Guidelines refer to the implementation of United Nations Conventions and Declarations and underscore the importance of taking full account of human rights in both these processes. The CCA thus helps to facilitate efforts for coherent, integrated and coordinated UN support to government follow-up to the Conferences and the implementation of Conventions at the field level.

This parallels the principles enunciated in the World Bank's Comprehensive Development Framework (CDF), the joint WorldBank/IMF Poverty Reduction Strategy Paper (PRSP) initiative, the formal design of which reflects human rights concepts and standards.

A project of the OHCHR to produce guidelines for the integration of human rights in poverty reduction strategies, including Poverty Reduction Strategy Papers (HRPRS Guidelines), has highlighted the close correspondence between "the realities of poor people," as identified by Voices of the Poor and other poverty studies and the international human rights normative framework.

Thus, attention to human rights will help to ensure that the key concerns of poor people become, and remain, the key concerns of poverty reduction strategies. For example, the integration of human rights into anti-poverty strategies will help to ensure that vulnerable individuals and groups are not neglected; that the active and informed participation of the poor is provided for; that key sectoral issues (e.g.education, housing, health and food) receive due attention; that immediate and intermediate (as well as long-term) targets are identified; that effective monitoring methods (e.g. indicators and benchmarks) are established; and that accessible mechanisms of accountability, in relation to all parties, are instituted. Furthermore, human rights provide poverty reduction strategies with norms, standards and values that have a high level of global legitimacy.

Chapter 6
Freedom from Fear for Human Well-being: The Need for Humanitarian Medicine in the Prevention of Torture and the Treatment of its Survivors

Jaap A. Walkate LLD

Torture should not be considered and far from accepted as if it were a natural disaster which is caused by powers beyond our control. Torture is a political problem first of all. We are talking about a *man-made disaster* which causes tens of thousands of victims each year.

The *prohibition of torture* is unconditional: no exceptional circumstances whatsoever, whether a state of war or a threat of war, internal political stability or any other public emergency, may be invoked as a justification of torture.

Where *medical personnel have been and/or still are involved in the practice of torture*, the International Association for Humanitarian Medicine may consider it one of its objectives to be aware and vigilant of these breaches of medical ethics and violations of the right to health and to prevent any human degradation resulting therefrom.

Physicians have an important role to play in the prevention of torture and in the treatment of victims. In cases where they are called upon to examine persons who declare they have been tortured, and to verify their statement, the physician's role may be crucial in saving the accused from further detention or even conviction.

The extent to which medical personnel can play a decisive role in *fact-finding* and thus contribute to the *prevention of torture* and to the effective treatment of victims is impressive.

The International Association for Humanitarian Medicine could play a role in the dissemination of the Protocols Manual on a global scale. Also, and more obviously, *medical doctors will play a vital role in treating and curing victims of torture*. It takes special skills to assess their statements and to treat the sequelae of torture. The terrible *plight of those in Sierra Leone* who did not take the side of the rebellious troops that had overtaken part of the country and, who if they were not killed, were tortured and often lost one or more limbs by amputation, men, women and children alike, is a challenge par excellence to the International Association for Humanitarian Medicine and to professionals specialized in the field of orthopaedics.

It has been proposed among others by the Dutch Johannes Wier Foundation for Health and Human Rights to request the United Nations to appoint a *Special Rapporteur on Health Professionals and Human Rights* whose mandate would be to monitor and report on any violations of the right to health care. It is suggested that the International Association for Humanitarian Medicine sponsor this proposal and propagate it, after further study, among the Member States of the United Nations.

Possible objectives: The International Association, keeping in mind that there are already many non-governmental and intergovernmental organizations active in the field of humanitarian affairs, in the field of medicine, and in the field of rehabilitation of torture victims, should consider cooperation, therefore, with existing organizations as the most effective thing to do. It should try to:

- help decide on needs, priorities and strategies;
- use its good offices with governments;
- propagate the need for a Special Rapporteur of the United Nations on Health and Human Rights, establish a network of experts who are willing to render services in the field of humanitarian medicine (WOH), and
- function as a professional sounding board for the medical profession, for providers of humanitarian aid and medical help and all this in the framework of offering relief to victims, either collectively or individually, of both natural and man-made disasters, violations of human rights and of human dignity, thus safeguarding people from fear and therefore enhancing their human well-being.

6.1 Introduction

Torture—it is a practice from which we revolt and which we would prefer to deny exists. That is the easiest way out: to deny its existence or to belittle its scale and effects frees us from taking action to help and do something about it. What we know about torture and what appears in the media about torture is so abhorrent that it is hard to believe and therefore it "cannot be true." This is a general reaction—a very human reaction too among the public at large and one of the reasons why torture can be practised in many countries without getting too much public opposition. And this is also why so many governments in the world get away with *government-sponsored torture* or with, what I would call *government-tolerated torture*. Government-sponsored torture would be the systematic intimidation through the practice of torture as a policy of the government (examples are found among the past governments of some countries in the southern cone of Latin America), while government-tolerated torture would be the acceptance by the government, but not as a considered policy, of torture being committed down the lines of the law enforcement agencies of the State without taking action to do something about it (examples only too many). In their effects on the victims, both are equally pernicious and indeed unacceptable.

Let us remind ourselves constantly that torture should not be considered and far from accepted as if it were a natural disaster which is caused by powers beyond our control. It is not and it should not be, but unfortunately, often, for convenience' sake, it is. Torture is a political problem first of all. We are talking about a man-made disaster which causes tens of thousands of victims each year. The recent Amnesty International report (18 October 2000) in the framework of its campaign against torture states that torture is on the rise. The report finds fault with some 150 countries where to some degree or other torture is being practised over the past 3 years. It finds that in more than 70 countries, torture or ill-treatment by state officials was widespread, and in over 80 countries people reportedly died as a result.

We should try to muster all the political support we can find, and we should undertake everything in our power to prevent the disaster from happening in the first place. Here lies a task ahead for the International Association for Humanitarian Medicine.

The violation of human dignity and physical integrity which torture and, in its lesser form, cruel, inhuman and degrading treatment and punishment constitute is a *symptom of a sick society*. Its consequences in terms of human suffering, rupture of social fabric and duration of rehabilitation—if at all fully feasible—are unacceptable from a moral or ethical point of view but equally from a legal, political, medical or financial point of view.

6.2 The Prohibition of Torture Under All Circumstances

Article 5 of that famous Universal Declaration of Human Rights (1948) is the basis of the general prohibition of torture under international law. From this Declaration, many international instruments have originated, such as treaties and declarations adopted by the General Assembly of the United Nations and regional organizations, such as the Council of Europe and the Organization of American States, which incorporate and elaborate that unconditional prohibition, thus adding to the strength of the prohibition under international law and culminating in the UN Convention against Torture (1984). Torture in the definition of that convention (Article 1 paragraph I) is

> any act by which severe pain or suffering, whether physical or mental, is intentionally, inflicted on a person for such purposes as obtaining from him or a third person information or a confession, punishing him for an act he or a third person has committed or is suspected of having committed, or intimidating or coercing him or a third person, or any for reason based on discrimination of any kind, when such pain or suffering is inflicted by or at the instigation of or with the consent or acquiescence of a public official or other person acting in an official capacity. It does not include pain or suffering arising only from, inherent in or incidental to lawful sanctions.

In legal interpretations of this definition, it is assumed that torture is an aggravated form of cruel, inhuman or degrading treatment or punishment (see Article 16). What distinguishes torture from the common crime of maltreatment in whatever degree is the involvement of a "public official" and a third person (detainee, prisoner) being at his mercy. The prohibition is unconditional: no exceptional circumstances whatsoever, whether a state of war or a threat of war, internal political stability or any other public emergency, may be invoked as a justification of torture (Article 2 paragraph 2 of the Convention; see also for armed conflicts of an international character various articles of the four Conventions of Geneva of 1949 and for armed conflicts not of an international character, Article 3 common to these Conventions and see for public emergency, Article 4 of the UN Covenant on Civil and Political Rights of 1966).

The exception at the end of the definition of the Convention against Torture is subject to different interpretations: some countries, such as some Islamic states, where corporal and capital punishment is a lawful sanction, maintain that the definition does not apply to such punishment. It is, however, difficult to accept any interpretation which would rule out corporal punishment from the applicability of the definition, for how could one consider corporal punishment not a form of "cruel, inhuman or degrading punishment," not to mention in this context the death penalty. It is therefore the considered opinion of many that the exception for lawful sanctions only refers to the inherent inconvenience which a prison sentence brings upon a detainee.

6.3 Torture Is a Political Problem

For the victim of torture, it makes no difference whether he is being tortured because of an explicit, maybe ideological, policy of the government or those wielding power or he is being victimized by a law enforcement system which is corrupt, unprofessional and unethical, but which the government is unable to guide out of its unlawful practices. The survivor will suffer the same physical and mental wounds.

Experience shows that law enforcement personnel in many countries are not always and not under all circumstances (and this is an understatement) competent to apply the legal rules concerning arrest, detention and imprisonment properly and, therefore, often fail to assist in the administration of justice. This may lead under certain conditions, such as corruption or the need to produce a suspect or get a promotion, to the commission of or participation in acts of torture. If at the political level torture is accepted as an instrument to reach certain unlawful goals or is condoned as some form of unavoidable behaviour of law enforcement personnel, what hope do we have that whatever efforts undertaken at lower levels in the hierarchy to eradicate the evil of torture will be successful? All instructions and training programmes which may be devised for civil police, armed forces and prison personnel to instil the necessity of refraining from such practices will be most likely not effective, if they are sanctioned, either explicitly or tacitly, by the political leaders of the land. Although, under international law, an order from a superior officer or a public authority may never be invoked as a justification of torture, in reality this rule is being violated on a wide scale. Therefore, a *precondition* to all the work we are undertaking in our own national contexts is to ensure that at the *political level* the will exists to *publicly reject torture as unacceptable*. At the same time, there should be left no doubt about the political will to prosecute and bring to justice all those who are involved in acts of torture, either by committing them or by condoning them.

6.4 The Involvement of Medical Personnel in Torture

Where the practices of torture or corporal punishment exist, often this implies some form of cooperation of medical personnel, physicians or paramedical staff connected to institutions of detention. Unfortunately, there are too many reports, however incredible it may sound, that medical personnel have been and/or still are involved in the practice of torture: sometimes by devising methods of torture which do not leave visible scars on the victim, sometimes by preventing torturers going too far and losing a valuable detainee who still should disclose more information, sometimes by reviving victims to prepare them for another round of beatings, sometimes by falsely certifying a mental illness.

Such reports have been at the basis of the "Principles of Medical Ethics relevant to the Role of Health Personnel, particularly Physicians, in the Protection of Prisoners and Detainees against Torture and other Cruel, Inhuman or Degrading Treatment or Punishment" adopted by the UN General Assembly in 1982 (Resolution 37/194 of 18 December 1982). These principles were drafted on the basis of preparatory work undertaken in the WHO and the World Medical Association which had adopted already in 1975 a comprehensive declaration (Declaration of Tokyo) on the role of the medical profession in the case of torture. There are more texts adopted by the medical and paramedical profession in relation to the treatment of detainees, such as national codes of medical ethics and statements on nurses in relation to detainees and violations of human rights, such as torture.

What the UN principles do is put the subject in a legal and intergovernmental context and qualify violations as (gross) contraventions of medical ethics and as *offences under international law.*

Participation or complicity in torture by health personnel has been declared illegal and punishable as a "gross contravention of medical ethics" (principle 2).

The same Principles also declare inadmissible and a contravention of medical ethics the certification or participation in the *certification of the fitness* of prisoners or detainees for any form of treatment or punishment that may adversely affect their physical or mental health, nor to participate in any way in the infliction of any such treatment or punishment (principle 4). This is a reference to participation of medical doctors in the application of corporal punishment, be they beatings, floggings or amputations (still a current form of punishment in half a dozen countries according to the Amnesty International report), a participation which should be refused under any circumstance except in the cases where the physician is called upon to treat the wounds.

The International Association for Humanitarian Medicine may consider it one of its objectives to be aware and vigilant of these breaches of medical ethics and violations of the right to health and to prevent any human degradation resulting therefrom.

6.5 The Role of Physicians in the Prevention of Torture

Physicians have an important role to play in the prevention of torture and in the treatment of victims. In cases where they are called upon to examine persons who declare they have been tortured, and to verify their statement, the physician's role may be crucial in saving the accused from further detention or even conviction. A good medical examination when an arrested person arrives in the place of detention may offer some protection from torture because signs of it may be noticed immediately and the proof that torture took place—often difficult to prove—is so much easier to provide.

In this context, I would like to refer to the Principles and Manual on the Effective Investigation and Documentation of Torture and Other Cruel, Inhuman or Degrading Treatment or Punishment. This extraordinary document of *c*. 80 pages was drafted over a period of 3 years by more than 75 experts in law, health and human rights representing 41 organizations or institutions from 15 countries—among which the International Association for Humanitarian Medicine, had it actively existed, certainly should have appeared. Since the final text was adopted at a meeting in Istanbul, March 1999, the document is referred to as the Istanbul Protocol. The protocol was submitted later that year by the group to the United Nations of the High Commissioner for Human Rights.

The Special Rapporteur of the United Nations on Torture, Prof. Sir Nigel Rodley, who had participated in the drafting, annexed the Principles (not the Manual) to his report to the UN Commission on Human Rights at its spring session in Geneva. This brought the Protocol to the attention of the general membership of the UN (UN doc. E/CN.4/2000/9, Annex, of date 2 February 2000). The Principles outline minimum standards for State adherence to ensure the effective documentation of torture. They also hold guidelines for "medical experts involved in the investigation of torture or ill-treatment" who "should behave at all times in conformity with the highest ethical standards and in particular shall obtain informed consent before any examination is undertaken" (principle 6 (a)). The Manual contains more detailed guidelines for the assessment of persons who allege torture and ill-treatment, for investigating cases of torture, and for reporting such findings to the judiciary and other investigative bodies.

The extent to which medical personnel can play a decisive role in the fact-finding and thus contribute to the prevention of torture and to the effective treatment of victims as foreseen by the Manual is impressive. The International Association for Humanitarian Medicine could play a role in the dissemination of the Manual on a global scale.

Where medical help comes too late for a person presumed to be a victim of torture, it still is of great importance to determine under what kind of circumstances the person died and whether death was a result of torture. In some countries, it is not uncommon that in the case of custodial death, for example in police offices, police or prison doctors are under pressure to cover up any evidence of torture. Sometimes they are forced to sign autopsy reports where no autopsy had taken place, some of these doctors finding it difficult to oppose authorities that resort to torture. In such cases, the physician may be victim of the system as well. Like torture in general, custodial deaths seen to be on the rise.

For cases where, especially in developing countries, a doctor is not able to get the necessary evidence to authoritatively decide on the cause of death due to the lack of basic equipment with which to perform an adequate investigative autopsy, a special kit has been developed by two forensic experts under auspices of the Commission for Human Rights of India (see CHRI News, Autumn 1999, p. 9). The kit was presented at the VIII International Symposium on Torture, held in New Delhi, September 1999, and shows that it is possible to put together a set of basic tools for autopsy with relatively modest means (ca. US $60). It will provide physicians with a last resort in the continuing fight against torture.

6.6 The Role of Physicians in the Treatment of Victims

Also and more obviously, medical doctors will play a vital role in treating and curing victims of torture. It takes special skills to assess their statements and to treat the sequelae of torture. In the first place, often very refined means of torture have been used so as to leave no physical scars. But the deepest are the wounds of the mind and the soul. To ascertain a broken arm or leg is easier than to determine that the person has undergone electric shocks. Modern torture technology is developed with an eye on medical scientific publications on the subject. In the second place, victims or survivors do not necessarily say they have been tortured, not seldom ashamed of what has happened to them (especially sexual torture can reach intimate places) or of the fact that they were forced to give up and "confess." A physician must have special experience or get special training to find out what happened, and he must do so gently without scaring the patient who is often reminded of the past by the cell-like treatment room and the traditional white doctor's garb. Moreover, the physician and his staff must know that they are in for some gruelling sessions when survivors of torture tell their mind-boggling stories, during which sometimes both victim and physician break down. It happens that such physicians seek expert help from colleagues as if they were indirect victims. Health personnel engaged in the treatment of victims of torture in some countries may fall victim to the authorities when they are harassed and pressured to disclose the names of those they have been treating, and when refusing to do so, while invoking their professional oath, are arrested and subjected to acts of torture themselves. A vicious circle . . .

It is a sad but inevitable conclusion that probably no victim of torture will ever recover completely from what he or she has suffered. In many cases, the only thing we can hope for is that the victim will be able to live with his past and play a useful role again in society.

In this respect, I draw your attention to the terrible plight of those in Sierra Leone who did not take the side of the rebellious troops that had overtaken part of the country and who, if they were not killed, were tortured and often lost one or more limbs by amputation—men, women and children alike. The plight of these amputees is a challenge par excellence to the International Association for Humanitarian Medicine and to professionals specialized in the field of orthopaedics. Let me add that the Board of Trustees of the UN Fund for Victims of Torture has made special provisions for financially assisting these survivors, especially children, who have such immense problems to overcome. If the Association takes action, the Fund may help.

6.7 The Need for a UN Special Rapporteur on Health Professionals and Human Rights

It has been proposed among others by the Dutch Johannes Wier Foundation for Health and Human Rights to request the United Nations to appoint a Special Rapporteur on Health Professionals and Human Rights whose mandate would be to monitor and report on any violations of the right to health care. The mandate could be drafted along the lines of existing UN Special Rapporteurs appointed by the UN Commission for Human Rights, such as the Special Rapporteurs on Summary of Arbitrary Executions on Torture, among many others. Such a mandate, and I quote from a report by the Dutch Foundation from November 1996 on the matter, "should focus primarily on violations of the right to health care in areas of armed conflict and prison situation, since most of the violations occur in these contexts. In these situations the Special Rapporteur should be aware of the two main aspects of the right to health care: the right to medical care and the independence, inviolability and protection of medical personnel, facilities and patients." (Report no. 14, p. 13) May I suggest that the International Association for Humanitarian Medicine sponsor this proposal and propagate it, after further study, among the Member States of the United Nations.

6.8 Financial Implications

The number of victims of torture—and let us not forget their families—in need of treatment is of course not known, but the number probably runs in the hundreds of thousands all over the world. By far, the majority do not get any treatment at all, the rest of them are lucky if they find specialized centres for rehabilitation which are on the rise in all parts of the world, especially in the western countries because of the many refugees who find a place to stay there. We do not know the exact amount of money which is needed to provide the necessary help and support. According to the Convention against Torture (Article 14), States are under an obligation to ensure in its legal system that the victim of torture obtains redress and has an enforceable right to fair and adequate compensation, including the means for as full rehabilitation as possible. In reality, however, victims do not and often are not in a position to sue governments for payment of any such compensation.

One may argue that the UN General Assembly has assumed a form of collective responsibility for the rehabilitation of torture victims by establishing a Voluntary Fund for Victims of Torture in 1981 to receive contributions for the distribution, through established channels of assistance and of humanitarian, legal and financial aid (Res. 36/151 of 16 December 1981).

The Fund depends entirely on voluntary contributions from governments, private organizations and/or individuals. It does not receive any financial support from the regular UN budget.

Over the past two decades, between 30 and 40 Member States of the UN have become loyal and generous donors that enable the Fund to support a steadily

increasing number of over 100 non-governmental organizations, centres for rehabilitation and single projects in some 50 countries to the extent of some US $7
million this year only, while the requests this year totalled some US$ 10 million.
More contributions will be needed.

The Fund is administered on behalf of the Secretary General by the High Commissioner for Human Rights, assisted and advised by a Board of Trustees of five
experts in the field of human rights, each from one of the geographical regions in
the United Nations. In medical matters, the Board is assured of the expert opinion
of Dr William Gunn and Dr Adriaan van Es.

When Amnesty International says that torture is on the rise, I am disappointed
but not surprised: the Board of Trustees is every year confronted with more requests
from an increasing number of centres for rehabilitation of an increasing number of
victims.

Will it ever end, the violence, the brutality, the bloodshed, the infringement of
human dignity, will we be ever able to allay the fears of individuals, can we, in short,
with all our expertise cure a sick society when it is affected by the phenomenon of
torture?

6.9 Possible Objectives of the International Association for Humanitarian Medicine

The International Association, keeping in mind that there are already many (non-
governmental and intergovernmental) organizations active in the field of humanitarian affairs, in the field of medicine and in the field of rehabilitation of torture
victims, should consider cooperation, therefore, with existing organizations as the
most effective thing to do.

In the beginning of its existence, it should try to

- help decide on needs, priorities and strategies;
- use its good offices with governments;
- propagate the need for a Special Rapporteur of the United Nations on Health
  Professionals and Human Rights;
- establish a network of experts who are willing to render services in the field of
  humanitarian medicine; and
- function as a professional sounding board for the medical profession, for providers
  of humanitarian aid and medical help and all this in the framework of offering
  relief to victims, either collectively or individually, of both natural and man-made
  disasters, violations of human rights and of human dignity, thus safeguarding
  people from fear and therefore enhancing their human well-being.

Part II
Humanitarian Medicine

Chapter 7
Humanitarian Medicine: A Vision and Action

M. Masellis, MD and S.W.A. Gunn, MD, FRCSC

At first sight, it may seem pleonastic to define medicine as humanitarian, since its principal aim lies precisely in human relationships, and rather enigmatic to talk of humanitarian medicine today, as if we were almost obliged to think of a new concept of humanity or medicine.

As physicians, we have to bear in mind that the canons handed down in the Hippocratic Oath have for decades constituted ample testimony of medical action in a humanitarian sense, where—establishing the duties of those who exercise the medical profession—they state "...I will regulate my patients' treatment to their advantage, according to my capacities and judgement, and I will abstain from every evil action and from every injustice ..." and they underline the fundamental principles of solidarity and devotion for all those who suffer. And even modern-day deontology, which has progressively become enriched with new contents and demands in relation to medicine's ever-growing ethical and social dimension, requires a profession of faith by those who undertake the medical profession: "I swear to treat all my patients with the same application and commitment independently of any feelings that they may inspire in me and ignoring every difference of race, religion, nationality, social condition, and political ideology ...."

The physician's oath therefore continues to reflect the foundations of a medical ethic that is still based on human solidarity as the basis of medical assistance.

From the viewpoint of the average person, the humanitarian aspect of medicine has always coincided with the traditional form of charity, originally practised on the basis of religious principles and performed only for those belonging to the same faith and the same creed, and later becoming, as lay opinion began to spread, a need of the community to support its own members.

In what way has the exercise of medicine changed? We do not think that it has changed in its deontology but rather in the concept of solidarity, understood as commonality with other persons. "Do unto others as you would have others do unto you" has become the golden rule of the modern humanitarian approach, subsequent to the universality of the principle that considers every person as different from every other, a principle that the more advanced countries have incorporated into their ever more democratic constitutional order. Following this line, humanitarianism has also begun to cross the border of the individual state, with the result that the question of its own sovereignty becomes involved.

While until just a few decades ago, health was seen as a prevalently personal matter, a reciprocal bond between physician and patient as codified in the Hippocratic Oath, today it is considered a universal human right, with complex implications that are not only medical but also philosophical, ethical, socio-economic, political, and legal. If we consider how the fundamental rights of children, the handicapped, and persons injured and killed in disasters have been universally recognized, we can say that the problem of health has become a global problem, regulated by international humanitarian legislation.

The Charter of the United Nations in 1945 was an event of great importance not only in the field of global geopolitics but also in that of health. The San Francisco Conference, where the UN Charter was signed, deemed it useful to institute an international organization for health, which was created on 7 April 1948 with the name *World Health Organization* (WHO), under the leadership of Dr Brock Chisholm. The guiding principle of the new organization, totally revolutionary and controversial, was *man's right to health.*

On 10 December 1948, the General Assembly of the United Nations adopted and approved the *Universal Declaration of Human Rights*, of which Article 25 states

> everyone has the right to a living standard adequate to maintain his own health and well-being as well as that of his family, including food, clothing, housing, medical care, and necessary services; everyone has the right to security in the event of unemployment, illness, incapacity, widowhood, old age, and every other lack of support, due to circumstances beyond the person's control.

The *Declaration of the Rights of the Child*, subsequently approved by the UN states, inter alia:

> all children have the right to the benefits of social security. All children have the right to a living standard that allows their physical, mental, spiritual, moral, and social development. Mothers and children must be guaranteed adequate pre- and post-natal care. Children are entitled to rest and free time to be devoted to play and the recreational activities of childhood.

Further support was guaranteed to children by the *Universal Declaration on the Eradication of Hunger and Malnutrition*, approved by the UN Assembly in December 1974. This solemnly proclaims that

> every child has the inalienable right to be freed from hunger and malnutrition

Thus were born *International Medical Precepts* and *International Humanitarian Law* to safeguard rights and guarantee duties.

On the one hand,

> stricken communities cry out for help as a right to which they are entitled, and not just as a form of charity;
> those who provide aid are beginning to regard it not just as an act of charity to help others in difficulty but as a duty based on reciprocal help. Organized aid, in the event of a grave emergency is not regarded only as an isolated episode but also an essential factor in the long-term development of the community affected.

On the other hand,

on the basis of international agreements that are continuously being updated, intervention is performed by international organizations (International Red Cross), intergovernmental organizations (UN, etc.), and non-governmental organizations (NGOs) that mobilize either spontaneously or at the request of countries and are already active, always for humanitarian purposes, in the areas affected.

Humanitarian Medicine can thus be defined as follows:

While all medical intervention to reduce a person's sickness and suffering is in essence humanitarian, Humanitarian Medicine goes beyond the usual therapeutic act and promotes, provides, teaches, supports, and delivers people's health as a human right, in conformity with the ethics of Hippocratic teaching, the principles of the World Health Organization, the Charter of the United Nations, the Universal Declaration of Human Rights, the Red Cross Conventions and other covenants and practices that ensure the most humane and best possible level of care, without any discrimination or consideration of material gain.

—Gunn

Generally, medical practice has been competitive, while humanitarian medicine is co-operative. These considerations imply that humanitarian medicine is mainly directed at people who live in especially precarious conditions, as in the emerging or developing countries, and that humanitarian medicine is fired by a spirit of human solidarity.

In these countries, economic progress and continuous cultural growth have increased the demand for medical care, parallel to an increased respect for the human individual and for the training of a more specialized medical sector. The evolution of globalization, with the excessive use of information technology, may have led to a continuous cultural and scientific levelling of the industrialized countries, but it has also enabled emerging countries to look at a more advanced, predominantly techno-economical model of society that has also affected the demand for health aid.

The concept of international aid has therefore been modified, and all humanitarian action has inevitably adapted itself to this new way of "providing help." Voluntary action has been replaced by specific requests for co-operation, capable of guaranteeing, in the local territory, more effective medical action, more rigorous post-operative care and long-term checkups, greater responsibility at the level of the training of medical, nursing, and technical staff, a programmed technological updating of health structures, and better co-ordination of rescue operations in the event of disasters. Humanitarian NGOs that work in developing countries have to operate with competence, willingness, responsibility, and continuity in close co-operation with local medical teams. They receive from these adequate information about diseases that may at times be unusual and opinions on what type of medical action is advisable not only in relation to the final outcome but also as regards cultural and religious aspects. Co-operation also permits better operational support, greater integration in their activities, a more advantageous exchange of technical and scientific know-how, and the replacement of the figure of the foreign doctor – who is sometimes seen as a dominator and/or cultural colonizer—by a person seen as one who collaborates, helps, advises, and participates in the same working conditions. Last but not least, this relationship helps to reduce the suspicion of speculative behaviour with regard to management of the patients and to avoid conflict with local physicians due to jealousy, unfair competition, and violation of other interests.

Unfortunately, even if—parallel to spectacular and beneficial progress in saving life—the health sciences have expanded in the sector of social engagement and humanitarian action, the current inequalities, conflicts, and tensions continue to penalize the health and well-being of an unacceptable percentage of the world community in developing countries, in unhealthy environments, disasters, or in chronic conditions of poverty. The numerous intergovernmental and non-governmental organizations face the problem with great determination, but the problem exists and in certain ways is growing more serious.

7.1 IAHM: International Association for Humanitarian Medicine Brock Chisholm

In 1998, a group of professionals of various disciplines sensitive to these problems registered in Palermo the International Association for Humanitarian Medicine to support human rights and the principles of humanitarian medicine in favour of health for all. This was an extension of the Brock Chisholm Memorial Trust, founded[1] in WHO, Geneva in 1984 to keep alive the ideals of Dr Brock Chisholm, first director-general of the World Health Organization, now incorporated as the International Association for Humanitarian Medicine Brock Chisholm (IAHM).

The International Association for Humanitarian Medicine Brock Chisholm, as an instrument for realistic international humanitarian medical aid, proposes to promote initiatives more in line with the real demands of a humanity that asks for help.

The objectives of the Association are

to promote, provide, deliver, and support peoples' health as a human right in conformity with medical ethics and humanitarian practices based on the above-mentioned principles and the Charters of the United Nations, the Universal Declaration of Human Rights, the Red Cross Conventions, the mandate of the WHO Collaborating Centre for Burns and Fire Disasters—in Special Consultative Status with the Economic and Social Council of United Nations, and the Brock Chisholm Trust.

The aims of the Association are uniquely humanitarian, scientific, and social, with commitment to the provision of health for all, social justice, peace, and the dignity of man. Advocacy of health as a human right is paramount.

The action of the Association is

a) in practical terms:

  – to provide medical, surgical, and nursing care to patients in or from developing countries deficient in the necessary specialized expertise;
  – to provide relief to victims of disasters where health aid is lacking;

---

[1] By Mrs Grace Brock Chisholm and Dr S. William A. Gunn

- to mobilize hospitals and health specialists in developed countries to receive and treat such patients on a humanitarian basis;
- to collaborate with other institutions pursuing similar objectives.

b) in conceptual terms:

- to promote the concept of health as a human right;
- to encourage the practice of health as a bridge to peace;
- to advocate humanitarian law and humanitarian principles in the practice of medicine;
- to promote the availability of health for all.

7.2 WOH: World Open Hospital

Besides its principal action of promoting the right to health, the Association has also established a mechanism for relief. The operational instruments to develop assistance can be summarized as follows:

- professional contacts with the authorities and organizations in industrialized countries, in order to set up, in major hospitals, specialized sections dedicated to hospitalization and medical, surgical, and rehabilitation treatment, free of charge, for patients coming from developing countries and needy populations;
- linkups and relationships of co-operation with other humanitarian aid organizations that operate around the world, particularly in emerging countries, so that these can work with the appropriate authorities to transfer complex medical and surgical cases requiring specialist assistance that cannot be resolved in their own countries, to be treated in hospitals possessing sections for humanitarian medicine;
- the creation of a network of such specialized sections that would thus constitute a virtual network of World Open Hospital (WOH);
- the offer to physicians, nurses, and technicians in the health sector of the possibility to attend professional training courses in university and hospital facilities in the industrialized countries;
- the constitution of Specialist teams which on the request of hospitals or health structures in the emerging or developing countries are able to transfer abroad, provide medical and surgical aid, or hold technical and professional training courses, with a view to assuring the necessary assistance (Figure 7.1).

To date, besides its advocacy of human rights, IAHM has principally been active in the management of patients coming from developing countries who need highly specialized treatment that cannot be provided in the patients' countries.

The following algorithms outline IAHM's sectors of activity within the WOH network:

SPECIALIZED ASSISTANCE

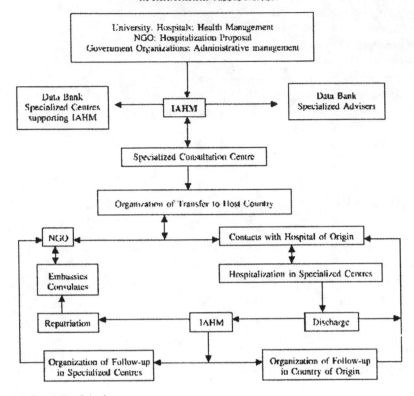

Fig. 7.1 Specialized Assistance

7.3 Health Assistance

Collaborating with the humanitarian NGOs, IAHM uses the following operative working procedures for health assistance:

– Contacts with local health structures;
– Selection of the difficult condition needing treatment;
– Evaluation of type of action;
– Possibility of providing the treatment on site, locally;
– Analysis of degree of post-operative assistance available locally;
– Contacts with IAHM network;
– Clearance of formalities for transfer;
– Hospitalization in specialized centre;
– Treatment and rehabilitation;
– Repatriation and follow-up.

Two aspects are especially important in this system: (1) the individual selection of the patients and (2) the contact with the health structures. *The individual selection of the patients*, in this early phase, is the task of doctors and NGOs operating locally, true witnesses of the real needs of persons who are suffering and whose right to health and care it is their duty to safeguard. Their action makes the WOH programme more concrete and rapid. Through their contacts with the international professional organizations, they identify the specialized facility where the patient will be treated and see to his transfer. Many problems are thus overcome, for example, travel expenses, entry visas, residence permits, and repatriation formalities.

The patients, especially children, are thus more protected in their traumatic transfer to hospital structures in often very different countries and cultures, and better safeguarded in the therapy they will have to face, which can be very long.

Contacts with local health structures: this refers to local organizations, university or other hospital facilities in the individual countries that are the first to clinically evaluate the patients, draw up the relative therapeutic proposals, analyse the shortages of treatment locally, and thus, more rationally request transfer to specialized foreign structures.

In this phase contacts are created with the receiving structure, using, where possible, advanced information technology, such as the Internet or teleconsultation, therapy protocols are prepared and the treatment to be followed by the patient on his or her return home. Thus, the foundations are laid for a profitable dialogue and a real co-operation between the local physicians and those in the specialized centres abroad, and for the initiation of a technical and cultural exchange, that is, the premises for a more useful programme of treatment and training lacking in that particular country.

7.4 Assistance in Disasters

In disasters, whether natural or man-made, war or terrorism, IAHM's action is subject to a specific request by the local authorities. The action may consist of direct intervention in *loco* by specialist teams sent to the scene, or of transfer to specialized centres of patients in the acute phase (e.g. burn victims) or patients with serious invalidating sequelae (Figure 7.2).

7.5 Relevant Training

In a continuously evolving world, where respect for the person and the duty to help others are taking on ever more value, no form of scientific or professional colonialism has any right of asylum. The treatment of persons who are suffering must be global: in all phases of prevention, therapy, and post-operative, if possible in their own customary family environment, with relief of both physical and psychological suffering. This requires commitment and professional training of physicians and

The activity is articulated as follows:

DISASTERS

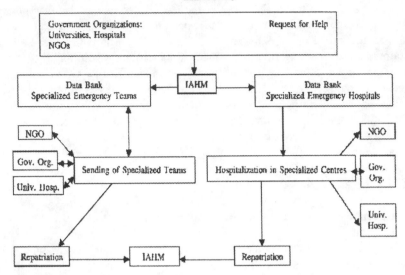

Fig. 7.2 Disasters

nursing staff both in and for the developing countries. IAHM is strongly committed to this activity, as shown in Figure 7.3.

Currently, 32 hospitals in 13 industrialized countries have joined the IAHM network. The virtual WOH has now in real terms more than 40 beds in high-level medical and surgical specialities.

So far 23 patients have been treated, suffering from serious pathologies requiring neurosurgery, pulmonary surgery, burns, reconstructive surgery, and orthopaedic surgery.

7.6 Conclusions

7.6.1 The Prospects of Humanitarian Medicine

All projects aimed at the relief of other people's suffering require strong commitment on the part of the persons who propose them and those who become aware and get directly involved. To be productive, credible, and impartial, all action must be planned, competent, and carried out with absolute respect and irreprehensible observation of international precepts; this is essential in order to avoid abuses, excesses, or excuses. For these reasons, *humanitarian action must not become a new form of cultural or professional colonialism; it must be seen as a voluntary request by persons suffering, who have the right to be helped, directed to those who have the duty to do so.* If all operators in the field of individual and collective health succeed in getting the old and the new to integrate positively, with honesty, competence,

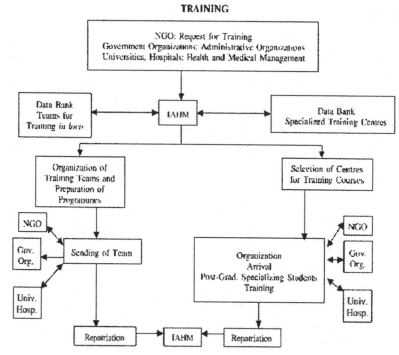

Fig. 7.3 Training

and, above all, humility, they will certainly contribute to make suffering take a step backward and human rights a step forward.

7.6.2 IAHM'S Vision

The favourable welcome received from many in the scientific, political, and cultural world and the support of numerous countries for the proposal at once conceptual and operational, launched in November 2000, constitute a concrete demonstration of the validity of the principles that the International Association for Humanitarian Medicine Brock Chisholm aims to pursue no longer just a voluntary and simple medical act to reduce illness and suffering in a spirit of human sympathy, but rather a commitment that goes beyond the usual therapeutic intervention, promoting, providing, teaching, and supporting health as the right of the individual. IAHM, with its requests to industrialized countries to constitute a network of Specialized Centres, thus becomes the operative centre of a virtual world open hospital, ready to meet the requests of countries that apply. These countries are also offered the possibility to take advantage of specialized teams that are ready to act locally in case of need and to provide all support in professional training.

All this is done in the context of health as a human right, and in a spirit of human solidarity and peace that honours the medical profession.

Bibliography

Bernier P., Fonrouge J.M., Gunn S.W.A.: Legal, diplomatic and geopolitical concepts that physicians on international humanitarian missions should know. Prehosp. Disaster Med., 14: S87, 1999.

Butros-Ghali B.: From peace-keeping to peace-building. Lecture by the Secretary General. UN document PR/SG/SM 1330, May 1992.

Diamond J.: The Rise and Fall of the Third Chimpanzee. Vintage, London, 1992.

Gunn S.W.A.: The right to health. Cemec Monographs No. 2, European Centre for Disaster Medicine, San Marino, 1989.

Gunn S.W.A.: Multilingual Dictionary of Disaster Medicine and International Relief. Kluwer Academic Publishers, Dordrecht, London, 1990.

Gunn S.W.A.: The scientific basis of disasters management. Disaster Prev. Manage. J., 1 (3): 16–21, 1992.

Gunn S.W.A.: Il presupposto umanitario nel soccorso a livello internazionale. Oplitai, Ital. J. Emerg., 5: 7–11, 1993.

Gunn S.W.A.: A humanitarian non-combat role for the military. Prehosp. Disaster Med., 9 (2), Suppl.: 46–8, 1994.

Gunn S.W.A.: The right to health through international cooperation. J. Humanitarian Med., 1: 1–3, 2000.

Gunn S.W.A.: On man-conceived disasters. J. Humanitarian Med., 1: 7–8, 2001.

Gunn S.W.A.: Disasters and conflicts. Encyclopaedia of Life Support Systems, UNESCO, Paris, 2002.

Gunn S.W.A., Masellis M.: World Health Organization Centre for Prevention and Treatment of Burn and Fire Disasters: The Mediterranean Club for burns and fire disasters. Ann. Burns Fire Disasters, 11: 3–6, 1998.

Magnusson G.: Health and human rights—a public health perspective. J. Humanitarian Med., 2: 1–3. 2002.

United Nations: Human Rights—A Compilation of International Instruments. United Nations, New York, 1988.

World Health Organization: Basic Documents, WHO, Geneva, 2005.

Chapter 8
Ethical Principles for Everyone in Health Care

C. Rollins Hanlon, MD, FACS

This paper reports on an April 2000 conference in Cambridge, MA, to discuss a "Shared Statement of Ethical Principles for Everyone in Health Care." The "Statement" was actually a series of six propositions, each with two to five subpropositions designed to establish a shared ethical code ". . . that might bring all stakeholders in health care into a more consistent moral framework."

The background of the conference was set out in a December 1997 editorial in the *British Medical Journal* (*BMJ*) entitled "An ethical code for everybody in health care." It was the premise of the editorial that care of patients was now influenced by so many complex interactions that an ethical code generated by a single profession was no longer "a sufficient moral compass."

The authors of the 1997 *BMJ* editorial included three representatives from the Boston complex of health care institutions. They were Donald Berwick, MD, President, Institute for Health Care Improvement; Howard Hiatt, MD, Professor of Medicine, Harvard Medical School; and Ms Penny Janeway, Executive Director, Initiatives for Children, American Academy of Arts and Science in Cambridge, MA. The fourth author, from London, England, was Richard Smith, Editor, *BMJ*.

The editorialists asserted that no single profession could credibly declare that its own ethical code was adequate. As a result, they had embarked on the search for "an ethical code to cover everybody involved in health care."

After presenting a series of ethical dilemmas involving individual and organizational case studies from Great Britain and the United States, the editorialists cited a number of current initiatives to address these questions from the standpoint of organizations such as the American Hospital Association, the American Medical Association, the British Medical Association, and a group of clinicians in Massachusetts. They judged all such efforts inadequate because they did not bind and guide equally such diverse stakeholders as ". . . doctors, nurses, other health professionals, healthcare managers and executives, regulators of care, and private and public players".

To begin the process of creating a more ecumenical code of ethics, they had earlier written letters to more than 100 health care leaders and academicians in a dozen countries. Replies indicated the existence of many related ethical initiatives, but nearly all involved professions and disciplines rather than the system of care as a whole.

Acting on many encouraging responses, and with foundation support, a group of 15 leaders with diverse backgrounds assembled in February 1998 to survey the need and write an initial draft code of ethics. This "Tavistock Group" (so called because of its initial meeting at the British Medical Association's House in London's Tavistock Square) included ethicists, members from medicine and nursing, health care executives, and a jurist, an economist, and a philosopher. They soon decided that a "code of ethics" was too restrictive to fit the prevailing circumstances both within and among nations. Instead, they constructed a draft to embody generic statements of ethical principles that might be helpful throughout the entire world of health care settings.

Attached to the initial progress report of the Tavistock Group was "A Shared Statement of Ethical Principles for those who Shape and Give Health Care." In its original form, the statement contained five principles and interpretative statements, but before the April 2000 conference in Cambridge, the conveners added a sixth principle, well recognized by generations of health care ethicists: "Do no harm."

A draft of the six major principles that should govern health care was placed on the agenda at the April 2000 conference as follows:

1. Health care is a human right.
2. The care of the individual is at the centre of health care, but the whole system needs to work to improve the health of populations.
3. The health care system must treat illness, alleviate suffering and disability, and promote health.
4. Co-operation with each other, those served, and those in other sectors are essential for all who work in health care.
5. All who provide health care must work to improve it.
6. Do no harm.

Each principle was presented by a main speaker, followed by a designated commentator before open discussion from an audience of more than 100 participants. On the second day of the conference, small group discussions allowed more intensive exchanges between participants, and the results of these group discussions were reported to the assembly by the moderators.

Among the participants were representatives of several health care institutions that had undertaken to test under practical conditions the use of the six principles of the draft statement. They presented reports of their experiences under what was known as a "fast track" testing, while recognizing that the six principles were still subject to modification. These reports elicited spirited discussion of practical issues in implementation.

Two major issues underlay all the discussions. The first concerned construction and phrasing of the six principles that should govern health care; the second, if the principles were drawn up satisfactorily, how they would be widely distributed and implemented to guide everyone concerned in the provision of health care.

The magnitude of these two issues was well recognized by the Tavistock Group during its early deliberations. To bring the geographic scope of application into a more manageable dimension, the decision was made before the current conference to focus on Great Britain and the United States as a binational rather than a multinational or global sphere of action. These two geographic zones show strong disparities in recent and remote approaches to the provision of health care. Difficult as it may be to establish and implement a common set of principles applicable on this binational basis, it is clearly more feasible than to attempt the task with polities having more radically different cultures and languages. So the ecumenical goal was scaled back to two nations.

8.1 Principle 1: Health Care Is a Human Right

The keynote address on the first principle, health care is a human right, was given by Amartya Sen, PhD, Master, Trinity College of Cambridge University, UK, and a Nobel Laureate in economics. The general nature of the conference was briefly noted, before Dr Sen's presentation, to indicate that the six principles were not to be thought of as "non-negotiable," but rather as statements that might need ongoing modification.

Dr Sen then discussed the concept of rights, including the question of a moral claim for human rights in the absence of legal validation or authority. He noted a critical issue that would surface repeatedly in later discussions: the relation of health as a human right as contrasted with health care as a human right. He noted as well that many things other than health care affect health, but we must not carry this to the point of suggesting that health care does not matter in the equation. He also touched on the difficulty of defining a "minimal level" of health care and the role of class structure as a determinant of health.

Discussion was opened by Marilyn Gaston, MD, Director of the Bureau of Primary Health Care in the US Department of Health and Human Services. Dr Gaston expressed doubt that everyone in the United States believes in the principle of health care as a right. She noted that the programme she administers exists because of legislation, and that legislators commonly adopt an incremental approach to problems. There is clearly difference of opinion about the definition of "basic services" in health care.

Various other discussants focused on differences among nations, the importance of health promotion strategies, and the capacity of economically favoured individuals to buy health care coverage in addition to the "basic" package. It was noted that legislation more than three decades old had characterized health care as a right in the United States.

To move briskly through the basic aspects of the six principles on the first day of the conference, issues of implementation were scheduled for the second day. Although each major principle was accompanied by two to five subprinciples for elucidation, the time allotted did not permit extended discussion of these subprinciples. Concepts such as providing care "regardless of inability to pay" and the obligation of "care providers" to teach, publish, and co-operate with their colleagues, "regardless of organizational affiliation," were not discussed.

These knotty problems were held over for the sessions on implementation, and even there they were bypassed rather than fully resolved.

8.2 Principle 2: Care of the Individual Is at the Centre of Health Care, but the Whole System Needs to Work to Improve the Health of Populations

The initial speaker was Dr Paul Farmer, MD, PhD, Director of the Program in Infectious Disease and Social Change in the Harvard Medical School Department of Social Medicine. He pointed out how infectious diseases illustrate the "false dichotomy" between patient care and preventive medicine and that one should think of these aspects in concert. But in the realities of practice, he conceded the impracticality of trying to instruct nurses at work in the intensive care unit about the social aspects of care. But attention to global equity in health care becomes an ethical question when there is an effective form of treatment and one confronts how to apply it worldwide. In opening the discussion, Sir Brian Jarman, MD, Professor Emeritus of Primary Health Care at St Mary's Medical School in London, reviewed the introduction of the National Health Service in Great Britain in 1948. He stated that we cannot have health care as a human right if it is tied to ability to pay.

Others pointed out that the second principle put care of the individual in contrast or even opposition to the health care for populations. One suggestion favoured elimination of the world "but" separating the individual- and population-based parts of care so that they would not appear antithetical. Sir Brian noted that guidelines on doing one's best for the individual patient had to work within the realities of what was feasible. Dr Farmer expressed the hope that our binational focus would not erase consideration of third-world populations. He had noted earlier that 70 % of all tuberculosis patients in the United States are foreign-born. Infectious diseases constrain us towards a transnational viewpoint.

8.3 Principle 3: The Health Care System Must Treat Illness, Alleviate Suffering and Disability, and Promote Health

William Foege, MD, Distinguished Professor of International Health at Rollins School of Public Health at Emory University in Atlanta, emphasized the interdependence of all those working in the health care system. During his own hip replacement operation, he observed multiple individuals in the operating suite. Any one of these participants could have adversely affected his care had they not been working together towards a shared goal. He stated that our capacity for superior care depends on how much we bring to the task from outside our narrow band of technical competence. If we understand that care is a continuum, we will not make an artificial distinction between prevention and treatment. The surgeon who performed a pulmonary lobectomy on his father at age 78 was carrying out preventive care that allowed the patient to live another 17 years.

Dr Foege stressed two other aspects of continuity. First, any health care activity carried out in Boston affects individuals in Haiti and in Zimbabwe, whether or not we are aware of it. Our teaching and mentorship extends our influence to unknown generations. The vast majority of people "served" by existing health care practitioners have not yet been born or may come from a country remote from the present locale of practice.

The opening discussant was Barbara Stocking, a regional director in the National Health Service in London, England. She emphasized that all the various performers in Britain's national health service must work together despite their different perspectives. She felt that major problems such as teenage pregnancy, smoking, and drugs have a greater role in patient self-esteem than does health care. During a recent hard winter in Britain, the technical care of old people was quite adequate but the preservation of their dignity as individuals was insufficiently addressed. Addressing the issue of adequate governmental funding, she predicted that a 3 % diminution in the £5.5 billion spent on 8.5 million people would show striking adverse effects in Great Britain. Various other speakers stressed the importance of precise definition and measurements to clarify what it is we are guaranteeing in an ideal health care system.

8.4 Principle 4: Co-operation with Each Other, Those Served, and Those in Other Sectors Is Essential for All Who Work in Health Care

The initial speaker was Rabbi Julia Neuberger, Chief Executive of the King's Fund in London. Rabbi Neuberger works with six health care organizations in the United Kingdom. She has written on the importance of co-operation among the health care delivery systems, those who work in them, and those who use them. Perhaps a more critical objective was to address illness at its start and to stress the importance of patients' being in control as a factor conducive to good health.

How we can affect the determinants of health increasingly is a matter of international concern. There is growing acceptance of nontraditional and complementary therapy in Great Britain. The economics incident to such therapy underline the essentiality of rationing in any system, however defined. Letting the patient select the type of therapy is threatening to conventional Western medicine. It is apparent that physicians are increasingly subject to scrutiny, and that self-regulation is being supplanted by outside regulation.

Rabbi Neuberger observed that the usefulness of partnership as a goal can be defeated if too much time is spent in meetings seeking "togetherness."

It is important but difficult for many caregivers to share the decision-making with patients. Patients must understand why they are unwell and what the prognosis is. She thinks this education is done better in the United States than in Britain.

Initial comments were made by Howard Raiffa, Emeritus Professor of Economics at Harvard University. As a decision analyst, he largely agreed with Rabbi Neuberger, though he might subject some of the terms to a more formulaic approach. He raised critical questions regarding precise definition of the problem, including objectives, alternatives, and the consequences of a given action. A satisfactory treatment solution will usually involve trade-offs. Professor Raiffa presented a mnemonic, FOTE, which stood for "full, open, truthful exchange" with the patient. This contrasted with partial exchange, where one might hold back some of the truth. His view focused on alternative dispute resolution, in which a pledge of collaboration among the parties might be followed by "collaborative lawyering" and the use of facilitators, mediators, and arbitrators.

Other discussants brought up issues of "transparency" in negotiations between unions and employers over the cost and value of insurance viewed as a part of wages.

8.5 Principle 5: All Who Provide Health Care Must Work to Improve It

The initial presentation was made by Maureen Bisognano, Executive Vice-President and Chief Operating Officer of the Institute for Healthcare Improvement. Ms Bisognano reviewed many of the principles and quality performance factors that Dr Donald Berwick had stressed on the way to establishing the Institute for Healthcare Improvement. The need for improved quality is driven by escalating knowledge, innovations in technology, and increasing patient expectations. The challenge is to execute change and diffuse it widely across the delivery system. Faults to be addressed include overuse, underuse, misuse, difficulties in access, and service problems. There may be variations in cost and quality, and these are being affected by third-party intervention and regulation.

In general, improvements in the system may be effected by a team effort to modify the causes of low quality, drive out waste, make the pattern of improvement a never-ending part of the professional repertoire, and modify the educational curriculum so that these principles are incorporated.

The discussion was opened by Helen Bevan, MD, Director of Redesign, The National Patient's Access Team, from Leicester, UK. She emphasized the need to define "improvement" in care, keeping in mind that up to 70% of our professional ministrations may not benefit the patient. Some attempts at improved care may actually worsen it.

Other discussants seconded the notion that you cannot improve what you are unable to define. We must agree on a systems-based practice; ultimately this may be externally imposed.

8.6 Principle 6: Do No Harm

The opening presentation was made by Uwe Reinhardt, PhD, James Madison Professor of Political Economy at Princeton University. Professor Reinhardt spoke of the Hippocratic Oath and the significant revisions that have been made in recent years to the conventional ideas of the oath's background and significance. Today's criteria for adherence to a Hippocratic standard would call for continuing education, recertification, work on systems to minimize errors, and funding to facilitate dispersion of widely accepted best practices.

He spoke vigorously against the "securitization" of patients, by which he referred to the sale of a physician practice to an investor-owned company so that the company might profit in the future from the cash flow derived from these patients. Physicians who have turned their practices into "securities" that could be traded like any equity on the stock market should not complain over commercial strictures after they voluntarily entered into a purely financial venture with the management company. In a reference to a 1997 article on this topic, Reinhard asked if the patients had been fully aware of the implications related to transfer of the future cash flow from their care. He also spoke critically of unions that might be formed by physicians to increase their leverage with the companies to which they have sold their patients.

At the end of specific discussion of the six principles, there was a talk by Jo Ivey Boufford, MD, Dean of the Robert F. Wagner Graduate School of Public Service at New York University. Dr Boufford spoke to the general topic of "Tough Problems" focusing on the conflicts between personal care of individual patients and the push for overall changes in the system. She diagrammed the "targets of intervention" in going from an individual's illness to a desirable level of health in the community.

One could begin with clinical care of the individual, moving on to health promotion and preventive service. When this progresses to public advocacy, there is some concern about the propriety of this as a function of the medical profession, with the concern increasing as one pushes for improvement in jobs, education, and housing as targets in aiming at better health. Where should we terminate the role of the medical profession along the spectrum of responsibility for health care of the public?

The major factors in premature mortality are behavioural in 50%, genetic in 20%, and inadequate access in only 10%. There is a practical problem in bringing research findings to the bedside for implementation. Markets tend to go in the direction of the money, and education through the Internet may be promising but it is largely uncontrolled.

With regard to the role of patients in effecting improvement in their own health, the word "co-operation" seems too weak. The patient rightly expects the physician to be a patient advocate, while retaining the right to define a personal quality of life. The recent focus on a "patient-centred" practice might well be replaced, according to Boufford, by a "patient-driven" practice, captured in the phrase ". . . nothing about me without me."

She questioned how such a system is to be operationalized. A union-sponsored participant suggested that the system be made more "transparent", so that everyone might judge whether the care is good or bad. When Dr Berwick asked what patients might want from their caretakers, the answer from Dr Boufford was to build trust by way of documentable reassurance.

The task of summarizing the first day had been assigned to David Garvin, PhD, Professor of Business Administration at the Harvard Business School. He compared his state of mind to that of the famous frontiersman Jim Bowie, responding to the question whether he had ever been lost. Bowie denied that characterization but admitted that on one occasion he had been "bewildered for three days."

Professor Garvin viewed the aim of meeting as the setting of a moral compass, directed to individual or organizational audiences. The organizations might be scholastic or health care related and the ultimate action could be regulatory or legislative. For individuals, the six statements might be an aid to decision-making.

The process of seeking certain human rights such as life, liberty, and the pursuit of happiness has occupied workers in case law for hundreds of years and is a continuing effort. The six principles under examination here are an open door to public discourse. In that discourse, we must set priorities based on the importance of different objectives. This focuses the issues of rationing services and the level of "basic services," suspended between too little and too much.

Regarding principle 2, concerning the relation between individual care and care of the total population, the emphasis should be on supplying both rather than viewing them as antithetical. With finite resources, rationing of services in both categories may be necessary.

In the third objective, we see different emphases in the United States and the United Kingdom, with the latter stressing health promotion rather than alleviation of individual illness, suffering, and disability.

For the fourth principle of co-operation among patients, caregivers, and those in other sectors of the health care system, the focus is on where autonomy ends and co-operation begins. Can the national administration overrule the opinions of the professionals? How to decide when experts disagree? And if co-operation fails to occur, what part will Professor Raiffa's "collaborative lawyering" play in the dispute resolution?

Regarding the fifth principle of responsibility of all parts of the system to work at improving it, one faces again the issue of whose priority has primacy, that of the individual or that of the system.

As to the stark principle 6, to do no harm, which has long been considered basic to many in medicine, we need to define the issue. Is it simply minimizing errors, establishing correct processes, and avoiding conflict of interest while recognizing the limits of technical feasibility? Is there an even higher standard than doing no harm, such as truth in public debate that goes along with a "transparent" system? These questions closed the formal sessions for the day and led on to the dinner speaker, Kenneth Roth, Executive Director of Human Rights Watch.

Roth spoke on "Other Experiences with Codes," based on the work of his organization in its worldwide activities. He cited books with a plethora of human rights documents in both peace and war, but noted that implementation depended more on a situational approach than on a literal application of the texts. Enforcement of human rights statements is hindered by the absence of a global police apparatus or court, and the inadequacy of moral suasion. The propriety of specific policies in war may be viewed differently even by different governments in an alliance. Enforcement may rely on four different types of codes, namely, legal, aspirational, rhetorical, and a "shaming" code.

The legal code may hark back to a theistic authority in Western or Eastern religions. Or it may look to a secular authority such as judges or legislators, whose actions must then be interpreted by "expert" bodies. Effectiveness of such mechanisms varies with geography; for example, they work better in Europe than in Asia or Africa.

The "aspirational" code assumes a degree of good faith and will to co-operate; it relies for its legitimacy on faith in a process, established by the originating bodies with details hammered out in a venue such as Geneva. If a council in Europe sets guidelines for what it means to be ethical, a number of countries outside Europe may consider it desirable to join the effort, despite cultural problems that impede their participation.

The third type of code is political or rhetorical. It assumes there are people with an opposing viewpoint and it tries to equip its proponents to deal with contrary views, using arguments to show that "rights" on one side overpower mere "interests" on the other side. It may be necessary to enlist some "outside" arbiter to deal with ethical conflicts. The need to find a powerful adjudicator explains why few people are satisfied with aspirational or rhetorical codes.

The fourth mechanism, a "shaming" code, is a strong weapon of human rights organizations. Such groups work mainly to investigate and publicize violations of a moral code, so that a worldwide public will respond by labelling the action in question as "wrong." Governments are moved by the need to maintain favour with other governments or with a wide range of populations joined in an electronic communications network.

By publicly accepted opinions on well-known concrete instances, principles can be developed. Although there may be ambiguity in defining certain activities such as the definition of torture, much human rights work is directed, for instance, at generating shame on the part of multinational corporations over discriminatory labour practices. Impressive results have been achieved by merely calling such violations to the attention of corporate headquarters.

Despite the provisional nature of the six principles, and the need for ongoing review of how they are stated, several health care groups were enlisted to field-test the principle under conditions of practice. Because these practice experiments were conducted for only a few months, the results were presented to the conference as provisional or "fast track" reports.

The reports related to practice organizations in the US; no United Kingdom groups or investor groups were represented. The initial presentation concerned a group with 200 physicians, 185 in the primary care category. They involved 1,25,000 "covered lives"; last year there were 84,000 patient encounters among the group. After acceptance of the principles by the executive committee of the group, they followed a six-point strategy to incorporate them into their practice: (1) get wide acceptance of the principles by everyone in the system; (2) integrate the principles into the practice; (3) communicate these ideas to the patients; (4) measure and quantify the results; (5) set up benchmarks; and (6) use feedback from patients and caregivers. Information in this group is spread by a web site, by the Medical Director's Newsletter, by semi-annual corporate meetings, and by patient satisfaction surveys. The incorporation of the ethical principles into day-to-day practice highlighted a number of practical issues. For example, solvency of the group could be threatened by overly permissive agreement with the patients' desire for unwarranted diagnostic tests. This dilemma is captured in the phrase "no margin, no mission," indicating that a certain margin of profit is essential or the survival of the group practice is in jeopardy.

This conflict between adherence to strict ethical principles and the financial well-being of a group practice was evident in the presentations of other "fast track" organizations working to incorporate the six principles into their practice. Closely tied to the question of financial feasibility was the determination of a "basic level of service." Setting the level too low runs the risk of lowering quality of care, while being overly expansive about allowable procedures might fatally influence the bottom line.

A presentation by the chief executive of a small insurance company highlighted financial risks of such companies in providing health insurance while conforming to guidelines of the Health Care Financing Administration (HCFA). As an unusual aspect of following the mandate of principle 6 ("Do no harm"), the insurance administrator suggested that this injunction might be applied with comparable validity to the preservation of the insurance financing system.

One administrative participant in a health care system, addressing the previously discussed contrast between a primary focus on the individual patient versus a population-based emphasis, raised the arresting question of whether the care of the individual should be the primary concern. This unusual viewpoint would put public health into a dominant position in the second principle.

The small group sessions allowed close argument over working details experienced in applying the six principles to real-life situations. Broader issues were also raised, such as the question of whether the thrust of a conference like this was a move towards universal health care. Previous attempts at a widely applicable code of ethics for health care were reviewed, including the Colorado experience of 1998, which produced a clearly written pamphlet describing the effort to involve all segments of the community in ethical guidelines. Also noted were organizational efforts by ethics institutes to develop measures of ethical quality, even in the absence of principles commanding universal agreement.

Follow-up activities to this conference would entail refinement of the principles and their widespread dissemination among organizations in the health field. Entry to medical educational facilities is also important, along with familiarity by medical faculties. Dispersal will require time and financial resources. There is not a widespread perception among professionals and patients that this is an urgent priority, especially because it does not appear to offer a clear, competitive advantage in an era where entrepreneurial health care is the norm.

Administrators of large health care plans cited the difficulty of finding common ground in groups with thousands of physicians. If the six principles are to find widespread acceptance, they will require clarifying statements rather than complicating subprinciples. Simplification rather than complexity is called for. Core studies exemplifying the principles would facilitate wider understanding. Despite the familiar attractiveness of the "Do no harm" principle, one must ask pragmatically whether it is possible to practice medicine with the available powerful tools without a certain modicum of harm as a realistic consequence.

There are immense problems with directing public attention to these ethical principles, much less having them widely accepted. If there is still room for professional debate over the contrast between health as a right and health care as a right, the issue cannot be simplistically put out for public consumption as a definitively settled issue. Does the general public equate health care with food and shelter? Is the public well informed about the real nature of problems in the health care system and about the options for remedy? Will the attitude of industry towards defined health benefits change when there is an inevitable downturn in the economy? And will health care be dominated more clearly by patients as medical information on the Internet increasingly captures their interest and facilitates personal decision-making?

To broaden institutional participation in furthering the process, the sponsors saw the need for involvement that would not call for complete agreement with the tentative principles as a condition of joining in the work. In other words, more people in more organizations would be urged to address seriously the underlying ethical issues of health care despite reservations about some of the phrasing in the "principles" discussed at the Cambridge meeting.

What is actually happening to move the discussion forward, in addition to potential changes in attitude of the conference participants? Editorial comments in their respective journals by the editor of the *British Medical Journal* and the editor of the *Annals of Internal Medicine* summarize the status of the project from the viewpoints of well-informed participants in the original Tavistock Group. How this enterprise will work out should be of interest to a wide spectrum of individuals and organizations in the broad field of health care. The April 2000 conference was a significant event, but there is clearly a great deal of work yet to be done.

Bibliography

Berwick D., Hiatt H., Janeway P., Smith R.: An ethical code for everybody in health care. Br. Med. J., 315: 1633–4, 1997.

Colorado Code of Ethics for Healthcare: A Guide for Consumer Patients, Providers, Physicians, Practitioners, Purchasers, Employer and Health Plans. Denver, CO: Rocky Mountain Center to Healthcare Ethics, 1998.

Davidoff F.: Changing the Subject: Ethical Principles for Everyone in Health Care. Ann. Intern. Med., 133: 386–9, 2000.

Smith R.: Editorial. Br. Med. J., 1999.

Smith R., Hiatt H., Berwick D.: A shared statement of ethical principles for those who shape and give health care: A working draft from the Tavistock Group. Ann. Intern. Med., 130: 143–7, 1999.

Reinhardt U.: Hippocrates and the "securitization" of patients. JAMA, 227: 1850–1, 1997.

Reproduced by kind permission of the American College of Surgeons and Elsevier Science, Inc. from *Journal.of American College of Surgeons*, 192: 1–8, 2001. The author is a Regent of IAHM.

Chapter 9
Quality of Life and Medical Practice

Radana Königová, MD, CSc

The concept of "quality of life" as it figures in medical decisions has been explored in interdisciplinary discussions between doctors, philosophers, theologians, and other interested parties since 1985 and, indeed, both the Czech Burn Association and the International Association for Humanitarian Medicine conducted two symposia on the subject.

The expression "quality of life" is now being increasingly used not only in the medical and legal literature but also by patients.

Technological advances have enabled patients to be saved from conditions that would previously have brought about their death. The growth of medicine's power to sustain life in the face of critical, terminal, or debilitating illness has been so rapid that it has caught our society unawares, leaving us unsure of how to deal with the choices with which we are presented. A conflict occurs in the treatment of an individual patient between the aim of prolonging life (quantity of life) and the aim of promoting quality of life.

Can quality of life be measured? Quality of life is what successful treatment aims at, other than extension of life. It is best estimated under the following five headings:

1. degree of pain, distress, or discomfort experienced, whether physical or emotional;
2. degree of normal activity attainable;
3. nature of personal relationships achievable;
4. extent of capacity to undertake and complete projects;
5. extent to which hopes and ambitions can be fulfilled.

The first two items in the list seem "objective" when contrasted with the remaining three.

The doctor should be able to predict how much pain the patient is likely to experience from a given treatment and what degree of activity the treatment will allow. At least, in principle, this can be done, as patients differ in all sorts of respects.

The other three items (which might be called "subjective") are more difficult to forecast. Success in relation to them depends upon the character and personality of the patient and on his or her will power.

What really matters is what the individual feels as "subjective" satisfaction. In *competent* patients, quality of life should be assessed entirely by the individual person.

Medical practitioners have an important role to play in taking the decisions with which patients are confronted: quantity or quality of life? In *incompetent* patients (including young children and the mentally handicapped), there can be no question of discovering their preferences. By what standard is their quality of life to be assessed and who is to do it? Whose quality of life is to count when a choice has to be made between treatments that differ in the nature and extent of the burdens they place upon relatives and others who care for the patients?

Doctors and other health care professionals occupy a special sort of position in our society, facing life-and-death decisions. They all have a responsibility to take due care according to ethical principles: above all, not to injure or harm the trusting patient. A *duty of non-maleficence* is stronger than a duty of *beneficence*. It may be more harmful to patients that their lives should be extended in a way that prolongs suffering or entails a loss of dignity than that they should be allowed to die peacefully.

There is another principle within medical ethics, the *principle of autonomy*, implying that all decisions relating to treatment should be made by the patient, who must be well informed of possible benefits or risks when there are alternative treatment options (*doctrine of informed consent*). There can be a clash between autonomy and beneficence or non-maleficence when a patient requests treatment that is not as good as an alternative or is unnecessary, futile, or even harmful.

The doctor still has a responsibility to assist the patient in decision-making. Such assistance requires the doctor's sensibility to issues of quality of life and the reliability of studies of *quality of life under different treatments*, if the advice is to be useful.

The ethical principle of fairness is called *distributive justice*. Allocation of (scarce) medical resources is divided into macro-allocation problems and micro-allocation problems. The first one is what proportion of society's resources should go towards health care? The second one is whom to choose between competing candidates for some form of treatment that cannot be given to all who need it?

Principles of truthfulness and confidentiality arising in medical practice can be resolved only by a sensitive and determined effort to uncover the facts of the case; it is a process in which both the intuitions and the principles undergo a process of testing.

The attempt to measure quality of life is an attempt to make comparisons regarding the life of the same individual under different circumstances and to compare the different states of an individual's life to the lives of different individuals.

Although the right of patient autonomy was articulated in 1914 and the phrase "informed consent" was coined in 1957, it was not until 1985 that open discussion of explicit policies to limit medical care began. The quality of life can be as strong a *rationale for a DNR order (do-not-resuscitate) as futility of therapy*.

Different qualitative factors contributing to DNR decisions are encountered in *burn medicine*. Modern burn care often leads to the dilemma of what should or should not be done for patients with clinical deterioration and organ system failure with no response to therapy (Frantianne, 1992). The questions are "When is enough enough?" and "Who decides?"

A structured conference is recommended to address these issues and to help decide whether to continue invasive diagnostic and therapeutic intervention or to allow the patient to *"die with dignity"*.

Every life is different from any that has gone before it, and *so is every death*.

The uniqueness of each of us extends even to the way we die. Every one of death's diverse appearances is as distinctive as that singular face we each show the world during the days of life.

Chapter 10
Medical Contributors to Social Progress: A Significant Aspect of Humanitarian Medicine

William C. Gibson, MD, DPhil, FRCPC

Scientific discoveries in the field of medicine over the last four centuries have undoubtedly had social repercussions. Edward Jenner (1749–1823) saw cowpox protecting milkmaids from smallpox and launched an inspired generalization upon the world, bringing us vaccination (from "vacca" meaning cow). While there were, temporarily, wild political happenings following the enforcement of vaccination laws—such as the burning down of the city hall by a mob in Montreal—there were massive improvements of health in society and its instruments such as hospitals, libraries, and universities. Seven examples of social, humanitarian progress following medical contributions are described below.

One of the most interesting physicians in this remarkable field was the little general practitioner in London's east-end dockland—Dr *James Parkinson*. Today his name is on the lips of laymen and physicians alike, the result of his description, in 1817, of six cases of *paralysis agitans* seen in his practice, or taken from the sparse literature of the time.

While Parkinson is remembered for his classic medical description, and to some extent, for his early volumes on fossils, as well as the first description in English of perforation of the appendix, his contribution to social change is considerable. He began at the age of twenty-three with an attack on quacks! Moreover he struck a blow for freedom by piloting through the press the two-volume work of Tom Paine on *The Rights of Man*, after Paine had had to flee to France to escape arrest in London.

It was now Parkinson's turn to be arrested, along with all who sold Paine's work. Some were jailed for alleged "libel," others "transported" to Australia. But Parkinson, on being hailed before Pitt, the prime minister, and the Privy Council, stood his ground and successfully challenged their right to apprehend him. Pitt spat on democracy and what he called "that monstrous doctrine" of "the rights of man."

James Parkinson had been a pupil of the great surgeon John Hunter, whose lectures he took down in shorthand. His colleagues in the fight for democratically elected Parliament numbered, among others, writer Richard Brinsley Sheridan and Samuel Whitbread of the brewery family. The "underground" consisted of what were called "Corresponding Societies" that met in pubs—where information was exchanged and campaigns against a most corrupt British government were hatched. The problem was that while the great cities of Liverpool, Birmingham, and Manchester were denied even a single seat in the House of Commons, the unpopulated country, Cornwall, boasted 44 seats.

Parkinson lived a busy life as a general practitioner while, at the same time, discharging broadsides against the government. His pamphlet which the government found most disturbing was entitled *Revolution Without Bloodshed; or Reformation Preferable to Revolt*, though it put forward social legislation that is today on the books of all advanced countries. His targets were well chosen, for example, he said, "The present system of Excising (taxing) almost all the necessities of life, as soup, candles, starch, beer, etc. might be abolished," and "The unfortunate tradesmen, ruined perhaps by some swindler of rank, might not be consigned to the horrors of a dungeon, because oppressed by the heavy load of misfortune."

His books on gout and dangerous sports must have been fitted into a demanding life, along with works on chemistry and paediatrics. He served as a church trustee and went about establishing Sunday schools. The apostate Edmund Burke, once a supporter of parliamentary reform, went over to the Tory government and became its defender of corruption. He now shouted against reform. "Learning will be cast into the mire and trodden down under the hoofs of swinish multitude."

Parkinson, using a pen rather than a sword replied by one of his sixpenny pamphlets entitled: "An address to the Hon. Edmund Burke from the swinish multitude." He signed it "Old Hubert." This pseudonym he applied to other pamphlets and posters put up at great risk by "billstickers"—many of whom were thrown in prison. Nevertheless, Parkinson kept after Burke, the silver-tongued orator, in a further blast: "Pearls Cast Before Swine by Edmund Burke—Scraped Together by Old Hubert." In this masterpiece, Parkinson said it all in one phrase: "When bad men combine, the good must associate; else they will fall, one by one, an unpitied sacrifice in contemptible struggle."

We leave Parkinson, the physician, as we read the final words in his epoch-making *Essay on the Shaking Palsy:*

> Before concluding these pages, it may be proper to observe once more, that an important object proposed to be obtained by them is, the leading of the attention of those who humanely employ anatomical examination in detecting the causes and nature of diseases, particularly to his malady. By their benevolent labours it's real nature may be ascertained, and appropriate modes of relief, or even cure, pointed out. To such researches the healing art is already much indebted for the enlargement of its powers of lessening the evils of suffering humanity. Little is the public aware of the obligations it owes to those who, led by professional ardour, and the dictates of duty, have devoted themselves to these pursuits.

The year of Parkinson's death, 1824, saw a precocious and diminutive youth entering Harvard College. *Oliver Wendell Holmes* found it chilly and cheerless around the temples of the law and, fortunately for all women bearing children in bacterial polluted hospitals, he took up the study of medicine. As was the custom in Boston 150 years ago, Holmes with the sons of John Collins Warren, Nathaniel Bowditch, and James Jackson went off to Paris to walk the wards of La Pitié with the great clinician Pierre Louis (also once a law student) and the father of statistics in clinical medicine Gabriel Andral. The young Americans, upon examination, became members of the Society for Medical Observation, where no holds were barred.

Holmes prospered in this highly charged intellectual climate and developed two convictions that (a) most medicines being prescribed then were better thrown into the sea, though that would be harsh on the fishes; and (b) childbed or puerperal fever was demonstrably contagious. The rigorous discipline exercised by Louis over his foreign students was the making of Holmes as a penetrating analyst of medical causes of social distress.

On returning to graduate in medicine at Harvard in 1836, with a thesis on pericarditis, Holmes lost no time in joining The Boston Society for Medical Improvement. There he learned that a physician who had done an autopsy on a woman with childbed fever succumbed himself to the infection which he acquired at the post-mortem table—but not before he had infected a number of women he was still able to attend. This lit a fire under the receptive Holmes and he set out to collect the facts on this pestilence. He was already well known to the public for his widely admired poem "Old Ironsides," which caused the Secretary of the Navy to think twice before sending the famed frigate *Constitution* to the shipbreakers. In addition, at age 33, he had rallied the medical profession against quackery, as Parkinson's first paper had done. Holmes' essay on "Homeopathy and Its Kindred Delusions" convinced his readers that he had given up the levity of his days in the Hasty Pudding Club at Harvard, and was now waving a pen sharper than any bistouri.

A year later, he launched the rocket which assured his place in both medical and social history. He collected and analysed reports on dozens of deaths from childbed fever. If ever a man had been well prepared for this demanding task, it was Holmes, the student of Andral. As Pasteur used to say, "Fortune favours the prepared mind."

Of these stirring days of conflict with the obstetricians, Holmes wrote, years later, to William Osler:

> I have rarely been more pleased than by your allusions to an old paper of mine. There was a time, certainly, in which I would have said that the best page of my record was that in which I had fought my battle for the poor poisoned women (i.e., The Contagiousness of Puerperal Fever). I am reminded of that Essay from time to time, but it was published in a periodical which died after one year's life

General practitioners wrote sad letters to Holmes saying that they now realized how they had been transmitting infection to their maternity patients. However, the obstetricians tried to belittle the matter, while surreptitiously trying to have Holmes dismissed from his Chair of Anatomy of Harvard. To its everlasting credit, Harvard replied by making Holmes the Dean of Medicine.

Before we leave Holmes' contributions, it should be noted that he gave us the term "anaesthetics." He was also the founding president of the Boston Medical Library in 1875, which in its reincarnation today remains a beacon of enlightenment.

Nine years junior to Holmes "the poet" was *Ignaz Semmelweis* "the peasant." Boston and Budapest saw these two disparate young men studying law at first, but emerging as medical graduates. Semmelweis studied first in Pesth and then in Vienna, where he graduated in 1844, his thesis describing his experiments on pneumonic infection in animals. His degrees were Doctor of Medicine and Doctor of Midwifery.

Paralleling Holmes' first awakening to the possible cause of puerperal sepsis, Semmelweis grieved for the loss of one of his obstetrical colleagues, who had died of a small dissecting wound following an autopsy, and began to connect the large number of similar deaths on his obstetrical service with the examinations made by professors and students proceeding directly from the anatomy and the pathology dissecting rooms. By instituting the scrubbing of hands with calcium chloride, he was soon able to reduce the incidence of childbed fever to one-eighth of what it had been.

The conservative Vienna Medical Society, led by Scanzoni, heard this 29-year-old's views with alarm. Though the veterans Skoda and Hebra stood by Semmelweis, he was relieved of his post, and wisely returned to Budapest. There he found that his teaching wards were situated between the morgue and the cemetery. He soon changed this and was able to show that in 514 confinements on his service there were only two deaths. With this experience as his springboard he began, at age 39, to write his immortal book, "The Cause, Concept and Prophylaxis of Puerperal Fever."

What a clarion call to action it was:

> My Doctrine is not firmly established in order that the book expounding it may moulder in the dust of a library; my Doctrine has a mission and that is to bring blessings into practical social life. My Doctrine is produced in order that it may be disseminated by teachers of midwifery, until all who practise medicine, down to the last village doctor and the last village midwife, may act according to its principles; my Doctrine is produced in order to banish error from the lying-in hospitals, to preserve the wife to the husband, the mother to the child.

Alas, Semmelweis died at age 47, in a mental hospital, broken in spirit and in body after 20 years of suffering the ignorant abuse of his obstetrical colleagues. Society will remember him long after they are forgotten.

Three years younger than Semmelweis was *Rudolph Virchow*, the father of "cellular pathology." His war cry was "omnis cellula e cellula"—each cell arises from an antecedent cell. Virchow was an army medical student in Berlin, as was the forerunner of penicillin therapy, Ernest Duchesne in Lyons. As an undergradute, Virchow conducted research on the inflammation of the cornea in rabbits, which were sent to him by his father in Pomerania. After a post-graduate year in pathology, Virchow was sent by the German government to investigate the sudden appearance of typhus in Upper Silesia. His report was a "blockbuster"—which included his typhus findings, but much more. He advocated "full and unrestricted democracy . . . with freedom and prosperity".

He was already suspect for publishing at the age of 25, in the first volume of his *Archiv*, his credo:

> The role of pathological anatomy as a dogmatic science is at an end.

He prophesied that pathological physiology would henceforth be "recognized as the stronghold of scientific medicine to which pathological anatomy and clinical observation form but the outworks."

The Prussian government was already paranoid on the subject of social revolution. Karl Marx had been doing too much reading in the British Museum! (Another of our physician reformers, Sun Yat Sen the non-communist, was to do the same 50 years later.) The Communist Manifesto of 1848 had the crowned heads of Europe in an uproar. Virchow told his students that Prussia was being ruled by a family wherein the father had softening of the brain, the grandfather hardening of the brain and the grandson no brain at all.

This brought about Virchow's speedy dismissal from his post in Berlin, and luckily he found a most hospitable opening at the University of Wurzburg. Seven years later, this talented teacher was invited, by a unanimous vote of the faculty, to return as Professor of Pathology in Berlin, where an institute was built for him.

This creative man was soon elected to the Reichstag, and he remained there for 50 years, the sworn enemy of the dictatorial Bismarck. Virchow's greatest coup was, as chairman of the Reichstag's finance committee, to prevent Bismarck building a large German navy early in the 20th century. On a more positive side, Virchow was the supporter of his friend Schliemann in digging up another civilization at Troy in Asia Minor.

We leave Virchow, who was Osler's and Sherrington's teacher, with a glance at his far-sighted words written at age 30, so reminiscent of James Parkinson's. Virchow said:

> There are also those who, if they do not create the current, still give it its direction and force. These men are not always the happiest. Many go down in the movement, or by it. Many grow weary after they have given it their best forces. Much power and great tenacity are necessary if the individual shall not only live to see his triumph but also to enjoy it.

It has always seemed to me that there was at least one case of a "prepared mind"— to use Pasteur's phrase again—having the satisfaction of seeing his diagnosis and treatment of a social ill compressed into one week. *Dr John Snow* (1813–1858) at the age of 36 won a prize of 30,000 francs from the Institut de France for an essay on the spread of cholera. Suddenly, on the first day of September in 1854, people in the immediate neighbourhood of the Broad Street pump in London began dying. By 7 September, more than 500 were dead. On 8 September, Snow, with the informed permission of the Guardians of the Parish of St James, removed the pumphandle and the epidemic stopped. He was then able to go back to his practice as an anaesthetist. In that role, he twice attended Queen Victoria during confinement. He developed a pulmotor for infants on the point of asphyxia, and still had time to invent a trocar for draining the chest.

While these things were happening in the middle of the 19th century, war broke out between a French–British coalition on one side and the defending Russians on the other. The Crimean peninsular struggle on the Black Sea became one of the bloodiest shambles in history. You will ask: "How is that campaign related to doctors and social progress?" The answer is, of course, that despite the worst bureaucratic military medical martinets in history, *Florence Nightingale* (1823–1910) began the uphill battle to establish the profession of nursing. Without the congenital irascibility of Sir George Hall, the Inspector General of Hospitals during that war, which produced in the perceptive Miss Nightingale just the reverse, it is possible that military nursing, in fact all nursing, might have taken much longer to emerge as a respected and humane service. The story is too well known to require repetition here, but I want to mention the hospital at Scutari, just south of Constantinople (Istanbul today). The area is called locally, Uskudar. Her hospital had to be laboriously developed out of a rat-infested military barracks—a quadrangle, with each side the length of three city blocks.

So much for a triumph over doctors who tried to impede social progress. Even as Florence Nightingale was leaving Scutari to return to England, Dr Hall was spitefully writing in his diary: "Can any nonsense go beyond this?", referring to her distribution of remaining and unneeded rations to military stations, rather than to his medical establishment. Other gifts by her were, in his caustic words, "A matter of absurdity on the part of the kindhearted well-intentioned contributors, and a piece of silly ambitious vanity on her part to have the European reputation for being the guardian angel of the sick and wounded, but if she and her supporters could hear the commentary of our neighbours it would cool, if not cure, her officious intermeddling with other people's affairs." He certainly wore his liver on his sleeve.

A happier chapter in the history of social progress inspired by doctors is one which began in the spring of 1897 when a medical student, E.O. Huntington, at Columbia University took a long walk in New York with the Rev. Frederick Gates, who had been his pastor years before in a struggling Baptist church in Minneapolis. Gates asked the student if there was a textbook of medicine which would help a layman to understand the current position of medical science in the United States. The youth replied at once that William Osler's recent volume, "The Principles and Practice of Medicine," was just what he wanted. Thus Gates, the advisor to John D. Rockefeller, purchased Osler's well-written and truthful volume, along with a medical dictionary, and went off to the Catskills for his summer vacation.

Gates returned from his vacation an inspired man. He had, as the saying goes, "got religion"—this time in the form of medical research. He would have passed for an Old Testament prophet, thundering away against disease, sloth, malfeasance, and other crimes. Disease was his enemy and nothing less than a holy war would suffice. His retirement speech in 1923, according to one of his successors, Dr Alan Gregg of the Rockefeller Medical Sciences Division, as related in his biography by Wilder Penfield, is a masterpiece. Before the assembled and terrified Board of the Foundation, Gates roared:

> And when you die and come to approach the Judgment of Almighty God, what do you think he will demand of you—yes, each one of you? Do you for an instant presume to think he will inquire into your petty failures, your trivial sins, your paltry virtues? NO! He will ask you just one question: "WHAT did you do as a Trustee of The Rockefeller Foundation?"

The social progress fostered by the Rockefeller Foundation through medical research and education is well known, but from China, there is a story too rarely told. Planning for the Peking University Medical College project began in 1913, and this superior medical faculty operated until the Japanese invasion of China in 1937. For years thereafter, the fine granite buildings were used for hospital purposes, but in 1979, the PUMC, as it had been called since its inception, resumed its historic role in training scientist–clinicians and medical researchers. The competition for the 30 places in each year of study is intense, and one of the present students made the highest score in the entire country of one billion people, in any field of study, on his university entrance examinations.

This is all by way of introducing a physician who literally changed the world of one billion people and their successors. He was *Sun Yat Sen*, who was born in southeast China in 1866 in a poor farming family that lived in a forgotten hamlet euphemistically called "Blue Thriving Village," in an area known as "The Fragrant Hills." Before he died in 1925 of cancer of the liver in the PUMC Rockefeller Hospital just described, he, with his comrades, had finally freed his country from centuries of domination of the ruling Manchu line.

His fascinating life—much of it spent in exile—has been wonderfully chronicled by Abbie Lyon Sharman, an American who lived for years at Yenching University in China. Stanford University has reprinted her frank appraisal.

Now, in briefest form, the one-time theological student turned medical doctor received his first formal education at the Bishop's School in Hawaii, where his older brother was in the sugar trade, near Pearl Harbor. Sun Yat Sen mastered the English language and, in his third year, received a prize given by the king. However, the brother detected a preoccupation in the precocious young man: an interest in learning English, in the American Constitution, and in Christianity, so he shipped him back to the "Blue Thriving Village" not far from Canton. On being baptized by an American missionary in Canton, he proceeded with the good Dr Hager to evangelize the country villages, including those in his Fragrant Hills. He never forgot his humble origins, and years later made this clear when he said, in truth:

> I am a coolie, and the son of a coolie. I was born with the poor and I am still poor. My sympathies have always been with the struggling mass. (The Chinese words "koo lee" mean "bitter labour".)

It is reminiscent of Rudolph Virchow's credo, so much in keeping with humanitarian medicine:

> The physicians are the natural attorneys of the poor, and social problems fall to a large extent within their jurisdiction.

From the age of 18 until he was 20, this young Chinese was employed in the Anglo-American Mission Hospital in Canton, and there he developed an interest in medicine.

By the age of 20, Sun Yat Sen was convinced the recent history of dismemberment of his country by the Great Powers must cease and, axiomatically, the weak and pliant Manchu dynasty must be replaced by a republic.

Perhaps, because a doctor's expertise was easily portable and always in demand, he chose the medical career as his vehicle with which to accomplish the vast social transformation of China. After a year of medical education at the Canton Hospital, he transferred to the superior College of Medicine for Chinese in Hong Kong.

On graduation in 1892, at the head of his class, Dr Sun Yat Sen practised in clinics in Macao, the Portuguese island not far from Hong Kong, and then in Canton. His contact with endless indigent patients further strengthened his resolve to rid China of the Manchus.

From 1894 to 1911, he laboured to educate his people (a) as to the scandalous things happening to Mother China and (b) as to the type of genuine reconstruction needed. Each of the 10 times that uprisings against the Manchus failed, with frightful repression to follow, the masses came to heed what he was teaching them. He truly had a sense of mission and an evangelical approach to his eager audiences around the world.

Over and above these factors, however, was the stark reality of the butchery exhibited by imperialist powers such as Britain, France, Germany, and Japan. In fact, in the year in which he gave up medical practice, Sun Yat Sen was scandalized by incursions.

While this crude geographical surgery was going on, Sun Yat Sen was organizing expatriot Chinese wherever he could reach them. He stopped long enough in London to read voraciously in the library of the British Museum—where many revolutions had their beginning.

Sun Yat Sen's early message to his listeners at home and abroad consisted of three constant themes resulting from his reading at the British Museum, in addition to the "abolition of unequal treaties". These aims were

a. to achieve equality among the varied races within China and national independence and freedom without;

b. democracy—"to strive for the political liberty and equality of the people" through election, recall, initiative, and referendum;

c. "the people's livelihood—achieving economic equality of people by peaceful and evolutionary means."

I must not weary you with a litany of the frightful things which happened to Dr Sun Yat Sen and his movement after he was installed as the Provisional President of the Republic on 1 January 1912. As in many human activities, some join a good cause to see what they can do for it. Alas, there are others who join to see what the cause can do for them. Unbridled war lords went on the rampage, some with foreign backing it was felt, and, all told, the years between 1912 and 1925, in which year Sun Yat Sen died, were lost in turmoil.

Right up to the time of his death, he kept elaborating his writings on the reconstruction of China, on local and central government, foreign policy and national defence. He did all this despite the destruction of his valuable library in 1922 by a traitor.

However, these were the years in which the beleaguered statesman did his finest writing—*The First Step to Democracy*, and *A Plan for the Industrial Development of China*, as part of his major work, *The Plan of National Reconstruction*.

In January of 1925, he was operated upon for cancer of the liver at the Peking Union Medical College Hospital but died on 12 March. His body rests in a vast mausoleum on the slopes of the Purple Mountain near Nanjing. Few memorials in the world can compare with it in size or beauty.

Dr Sun Yat Sen's determination to "fight the good fight" goes on, his followers trying gradually to bring liberal democracy and good health to the world's most populous land.

This brings to the end a cursory review of the contributions of physicians to the world's progress. There are many, many others who could well have been discussed, but I hope that this sampling may give an increased pride in not only the medical but also the social achievements of this great profession, neatly summed up in the concept of Humanitarian Medicine.

Bibliography

Gibson W.C.: Young Endeavour: Contributions to Science by Medical Students of the Past Four Centuries. Ch. Thomas, Springfield, USA, 1958.

Gibson W.C.: Medical Comets: Scholarly Contributions by Medical Undergraduates. University of British Columbia Press, Vancouver, Canada, 1997.

Gibson W.C.: Old Endeavour: Scientific and Humanitarian Contributions by Physicians Over Age 65. Publisicula IAHM Publications, Palermo, Italy, 2007

Chapter 11
Humanitarian Medicine Applied in a Highly Specialized Field: Cardiovascular Surgery

Jan T. Christenson, MD, PhD, FETCS

11.1 Background

The key health issues faced by a number of developing and underdeveloped countries include, beside the burden of disease, a shortage of resources—financial, material and human, often aggravated by adverse economic conditions and loss of scarce trained personnel to other countries. Shortage of technology also is predominant in many such countries. Numerous governmental and non-governmental agencies have been providing excellent humanitarian medicine worldwide for a long time and for large populations in need. However, most of these actions have concentrated on aid during and immediately following national disasters and armed conflicts. Even though these interventions have often been excellent in providing acute medical and other aid, such programs are usually punctual, most often time-limited, with a specific purpose, and therefore do not result in local capacity building, something that is required for any degree of sustainable development.

The International Association for Humanitarian Medicine has established a valuable basic definition of Humanitarian Medicine. Thus, humanitarian medicine should be and is cooperative, in contrast to traditional medicine that is competitive. It sees no boundaries, political, cultural or religious. It does not work according to preset and unchangeable conditions. As various medical professional organizations have striven to achieve globalization of diagnostic as well as therapeutic modalities, including surgical techniques, with success, the time has now come to focus on how patients who need this expertise can best get it. There is enough room in this field for multiple individual approaches, even though open dialogue, consolidation of resources and coordination, together with some sort of monitoring, would possibly result in a higher degree of achievement. To this end, new frontiers and challenges have to be established.

11.2 The Dialogue

This is the focus for the Global Forum on Humanitarian Medicine in Cardiology and Cardiac Surgery in Geneva, providing a unique opportunity for all key players in humanitarian medicine (governments, governmental organizations, the UN system, the private sector, civil society and NGOs) to get together. The goal is to develop a better understanding of humanitarian medicine's future role in capacity building in underdeveloped countries and regions. Furthermore, the Forum addresses future visions and a dialogue on how best to deliver humanitarian medicine in the future. Last but not least, through the Forum, new partnerships are created and a network established as an aid to reach these set goals.

Many organizations are involved in humanitarian cardiovascular activities. These groups have various characteristics and goals; they may be recently founded or long established, some with few volunteers or as huge organizations, poor or rich, treating few or thousands of patients, and operating globally, regionally or just locally.

Various types of programs have been applied, and the most recent concept is focusing on transfer of medical knowledge and management skills.

11.3 The Challenge

Until recently, the coming generation, our children, have been the priority group of interest for many NGOs. Organizations such as "Terre des Hommes" have brought large numbers of children to specialized hospitals in the North. So has the University Hospital of Geneva, which for more than 30 years, has treated over 6,000 children suffering from congenital and acquired heart disease and other diseases.

However excellent these actions may be, unfortunately they focus on the few that can be helped and do not really participate in help for the many or in local capacity building for sustainable development.

However, a change in concept for humanitarian missions in the field of cardiology and cardiac surgery has been recently occurring. Instead of health care providers, we have taken the role of health care managers. Instead of transferring patients to highly specialized institutions, often far away from home, we now send teams and equipment to where they are needed. This has allowed the child to be treated in his/her local environment.

Numerous foundations and associations have thus organized missions in the field of cardiovascular disease treatment to various locations in the world each year.

The Geneva-based Association "Hearts for All" is just one such organization, the Paris-, London- and Brussels-based "Chain of Hope" or "Chaîne de l'Espoir" are other such examples. Teams of doctors, nurses and technicians have travelled to many countries with their equipment to save children with congenital heart disease. To a certain extent, such missions have also contributed to local capacity building, by training and education of local health personnel and drawing attention to future possibilities. Simplified techniques, use of biological materials and repair rather than replacement have been developed for this purpose.

Under such conditions, our cardiovascular mission's cost for open heart surgery is as low as 2,000 Swiss francs, compared to more than 25,000 SF if the surgery is performed in Europe.

The types of structures currently used in cardiovascular humanitarian medicine are shown in Figure 11.1. The "World Open Hospital" network of the International Association for

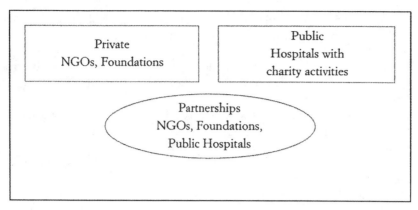

Fig. 11.1 Types of structure

Private NGOs, Foundations
Partnerships NGOs, Foundations, Public Hospitals
Hospitals with charity activities
The World Open Hospital network of IAHM

Medicine is yet another modern concept of providing specialized care to the needy populations.

11.4 The Goal

However, we are far from the ultimate goal. What should this goal be, even in a highly specialized field as cardiovascular medicine and cardiac surgery? The ultimate goal we wish to achieve is to train, educate and equip local teams and institutions to be self-sufficient so that our mission eventually is no longer needed, rather than the more short-sighted aim, where one sees no end to dependence.

What are the options, where are we today and why are cardiovascular diseases so important?

11.5 The Burden

A rapid increase in the number of patients suffering from cardiovascular disease in developing or underdeveloped countries, characterized by WHO as an emerging epidemic, has already started, placing an extra burden on the already limited health resources.

Cardiovascular disease is a group of disorders that affect the heart and the blood vessels and include hypertension, coronary artery disease, cerebrovascular disease, peripheral vascular disease, heart valve affections and congenital heart disease.

The majority of cardiovascular diseases are preventable. Cardiovascular disease is indeed of global concern because it sees no geographic, gender or socio-economic boundaries.

The North missed the opportunity to diminish the explosive threat of cardiovascular disease to the health care system by initially concentrating on diagnosis and treatment rather than prevention.

Treatment of cardiovascular disease is costly and long and requires expensive pharmaceutical therapies and/or surgical interventions; these are in contrast to prevention, which utilizes fewer resources at significantly lower cost.

The South still has the chance to meet the emerging epidemic of cardiovascular disease, by placing prevention as top priority in their population available for active and directed preventive programs.

11.6 A Futuristic View

Any local capacity building effort must include prevention, diagnosis and early treatment as well as diagnosis and treatment of already established cardiovascular disease in developing regions as joint humanitarian ventures between private donors, local governments, the pharmaco-technical industry, UN agencies and various other humanitarian organizations. The role of modern technologies, such as telemedicine, web-conferences, long-distance learning and so on, certainly is also important in this context.

One such example is the Maputo Heart Institute in Mozambique, created by five NGOs, ours included, which opened in June 2001. Long- and short-term fellowship training programs can be arranged at University hospitals in the North as well as at regional centres, which also provide local teaching programs covering all three fundamental aspects. Training and support should also be given to management.

Education and training locally, regionally and globally, promotion of local structures, development of more informed partners and transparency for donors are key elements. This structure was applied in the Maputo project with low treatment costs once the initial investments were covered.

A directed approach has been adopted concerning surgical treatment (selection) and surgical techniques focusing on local needs with focused teaching programs. Other such projects are already in the planning phase. Establishment of regional centres will also promote regional and international cooperation and understanding.

11.7 How Open Dialogue Can Allow Ideas to Branch

We NGOs in cardiology and cardiac surgery are like branches of a big tree, with some experience in new models for delivery of capacity building for humanitarian medicine. All such initiatives ought to be canalized into a common trunk, through open dialogue, which then could derive new ideas and concepts as how best to

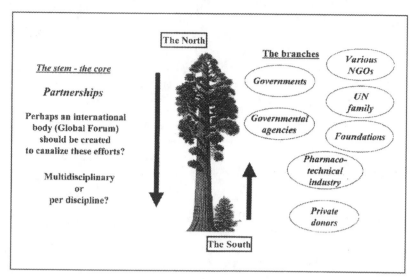

Fig. 11.2 The stem – the core

deliver humanitarian medicine in the future, with broad-based partnership with various global, regional and local key players (Figure 11.2).

As stated by Alexandre Dumas, "one for all and all for one", together, and by creating various types of partnerships, the future humanitarian goals can be reached more effectively. Together, we could envision the possibility for greater success, better health and satisfaction for all involved in humanitarian medicine.

Chapter 12
Humanitarian Medicine for a Developing Country: Outreach to Cuba

Paddy Dewan, PhD, MS, FRCS, FRACS

There are many ways to extend humanitarian assistance, and there are many countries where such action can be usefully applied. The Kind Cuts for Kids Foundation has been helping in providing pediatric surgical know-how in several developing countries, and the following concerns Cuba.

12.1 Kind Cuts for Kids Foundation

The Kind Cuts for Kids Foundation was established to assist Pediatric Surgeons in Australia and New Zealand to provide teaching and patient care in developing countries. The Foundation commenced on the back of an International Federation of Surgical Colleges initiative that recognized the need for improving the care for children with general surgical and urological disease, through the education of surgeons. The philosophy has been one of *teaching the teachers and developing sustainable programs in a number of developing countries*. The Foundation has a principle focus of targeting projects that will produce a sustainable outcome through skill transfer. Involvement in several countries has resulted in more than 65 visits since 1993, and surgery on over 2,000 children, with the establishment of the specialty of Pediatric Surgery in Papua New Guinea and Mauritius, and the advancement of Pediatric Surgery and Anesthesia in places as diverse as Monglia and Bangladesh. Not least of the unexpected outcomes has been the technical improvements that have come with the greater experience of those who are learning as they teach.

12.2 Pediatric Outreach to Cuba

Cuba has a rich history and unique place in the world, with an exciting mix of Latin American and African culture; known for its music, the old cars, cigars, Hemingway, Fidel Castro, the Bay of Pigs, and Guantanamo Bay. Cuba engenders a sense of fascination, excitement, and the unknown. The small country has been subjected to sanctions from its nearest neighbor, thus there are many material goods that are lacking, but there is no lack of courage, the spirit of life, and a warm welcome for humanitarian service.

Medical services, along with education, are important parts of the community support, thus there are many Cuban doctors who work both in their own country, or provide part of the international service provided by the Cuban government to countries in Africa, and as diverse as Timor and Venezuela. However, the lack of contact of the Cuban medical staff with the broader international community and the lack of medical equipment limit the developments of the specialties. Thus, an invitation to assist with training of the pediatric urology community was warmly received by the Kind Cuts for Kids Foundation.

The aim of the project is to provide sustainable assistance, with the expectation that well-trained pediatric urologists will readily make use of the lessons learnt during the tutorials, lectures, clinic, and intraoperative teaching. The aim has been realized, while a large number of children have been given an improved outcome for complex urological disease. Concurrently, education and clinical input have been given in theater nurse management, pediatric anesthesia, and pediatric uroradiology. Importantly, it should be recognized that, like any visit of medical professionals outside their own country, the learning is bidirectional.

12.3 The Project

The initial visit to Cuba was stimulated by contact between an Australian Council of Trade Union, Cuban Children's Fund, supported by the Ministry of Health in Cuba, Rotary Clubs, and several companies. The initial contact from Cuba was to help with equipment needs and to provide input into discussions about difficult cases. The first of five visits occurred in 2003 and have usually been with a focus on major pediatric urology, at the William Soler Hospital, particularly with patients requiring bladder extrophy redo surgery. The sixth visit coincided with a Urology conference in September 2007, as occurred in 2005.

The teams traveling to Cuba consisted of pediatric specialists in urology, anesthesia, radiology, and the theater nursing staff.

The initial visit was to the William Soler Hospital in Havana, with subsequent trips including clinics and operating at both the William Soler Hospital and the Juan Manuel Márques Hospital, with surgeons from the Havana Central Pediatric Hospital and other pediatric urology units in other parts of the country being involved. Despite the transportation difficulties of the pediatric urologists, most of those involved in the surgical program attended on most days. The importance of the training program was further highlighted by pediatric urologists from a peripheral center spending a week at the William Soler Hospital.

12.4 Surgical Consultations

There has been a strong trend to an increasing number of cases being seen in subsequent clinics in Cuba, which has stemmed from the awareness of medical staff of the nature of the improved options available for the complex cases, the awareness of the public of new solutions being offered, and the need for the pervious patients to be reviewed.

A total of 78 patients have been seen, but with a total of 186 consultations, as many of these patients have had repeat visits for a long-term plan of more than one stage surgery to overcome a complex anomaly and previous unsuccessful surgery. These include patients who have had two-stage hypospadias repairs and bladder than genital repairs.

The patients had been screened by the local staff, so that those with either complex pathology or difficult problems due to previous failed surgery were selected for consideration for surgery. Often, additional tests were arranged as part of the process to decide on the final intended intervention. The range of pathology included the two largest groups of patients (hypospadias 11, bladder extrophy complex 31), and intersex, anorectal anomalies, urethral obstruction and a range of other pathologies.

12.5 Operative Surgery

Lengthy sessions in the operating theater have been a feature of the pediatric urology visits to Cuba.

The total of 218 operations included mainly complex urological procedures in children and young adults with congenital anomalies, including Young Dees bladder neck reconstruction 7, wound revision 14, vaginovaginostomy 1, vesicotomy 3, vaginoplasty 6, urethrotomy 1, urethroplasty 5, urethroplasty—posterior 2, perineoplasty 6, osteotomy—bilateral posterior 10, osteotomy—bilateral anterior 15—omphaloplasty 12, transureteroureterostomy 5, bladder extrophy closure 5, bladder neck transaction/plication 10, inguinal herniotomies 8, Mitrofanoff 12, Cantwell Ransley epispadias repair 10, bladder augmentation with bowel 12, bladder augmentation with ureter 4, hypospadias repair 12, cystoscopy/urodynamics 10, urinary stone removal 4, Peno-anorectoplasty 3, cystectomy 2, nephrectomy 3, and a number of one only procedures on the urinary tract, with much of the complex surgery being for reconstruction of patients with bladder extrophy, with a total of 400 hours of surgical time in the 7 weeks of the team's working in Havana.

The operating sessions were long, and involving members of the local team as the assistants, and the providers of the pre- and postoperative care.

12.6 Bladder Extrophy Group Patients

Thirty-one children and young adults had some form of the bladder extrophy/epispadias complex, and most had undergone previous surgery.

The series of patients allowed for the demonstration of primary closure in the newborn period through to the treatment for incontinence with a continent division. In addition, one patient had the incorporation of a segment of bowel; another had a bladder neck reconstruction. The importance of the cosmetic outcome was highlighted by the wound revision, omphaloplasty, and perineoplasty osteotomies in brining the pelvic muscle together in the midline, while facilitating a secure closure and a good cosmetic result, was highlighted in six cases. Also, an important part of the care of these children was shown to be the postoperative care of the catheters, particularly the sequence of events for the removal of multiple urinary tract catheters. A detailed discussion on the last working day of each visit was ensured, and a written plan was in place for all those requiring ongoing treatment.

Many of the patients were complex bladder extrophy cases who had had a previous surgery. Those patients who were reviewed after previous complex operations had all had a satisfactory outcome.

Several bladder extrophy cases had been operated on previously, and had an outcome that was considered unsatisfactory, obviously being ideal cases for teaching and collaboration. The principle focus of the surgery was the establishment of continence in bladder extrophy patients, and managing complex genital anomalies in these patients. Two of the bladder extrophy cases are described in detail.

12.7 Surgical Teaching

Surgical teaching, as in any medical team visit to another country, has been a combination of clinics (including the participation of medical students) lectures, plus teaching during the operative sessions, including a wide range of topics. The idea is to leave a knowledgeable team behind, once the visiting group leaves.

With the relationship building and the coverage of topics on earlier visits, more time was available on subsequent trips for discussion of concepts related to the management of complex pediatric urological cases than had been available during earlier visits. Plans were put in place for the management of the surgical intervention of patients on the basis of these discussions.

Surgical teaching was enhanced by the involvement of two different Cuban institutions and participation in the National Urology conference in 2005. During the Urology conference at Varadaro in mid-2005, both members of the team participated in contributing during two round table presentations, and a presentation on the development of understanding of the anatomy and pathology of the posterior urethra in males. Participation in the urology conference in 2005 enabled lengthy discussion in both a formal and informal context, particularly related to the care of patients with hypospadias, vesicoureteric reflux and urethral obstruction. Surgical teaching was also assisted by the two visiting Australian nurses with Spanish as a first language, thus facilitating free flow of discussion during the ward rounds and operative sessions; communication is particularly important in overseas work.

12.8 Surgical Resource Limitations

The William Soler Hospital and the Juan Manuel Márques Hospital continue to provide most of what is required to give a good standard of care in pediatric urology, but within buildings that lack many of the "fancy" trimmings of an Australian

Hospital—light globes for many of the lights are missing. However, inventive solutions for many of the problems have been developed, such as modifying knives to make instruments with which to perform osteotomies. Unfortunately, inventiveness cannot solve all problems, and *the lack of suture material is a major cause of adverse surgical outcomes.* This simple note on a basic need shows the problems in a developing country, and highlights the value of humanitarian collaboration.

12.9 Anesthesia

There were a number of notable differences in the way patients were handled coming into theater compared to Australia. Preanesthetic assessment was often performed after arrival in the holding area, with no discussion of risks and complications, and no informed consent being obtained. The patients were often left alone in holding area, having been earlier separated from their parents upon arrival at theater, with little apparent effort to reduce preoperative anxiety.

Also, intravenous access was carried out in holding area by nursing staff, but with no local anesthetic cream available, with the concept of gas induction, and intravenous access after the patient was asleep, seemed to be an alien practice. The drug management also differed from Australia, with all patients, regardless of age or weight, given intravenous Atropine and Midazolam or Diazepam immediately prior to transfer to the operating theater.

Transfer of patients between the trolley and the table seemed haphazard, with no patient slide devise being available, there seeming to be little regard to staff health regarding back care with heavier patients. A lack of the facilities may have explained these differences.

12.10 Post-Operative Analgesia

Monitoring in recovery was rudimentary, often due to lack of equipment, with no pulse oximetry, sphygmomanometer, and other usual available equipment in Australia. Patients were often restrained in a crucifix position, with parents not able to be in attendance, and little, if any, effective analgesia, probably due to poor supplies of the drugs.

Despite the "historical" standard of care, compared with current "best-practice," the outcomes for children were good, there being no anesthetic morbidity or mortality.

An Australian anesthetist able to speak Spanish improved the skill transfer for the anesthetic part of the team. Lumbar epidural analgesia, caudal epidural analgesia, and laryngeal mask use were the principle techniques taught and also the issues mentioned earlier were discussed at length, to improve risk management and reduce patient stress.

12.11 Nursing

In 2005, an Australian–Spanish theater and ward nurse gave continuous input into the understanding of the preoperative, operative, and postoperative nursing and surgical management, and provided input to suggested changes in management of the theater complex. The Australian nurse involved in the program has also assisted with solving the problem of the very limited availability of sutures, by helping manage the meager supply.

A limitation of nurses in the ward resulted in families playing a major role in the care of the children, to the general advantage of the child, and with great enthusiasm of the parents. Catheter care required medical vigilance, particularly due to the tendency of the tubing to kink because of the "inventive" connections, and poor quality of some of the urine bags.

Certainly, there are a number of system issues in theaters that could be improved, including counting of items on and off the operative field, sterility, instrument care, and the handling of sharp objects during surgery. Still a scrub nurse is not used at the William Soler Hospital, and there appear to be somewhat rigid boundaries between the tasks performed by different staff groups. Further input is required to develop understanding of the processes and to facilitate change that would be "no cost" and an improvement.

12.12 Radiology

12.12.1 Introduction

The first visit of an Australian pediatric radiologist occurred during the third visit of the Kind Cuts for Kids Foundation, with the main aims to:

- evaluate the present status of equipment;
- assess the radiological staff arrangements, including radiologists and technicians;
- evaluate areas in which service, staffing equipment improvements would be desirable;
- teach pediatric radiology to surgical, technical, and radiological staff; and
- participate in the evaluation of urological cases.

Radiological input during the outpatient clinics, both pre- and postoperatively, and in-depth discussion of the surgical perspective gave a greater understanding and appreciation of what was required radiologically, and facilitated education of surgeons about the radiological investigations. The main investigations were ultrasounds, micturating cystourethrograms, and intravenous urograms.

12.12.2 Radiological Staff

Five Cuban trained radiologists work in the Radiology Department at the William Soler Hospital. In Havana, there are five training hospitals for radiologists, and other training schemes exist in provinces outside Havana.

After gaining the basic medical degree, there is a period of approximately 3–5 years internship where the junior doctors are classified as "family doctors," following which doctors can elect to specialize. The radiology training is 3 years, with an annual examination that is to be passed before proceeding to the next year. There is no specific subspecialty training in pediatric radiology.

There are approximately 10 radiographers/technicians and one nurse in the department at William Soler. The radiographers train though the School of Radiography and the William Soler Hospital is one of the training hospitals, with a training course of 3 years.

12.12.3 Postgraduate Radiological Training

The radiologists have limited access to postgraduate conferences or overseas fellowships, of which they are aware. Applications are directed to the Ministry, which then adjudicates as to who can attend, but most do not apply because of the high failure rate. Greater opportunities for continuing professional development would come from further visits to Cuba and greater opportunities for Cuban participation in international activities, which could be facilitated via the Internet and international grants.

12.12.4 Radiological Equipment

The Radiology Department is sparsely equipped, with only three plain radiography machines, three ultrasound machines, and fluoroscopy equipment: there is no CT or MRI machine in the William Soler Hospital. The level of equipment seems to reflect the standard in most hospitals.

12.12.5 Resource Deficiencies in Radiology

From discussion with radiologists, the perceived deficiencies are

1. lack of availability and access to radiology books and journals. The only available textbooks were out of date;
2. minimal access to Internet and Medline or other medical Internet sites;
3. poor equipment which frequently breaks down;

4. lack of access to MRI and CT. Neither is available in the William Soler Hospital, and they have very limited access to the few that are available within Cuba. There are three MRI scanners in Cuba and two were broken;
5. lack of ability to further their knowledge, both theoretical and practical, in pediatric radiology. All radiologists have been taught pediatric urology "on the job," which would be best supplemented by further training;
6. lack of ability or funding to travel overseas to radiological conferences/courses or to receive specialist training;
7. no Internet access in the Radiology Department;
8. inadequate radiation protection equipment.

12.13 Conclusion

Cuba is a country with a rich history, fascinating people and a strong focus on health care and education. Resource limitations have impacted on the ability of the senior medical staff to maximize their potential which can be overcome by humanitarian outreach. Most of the solutions to the difficult chronic problems can be addressed by "hand and heads" approach to system engineering. By that it is meant that clinical outcomes can be improved by those with additional educational opportunities in the past (the visitors) working with the team in the country being assisted, so that opportunities for improvements in care can be balanced with knowledge of the possible barriers.

This brief account shows the problems encountered in a developing country. Yet by general standards health conditions in Cuba are considered to be considerably better than in other, less fortunate developing countries. So the reader will realize the magnitude of the problem, and the need for "Kind Cuts" in all fields if health.

The invitation to assist with teaching related to pediatric urology in Cuba has opened the eyes and hearts of a group of Australian medical and nursing staff to the difficulties of health care in Cuba for a community that demonstrates compassion and resourcefulness. The Kind Cuts for Kids Foundation trusts we have improved the outcome for a small group of patients by our direct care and the coming generations of children through education.

Chapter 13
Humanitarian Basic Plastic Surgery

Bishara S. Atiyeh, MD, FACS

13.1 Introduction

Elsewhere in this book, several chapters abundantly demonstrate how the basic spirit of Health for All (Mahler, 2003) and the strategy of Primary Health Care, with its overriding principle of health as a human right (Gunn, 2000) underpin the philosophy and practice of humanitarian medicine. This, however, should not be interpreted as a second class medicine, reserved for simpler diseases and "cheaper" procedures. Indeed the right of the patient requires that, within all possibility, and barring irrelevant practices or frivolous demands, no life-saving or socially supportive needs be witheld. Thus, the accounts of essential cardiac surgery (Christenson, 2003) complicated urogenital reconstruction (Dewan, 1998) meticulous geriatric patient education (Assal, 2005) are concrete examples of extensive, scientific, necessary humanitarian medicine, as is humanitarian basic plastic surgery.

The spectrum of plastic surgery as seen by most people is based on television extreme makeover shows, thinking that this is what plastic surgery is all about (Dukes). Plastic surgery, however, is a well-defined specialty, which encompasses reconstructive surgery as well as cosmetic (aesthetic) procedures (Knipper), going from the very simple interventions up to the very complex micro-vascular reconstructive surgery (Dukes), sophisticated craniofacial surgery (American Academy), and management of burn injuries and their complications (McIndoe). It is far from being a luxury surgical service. Several branches of plastic surgery are deeply committed to humanitarian service with a great desire to enhance the quality of human life (American Academy). The term commonly used nowadays is "humanitarian plastic surgery" (Knipper).

However, several questions remain to be clearly answered. What is the place of plastic and reconstructive surgery within the field of general surgery in developing countries? (Micheau and Lauwers, 1999) Must the reparative motivation of plastic surgery intervention remain the only trace of a plastic surgeon's skill and humanity? During a plastic surgery humanitarian mission, can this surgery be aesthetic? Can aesthetic surgery be humanitarian (Knipper, 2003)?

13.2 Humanitarian Medicine

Disasters, unfortunately, and help, fortunately, are as old as humanity. As long as man has had a beating heart, some adrenaline, and a reflex for protection, he has had compassion and the urge to help. This is the natural and noble drive for humanitarian medicine (Gunn, 2000). And this was the drive that, in face of mounting natural disasters, conflicts, and social degradation, led a group of concerned citizens to establish, in 1984 at the World Health Organization, the Brock Chisholm Trust that was subsequently registered in Palermo, Italy, as the International Association for Humanitarian Medicine Brock Chisholm, to promote and support the right of health for all and access to appropriate medical care. To take the full measure and social significance of the concept of Humanitarian Medicine, it is worth to consider its formal definition (Gunn, 2000). Unfortunately, at present the "right to health," acclaimed, recognized and required everywhere, does not seem to get all the universal attention it deserves and is even precarious in terms of promotion, dissemination, and protection (ZENIT) (Masellis and Gunn 2002).

Historically, assistance in emergencies has evolved from early wound dressing and pain relief, to specialized techniques like emergency medical services and Disaster Medicine; to institutionalized mechanisms like the Red Cross, to concepts, like disaster prevention, and socio-political arrangements and Humanitarian Medicine (Gunn, 2000). The first "thorough study" of humanitarian intervention was published by Rougier in 1910: "Unfortunately, the conclusion which emerged from this study is that it is neither possible to separate the humanitarian from the political grounds for intervention nor to assure the complete disinterestedness of the intervening States." Whenever one power intervenes in the name of humanity in the domain of another power, it cannot but impose its concept of justice and public policy on the other State, by force if necessary (Boyle). Irrespective of this fact, international humanitarian law and human rights provide the normative context for those who try to deliver medical and emergency relief to war and disaster zones (Leaning, 1999) or to communities living in underprivileged areas. Unfortunately, unlike most professional activities, humanitarian relief is not subject to monitoring by professional bodies (JAMA, 2001) nevertheless, the key principles of international humanitarian law of relevance to physicians are neutrality, non-partisanship, independence, and humanitarianism with commitment to promoting the welfare of sick and injured people, treating everyone according to medical need. Physicians and other health care workers are protected from hostile action to the extent that they understand these principles and abide by the rules that flow from them. They must take no political sides in any conflict, be unarmed, and directed only by professional dictates (Bruderlein, 1999; Leaning 1999).

The practice of humanitarian medicine involves more than just the application of medicine or medical knowledge to the treatment of a patient as a person, who should not be viewed as a mere body requiring medical attention. Any physician practising humanitarian medicine must view the patient as someone possessing his own unique personal history and treat him in the context of being a member of a family even of a larger human family with neighbours and friends, not just in the context of being simply a patient (What is humanitarian medicine? http://www.medschoolchat.com/displayarticle65.html). Indeed, there is no need for a surgeon to go on a humanitarian mission in order to do humanitarian work. In principle, anything a physician does should be humanitarian, regardless of where in the world the treatment is being provided (Knipper). However, according to J. Habermas, the necessary conditions and limitations of humanitarian medicine and the main valid engagement should be a communicative action which means a true partnership with the local health care specialists (Montandon et al., 2004). Of paramount importance is the meaning of this commitment as well as the way in which the humanitarian action is perceived by the recipient country (Baudet et al., 1999; Gunn, 2000). Assistance and cooperation of local medical staff is essential in the pre-selection of cases to be operated while each single medical mission team provides all the necessary supplies for surgery, which invariably takes place in small hospitals provided by the local authorities (d'Agostino et al., 2001).

13.3 Humanitarian Action and Basic Plastic Surgery

Throughout the developing countries Primary Health Care is necessarily considered a priority, and hospitals used mainly for emergency operations are usually few in number and badly equipped; elective surgery is considered a luxury (d'Agostino et al., 2001). The demand for reconstructive surgery, however, is extremely high due to the high birth rate and consequently large number of patients, as well as the shortage of both medical staff and supplies (d'Agostino et al., 2001). Children, in particular, with congenital diseases and/or other non-congenital anomalies who are fortunate enough to reach a hospital will often be treated by general surgeons lacking specific training; those children suffering from disabling conditions are often neglected and left to live with their anomalies for the rest of their lives (d'Agostino et al., 2001).

Several humanitarian charitable organizations are sending at present plastic surgery teams to developing countries or areas (Dewan, 1998; Nicolai et al., 1998). In a humanitarian mission, plastic reconstructive surgery usually is only one modality, in a vast array of treatment approaches (Knipper). Accomplishment of humanitarian missions in plastic surgery, however, is stirring a lot of interest (Alfandari et al., 2004) and humanitarian plastic surgery is becoming much demanded so that more and more surgeons are attracted by this type of commitment (Montandon et al., 2004) which provides an opportunity of reflection about team training, the type of relation with the country where the mission is being conducted, and the type of right team required (Alfandari et al., 2004). Based on data collected from several missions and by consensus, the International Task Force on Volunteer Cleft Missions outlined recommendations for future volunteer cleft missions that are applicable to all plastic surgery humanitarian missions. These recommendations are related to (1) mission objectives, (2) organization, (3) personal health and liability, (4) funding, (5) trainees in volunteer cleft missions, and (6) public relations. The task force believed that all volunteer missions should have well-defined objectives, preferably with long-term plans. It decided also that it was impossible to achieve a successful mission without good organization and close coordination and advised that efforts should be made, and care taken, to ensure that there is minimal morbidity and no mortality (Yeow et al., 2002). The mission director must be an experienced surgeon in order to select the most reliable and the simplest procedure (Baudet et al., 1999). As ambassadors of goodwill and humanitarian aid, the participants in such missions must make every effort to understand and respect local customs and protocol while providing top-quality surgical service, training local doctors and staff, developing and nurturing fledgling reconstructive programs, and, finally, making new friends (Yeow et al., 2002).

In such humanitarian missions, plastic surgery is mostly practised in an unfamiliar and demanding environment and under challenging conditions and difficult circumstances (Knipper). Though some missionary hospitals tend to be well-equipped (d'Agostino et al., 2001), the facilities and working conditions for surgery are usually poor (Knipper). Moreover, the disorders and pathologies encountered may be far removed from the conditions seen in one's home country; the range of procedures to be performed may be vast (hand surgery, burn scar revision, orthopaedics and traumatology, maxillofacial surgery, etc.). The surgeon participating in such missions must be conversant with all aspects of plastic and reconstructive surgery (Knipper).

The technical and material limits, the constraints for the patients to travel to the hospital, to pay for costs, and the difficulties of follow-up require the selection of patients in whom the disease can be treated in a single stage procedure (Voche and Valenti, 1999). Three types of diseases are usually managed: (1) congenital anomalies, (2) post-burn, and (3) post-trauma sequelae. Due to the absence of hand rehabilitation locally, reconstructive tendon surgery is inadvisable to avoid disappointing poor results and discredit this part of hand surgery. For reason of complexity and unreliability of electromyographic examination, brachial plexus injuries as well cannot be treated except the simplest cases needing one or two tendon transfers. Concerning skin coverage and reconstructive surgery, experience has shown that pedicled local and loco-regional flaps and even micro-surgical transfers are adapted and reliable techniques due to the imperative of single stage procedure (Voche and Valenti, 1999).

13.4 Essential Aesthetic Surgery?

Aesthetic surgery is still considered as extravagant surgery undertaken to beautify patients who are not really ill, as opposed to the "real" surgery provided by the "humanitarian" surgeon whose aim is to help those in actual need. How can one envisage cosmetic surgery then when the object of a humanitarian mission is to meet the most basic demands for surgery (American Academy of Facial Plastic and Reconstructive Surgery)? How does one reconcile these two perceptions?

Even though many surgeons may feel that "humanitarian aesthetic surgery" is a contradiction in terms, any reconstructive surgery procedure must address the aesthetic dimension even when performed for "humanitarian" reasons (Knipper). It must be remembered that, barring frivolous demands, it is not for us to decide what is and what is not important to a given patient. The ultimate objective should always be the patient's well-being by meeting his/her needs.

Moreover, there is no need to "justify" aesthetic by reconstruction because aesthetic belongs, in itself to reparation and reconstruction. Only the very intention behind an intervention will decide whether it is an "unnecessary" aesthetic or a regular "plastic" intervention. There is nevertheless no reason to feel guilty whenever the technical gesture of a procedure is also aesthetic, since what really motivates the surgical intervention is not for us to decide (Knipper, 2003). Irrespective of the motivation, the surgical technique will be the same, and the surgeon will always try to do his very best achieving the best result. All this illustrates that our definitions are of minor importance, compared with the mere satisfaction we bring to the unfortunate patients, which, hopefully, will be a "beautiful" satisfaction (Knipper, 2003). In practical terms, and however paradoxical it may sound, we have learnt not to do aesthetic surgery, but to do surgery with a view to achieving an aesthetic result, even when working on a so-called humanitarian mission (Knipper; Knipper, 2003). The form reconstruction will take is very subjective and case-specific, and only the final result will have the last say. Hopefully, this surgical result will be aesthetically, functionally and humanly acceptable (Knipper, 2003). What a little girl with cleft lip wants is to look better with a more cosmetically appealing lip. In the final analysis, definitions of plastic, reconstructive or aesthetic procedures do not matter. Whether the cleft lip repair is undertaken for functional or aesthetic reasons, the needs and technical details remain unchanged, with the surgeon aiming at the best, useful pleasing result. What really counts is that the patient will be pleased and, as we hope, will be happy (Knipper, 2003, McIndoe, 1981).

Indeed these debates on justification become totally irrelevant when one considers the surgery needed for the disastrous and shocking facial disfigurements and totally dishonourable "honour amputations" that are inflicted in some countries as punishment on young women or helpless men in the name of honour, culture, or face-saving (what a misnomer!), as described so vividly and painfully by Mughese Amin (2007). Here surgery becomes truly humanitarian, and the problem a matter of human rights (Gunn, 1999)

13.5 Conclusion

Problems and/or questions often raised by humanitarian plastic surgery include the motives, sufficient training of the mission's team, choice of surgical techniques, post-operative follow-up, assessment of the results, availability of resources, and possible innovations (Montandon and Pittet, 1999). Various plastic surgery humanitarian missions have emphasized the importance of the long-term involvement of the same team, at the same site, with the same programme to pass on knowledge and, for the surgeon, to experience the richness of the people and area being visited (Dewan, 1998; Micheau and Lauwers, 1999).

Humanitarian plastic surgery missions are often a substitute, filling temporarily a gap in local capabilities. Plastic surgery missions should be training missions and are essential for the development of reconstructive surgery in developing countries. This training must be progressive and adapted to the country's needs. For that regard, several simple plastic surgery techniques are sufficient to treat a large number of patients (Saboye, 1999). Analysis of the type of operations required for any humanitarian plastic surgery mission shows that the techniques most frequently in demand are simple procedures (skin grafts, local flaps, etc.). This "basic" essential plastic surgery invariably is commensurate with local possibilities and corresponds to the population's real needs (Micheau and Lauwers, 1999) and well-being.

References

Alfandari B., Persichetti P., Pelissier P., Martin D., Baudet J.: Myanmar mission. Ann. Chir. Plast. Esthet. 49: 273–290, 2004.

American Academy of Facial Plastic and Reconstructive Surgery. http://www.ama-assn.org/ama/pub/category/print/15930.html.

Assal J.P. In: Understanding the Global Dimensions of Health. S.W. Gunn ed., Springer, 2005.

Atiyeh B.S., Al-Amm C.A., El-Musa K.A., Sawwaf A., Dham R.: Scar quality and physiologic barrier function restoration following moist and moist exposed dressings of partial thickness wounds. Dermatol. Surg., 29: 14–20, 2003b.

Baudet J., Martin D., Pelissier P., Genin Etcheberry T., Casoli V.: Humanitarian plastic surgery missions. Actions and considerations. Ann. Chir. Plast. Esthet., 44: 72–76, 1999.

Boyle F.A. The 2001 Dr. Irma Parhad Lecture. Humanitarian intervention and international law. http://www.ucalgary.ca/UofC/faculties/medicine/PARHAD/documents/BoyleLecture.pdf

Bruderlein C., Leaning J.: New challenges for humanitarian protection. *BMJ*, 319: 430–435, 1999.

Christenson J.T.: Humanitarian medicine applied in a highly specialized field: cardiovascular surgery. J. Humanitarian Med., 29–31, 2003.

d'Agostino S., Del Rossi C., Del Curto S., Attanasio A., et al.: Surgery of congenital malformations in developing countries: experience in 13 humanitarian missions during 9 years. Pediatr. Med. Chir., 23: 117–121, 2001.

Dewan P.: Surgeons overseas. Int. Fed. Surg. Colleges, 41–5, 1998.

Dukes M.E. Plastic surgery: most is necessary. http://www.armymedicine.army.mil/hc/healthtips/13/200409plasticsurgery.cfm.

Gunn S.W.A.: Female genital mutilation. World J. Surg, 23: 1087, 1999.

Gunn S.W.A.: Disaster medicine—humanitarian medicine. Prehosp: Disast. Med., 15:s53, 2000.

Improving standards in international humanitarian response: the Sphere project and beyond. JAMA, 286(5), 2001. http://jama.ama-assn.org/cgi/content/extract/286/5/531

Knipper P. Mission: Plastic surgery under challenging conditions, http://www.maitrise-orthop.com/corpusmaitri/orthopaedic/118 knipper/knipper us.shtml.

Knipper P.: Humanitarian aesthetic surgery. Ann. Chir. Plast. Esthet., 48: 288–294, 2003.

Leaning J.: Editorials: medicine and international humanitarian law. *BMJ*, 319:393–394, 1999.

McIndoe A: See Page G.: Tale of a Guinea Pig, Pelham Books, London and New York, 1981.

Mahler H.: Health for all or hell for all? The role of leadership in health equity. J. Humanitarian Med. 3: 43–45, 2003.

Masellis M. Gunn S.W.A.: Humanitarian medicine: a vision and action. J. Humanitarian Med., 2:33–39, 2002.

Micheau P., Lauwers F.: What are the objectives of a humanitarian plastic and reconstructive surgery mission? Ann. Chir. Plast. Esthet., 44:19–26, 1999.

Montandon D., Pittet B.: Humanitarian plastic surgery. Personal experience and reflections. Ann. Chir. Plast. Esthet., 44: 27–34, 1999.

Montandon D. Quinodoz P., Pittet B.: Questioning humanitarian plastic surgery. Ann. Chir. Plast. Esthet., 49: 314–319, 2004.

Mughese Amin M.: The dishonourable practice of "honour amputations" of noses and other body parts. J. Humanitarian Med., 7: 20–21, 2007.

Nicolai J.-P.A., Grieb N., Gruhl L., Schwabe K., Pressier P.: Interplast: five years of the Cochin project. Eur. J. Plast. Surg., 21: 77–81, 1998.

Saboye J.: Plastic surgery training missions in developing countries. A ten-year experience in Mali. Ann. Chir. Plast. Esthet., 44: 35–40, 1999.

Voche P., Valenti P.: Our experience of humanitarian hand surgery in Vietnam. Ann. Chir. Plast. Esthet., 44: 64–71, 1999.

What is humanitarian medicine? http://www.medschoolchat.com/displayarticle65.html.

Yeow V.K.L., Lee S.-T.T., Lambrecht T.J., Barnett J., et al. International task Force on volunteer cleft missions. J. Craniofacial. Surg. 13: 18–25, 2002.

ZENIT—The World Seen From Rome. Interview With Dr Michele Masellis. http://www.zenit.org/english/visualizza.phtml?sid=8480 2005.

Part III
International, UN
and WHO Cooperation

Chapter 14
Find New Unity

Kofi Annan

The thing that stands out when we review international engagement in countries affected by conflict is that no single approach has ever been adopted twice because no two conflicts or post-conflict situations are alike. Even the four recent cases of Afghanistan, Kosovo, Timor-Leste and Sierra Leone are very different from each other, in terms of the causes and consequences of the conflict, the United Nations previous involvement, the political and legal context governing the international community's response and the sheer size of the affected population and territory.

One of the most important lessons, when it comes to planning the international community's engagement in a new situation—such as the one we face now in Iraq— is the need, first, to reach a common understanding of what makes the crisis in question unique and then to develop our responses accordingly. We should draw on previous experiences to make our response as effective as possible, while bearing in mind that completely new approaches or forms of assistance may be required.

A few specific lessons stand out:

- The trust of the parties and the population can be fragile and cannot be taken for granted over time; their consent needs to be cultivated and preserved.
- The role of the international community is not to solve all of a country's problems but to help its people become self-reliant.
- Priorities must be set, starting with the essential humanitarian needs of the population, which includes the need for basic conditions of security, law and order. Meeting these needs will also make it easier to foster the conditions in which viable political processes can emerge and grow—for instance, by promoting reconciliation, good governance, the rule of law, human rights and transitional justice initiatives.
- Decisions on the reform of key State institutions and legal and political structures must, if they are to be sustainable in the long run, be taken by the people of the country themselves. Such a process can succeed only if all the main groups in the country or territory play a part in it and feel that it belongs to them, and do not perceive it as leading to a predetermined outcome. The pacing of the overall process and the sequence and timing of its component parts are also crucial to success. They need to take into account the political, security and socio-economic conditions in the country and the degree of support that can realistically be expected from interested members of the international community. Moving too

slowly risks losing momentum and fuelling frustration. But going too fast can be equally counterproductive, if it means taking hurried decisions whose effects are difficult to reverse.

- The regional dimension needs early and sustained attention.
- And lastly, there is direct correlation between United Nations success and Security Council unity—and between United Nations setbacks and divisions among Council members about the strategy to be pursued. The Council must be united in setting out the overall objectives for international assistance and a clear division of labour, and then maintain its unity in providing strong political support—both during rough periods when progress is at risk, and when the acute phase of the conflict has passed and no longer commands the attention of the world's media.

In the case of Iraq—which, of course, we all have in mind at the moment—the Council now has the chance to leave behind earlier disagreements and find unity of purpose in the post-war phase. Those decisions will not be easy. But they should not be impossible if you keep some shared principles firmly in mind. As you debate them, I would urge you to set aside past divisions and ask yourselves what will help the Iraqi people most. Their interests must come first. The overriding objective must be to enable the Iraqi people to take charge of their own destiny.

Already, in resolution 1472 (2003), you have reaffirmed your commitment to the sovereignty and territorial integrity of Iraq, your respect for the right of the people to determine their own political future and control their own natural resources, and your belief that all parties must abide by their obligations under international law, including the Fourth Geneva Convention.

I am sure you would all agree that sovereignty implies political independence, and that in order to determine their political future, the Iraqi people must be free to choose their own system of government and political leadership. What is needed is an impartial, representative and transparent process, leading to the choice by Iraqis themselves of a credible and legitimate Iraqi political authority to which sovereignty can be restored. I trust you would also agree on the need to put an end to Iraq's isolation and help the people of Iraq, as quickly as possible, to establish conditions for normal life.

The Council will have important decisions to take on existing mandates within the context of the new situation—notably on sanctions, the Oil-for-Food programme and weapons inspections. Beyond that, you will need to consider how best the international community can help Iraqis rebuild their country—and what part the United Nations might play in assisting that effort, and in the process, of restoring Iraqi sovereignty.

Courtesy, *UN Chronicle*, No 2, 2003.

Chapter 15
Health and Human Rights in International Legal Instruments

A WHO Compilation

The International Association for Humanitarian Medicine Brock Chisholm is dedicated to the inalienable principle of health as a human right. The following is a compilation of formal, international legal instruments, comprising Treaties, Declarations, Standards, Conventions, Constitutions, Conference documents and other Covenants relative to health and human rights. Listed in chronological order from 1930 to 2002 (Courtesy, World Health Organization).

I. International treaties, conventions and protocols

Convention (No. 29) concerning Forced Labour (1930); United Nations Charter (1945);

Convention on the Prevention and Punishment of the Crime of Genocide (1948);

Convention for the Suppression of the Traffic in Persons and of the Exploitation of the Prostitution of Others (1949);

Geneva Convention for the Amelioration of the Condition of the Wounded and Sick in Armed Forces in the Field (1949);

Geneva Convention for the Amelioration of the Condition of Wounded, Sick and Shipwrecked Members of Armed Forces at Sea (1949);

Geneva Convention relative to the Treatment of Prisoners of War (1949);

Geneva Convention relative to the Protection of Civilian Persons in Time of War (1949), and the Protocol Additional to the Geneva Conventions relating to the Protection of Victims of International Armed Conflicts (Protocol 1) (1977) and the Protocol relating to the Protection of Victims of Non-International Armed Conflicts (Protocol II) (1977);

Convention relating to the Status of Refugees (1950) and its Protocol (1967);

Convention (No. 105) on the Abolition of Forced Labour (1957);

International Convention on the Elimination of All Forms of Racial Discrimination (1963);

International Covenant on Economic, Social and Cultural Rights (1966); The right to the highest attainable standard of health (2000)

International Covenant on Civil and Political Rights (1966) and its two Protocols (1966 and 1989);

Convention on the Elimination of All Forms of Discrimination Against Women (1979) and its Protocol (1999);

Convention against Torture and Other Cruel, Inhuman or Degrading Treatment or Punishment (1984);

Convention on the Rights of the Child (1989);

Convention (No. 169) concerning Indigenous and Tribal Peoples in Independent Countries (1989);

International Convention on the Protection of the Rights of All Migrant Workers and Members of their Families (1990);

Convention to Combat Desertification in Countries Experiencing Serious Drought and/or Desertification, Particularly in Africa (1994);

Convention (No. 182) on the Prohibition and Immediate Action for the Elimination of the Worst Forms of Child Labour (1999);

Maternity Protection Convention (No. 183, 2000).

II. International declarations, principles and standards

Constitution of the World Health Organization (1948);

Universal Declaration of Human Rights (1948);

Declaration on the Use of Scientific and Technological Progress in the Interests of Peace and for the Benefit of Mankind (1975);

Declaration on the Rights of Disabled Persons (1975);

Principles of Medical Ethics relevant to the Role of Health Personnel, particularly Physicians, in the Protection of Prisoners and Detainees against Torture and Other Cruel, Inhuman or Degrading Treatment or Punishment (1982);

Declaration on the Right to Development (1986);

Principles for the Protection of Persons with Mental Illness and the Improvement of Mental Health Care (1991);

United Nations Principles for Older Persons (1991);

Declaration on the Rights of Persons Belonging to National or Ethnic, Religious and Linguistic Minorities (1992);

United Nations Standard Rules on the Equalization of Opportunities for Persons with Disabilities (1993);

Declaration on the Elimination of Violence Against Women (1993);

Universal Declaration on the Human Genome and Human Rights (1997);

Declaration on the Right and Responsibility of Individuals, Groups and Organs of Society to Promote and Protect Universally Recognized Human Rights and Fundamental Freedoms (1998);

Guiding Principles on Internal Displacement (1998);

Founding Principles of the International Association for Humanitarian Medicine Brock Chisholm (2000).

III. Regional legal instruments

American Declaration of the Rights and Duties of Man (1948);

European Convention for the Protection of Human Rights and Fundamental Freedoms (1950) and its Eleven Protocols (1952–94);

European Social Charter (1961) (revised 1996);

American Convention on Human Rights (1969);

African Charter on Human and Peoples' Rights (1981);

Inter-American Convention to Prevent and Punish Torture (1985);

Additional Protocol to the American Convention on Human Rights in the Area of Economic, Social and Cultural Rights—"Protocol of San Salvador" (1988);

Protocol to the American Convention on Human Rights to Abolish the Death Penalty (1990);

African Charter on the Rights and Welfare of the Child (1990);

Convention on the Prevention, Punishment and Eradication of Violence against Women (Convention of Belem do Para) (1994);

Arab Charter on Human Rights (1994);

European Convention on Human Rights and Dignity of the Human Being with regard to the Application of Biology and Medicine: Convention on Human Rights and Biomedicine (1997);

Inter-American Convention on the Elimination of All Forms of Discrimination Against Persons With Disabilities (1999).

IV. International conference documents

World Summit for Children, New York (1990): World Declaration on the Survival, Protection and Development of Children and Plan of Action for Implementing the World Declaration, and its follow-up, the United Nations General Assembly Special Session (UNGASS) on Children (2002): A World Fit for Children;

United Nations Conference on Environment and Development, Rio de Janeiro (1992): Rio Declaration on Environment and Development and Agenda 21;

World Conference on Human Rights, Vienna (1993): Vienna Declaration and Programme of Action;

International Conference on Population and Development, Cairo, 1994: Programme of Action;

World, Summit for Social Development, Copenhagen (1995): Copenhagen Declaration on Social Development and Programme of Action of the World Summit for Social Development, and its follow-up, Copenhagen Plus 5 (2000);

Fourth World Conference on Women, Beijing (1995): Beijing Declaration and Platform for Action, and its follow-up, Beijing Plus 5 (2000);

Second United Nations Conference on Human Settlements (Habitat II), Istanbul (1996); Istanbul Declaration on Human Settlements;

World Food Summit, Rome (1996): Rome Declaration on World Food Security and World Food Summit Plan of Action, and its follow-up, Declaration of the World Food Summit: Five Years Later, International Affiance Against Hunger (2002);

United Nations General Assembly Special Session (UNGASS) on AIDS (2001): Declaration of Commitment on HIV/AIDS "Global Crisis—Global Action";

World Conference Against Racism, Racial Discrimination Xenophobia and Related Intolerance, Durban (2001): Durban Declaration and Programme of Action;

Second World Assembly on Ageing (2002): Political Declaration and Madrid International Programme of Action on Ageing.

Chapter 16
The United Nations Today: Changes in Policies and Structures—The World Summit and UN Reform

Yves Beigbeder, LLD

You probably know the story: when he was appointed Secretary General of the United Nations in 1997, Kofi Annan complained that he was being accused of failing to reform the organization in 6 weeks. "But what are you complaining about," asked the Russian ambassador, "you have had more time than God." Annan replied: "But God had a big advantage; He worked alone, without a General Assembly, a Security Council, and all the Committees."

Indeed, an intergovernmental organization like the United Nations is totally dependent on its members, the governments, who decide on policy, programmes, and financing. The Secretary General has little power of his own. Reform of the United Nations is an uphill struggle. Reform has been a repeated slogan since the 1980s, with innumerable expert committees, intergovernmental commissions, international conferences and Summits, and resolutions of the General Assembly and of the Security Council. Among them: the 1985 report of Maurice Bertrand of the Joint Inspection Unit "Some Reflections on reform of the U.N."; the Group of 18's report of 1986 on financial and administrative functions; the 1988 Declaration on the Prevention and the Removal of Disputes and Situations Which May Threaten International Peace and Security and the Role of the United Nations in this Field (GA Res. 43/51); a UNITAR study of 1989 on "The future role of the U.N. in an interdependent world; several studies and initiatives in 1991 as the United Nations was approaching its fiftieth birthday: "The Stockholm Initiative on Global Security and Governance" and "The U.N. in Development Reform Issues in the Economic and Social Fields" by the Nordic UN Project, (1991) the "North South Roundtable Strengthening the U.N. for the 1990s"; General Assembly resolution 45/264 on "Restructuring and revitalizing of the U.N. in the economic, social and related fields" (May 1991); the Secretary General's Agenda for Peace of 1992, Annual Reports of the Secretary General; and other reports from the Joint Inspection Unit, national associations for the United Nations (USA, Canada, Italy), think-tanks, and scholars' studies.

UN reforms have generally focused on structure, management, budget, finances, personnel, audit, and programme and administrative co-ordination. While budget levels have attracted much attention, co-ordination between the United Nations and its agencies, and co-ordination of the many agencies in humanitarian emergencies, is an important, often neglected subject, sometimes called a "quixotic quest." Changes in policies have expanded the role of the United Nations through resolutions of the General Assembly and the Security Council, international treaties and conventions, new programmes, and initiatives by the Secretary General, not by formal reform. The UN Charter has only been revised three times to expand the composition of the Security Council from 11 to 15, and the composition of the Economic and Social Council from 18 to 27 and then to 54 (1963 and 1971).

The United Nations celebrated its 60th anniversary in October 2005, which offered an opening for new significant reforms. However, the World Summit held in New York on 14–16 September 2005 failed in its more ambitious goals. While some of its advances were praised, some diplomats and observers were dismissive.

In the most biting criticism, the Venezuelan President described the final document as being "conceived in darkness and brought forward from the shadows." The humanist musician, Bob Geldof, described the situation as "bloody outrageous, a scandal."

There has been no consensus on the main recommendations of the High Level Panel on Threats, Challenges and Change, of December 2004, nor on the proposals of Kofi Annan, the Secretary General, in his report of March 2005 entitled "In larger freedom: towards development, security and human rights for all."

The reputation of the United Nations and of Annan has been damaged by the devastating report of the Volcker Committee on the oil-for-food programme, which alleges failure of leadership and supervision, and corruption. The report said that the United Nations needs urgent reform.

The United Nations is still suffering from the deep division of the Security Council over the Iraq war.

National interest tends to prevail over the need for international agreement, co-operation, and understanding.

On security and humanitarian assistance, the United Nations is seen as unable to deal effectively with the tragedy in Darfur, Sudan: critics recall the UN incapacity to prevent the genocides in Cambodia and in Rwanda, the massacre of Srebrenica, and wars in general. There are charges of sexual misconduct by UN peacekeepers. The UN Secretariat is still accused of poor management, political appointments, lack of competence and dynamism, and even corruption, as in the 1950s.

16.1 The Outcome of the World Summit

The bargain almost achieved at the World Summit was to give some satisfaction to developed and developing countries:

- for Southern countries, the Millenium Development Goals (MDGs) to be reached by 2015 would be confirmed, with progress on disarmament; the composition of the Security Council would be expanded; more power to the General Assembly;
- for Western countries, a definition of terrorism; a responsibility of the international community "to protect" as a basis for collective action against genocide, ethnic cleansing, and crimes against humanity; a right to humanitarian

intervention; an effective, small Human Rights Council to replace the failed Human Rights Commission—a new peace-building commission; and management reform.

Unfortunately, this bargain was broken, through last-minute pressures by governments: no commitments were made and few firm decisions were taken. The final statement keeps to well-meaning generalities, with a few exceptions.

On development, developed countries were to commit themselves to the 0.7 % target of gross national income for official development aid by 2015. No such commitment was made: the achievement of the 0.7 % by "many" developed countries by 2015 was "welcome" but not given as a firm commitment by all countries, even though eight major MDGs were set.

This reflected the doubts of some Western governments as to the need for and the effectiveness of more aid, and more money to trigger development. Would more money be wasted by corrupt or incompetent governments?

An agreement would consider the cancellation of 100 % of the official multilateral and bilateral debt of heavily indebted poor countries.

On disarmament, the High-Level Panel had asked nuclear states to apply the reduction measures of the Treaty on the Non-proliferation of Nuclear Weapons, and nuclear states non-Parties to the Treaty to take other measures to reduce the risk of accidental nuclear war. They should also reaffirm their previous commitment not to use nuclear weapons against states without nuclear capacity. The Summit's final statement makes no reference to the dangers of *nuclear proliferation,* in view of the opposition of the nuclear powers to reducing their nuclear weapons. They do not accept any limitations to the use of their weapons. Annan said that we have allowed posturing to get in the way of results: "This is inexcusable, weapons of mass destruction pose a grave danger to us all."

On the preventive use of force, the Panel decided that force could be used to prevent a threat from becoming imminent. However, such decisions should be made collectively by the Security Council on the basis of five criteria:

- the seriousness of the threat;
- if the primary purpose was to avert the threat;
- if every non-military option had been explored;
- if the scale of the proposed military action was the minimum required;
- and if there was a reasonable chance of the action being successful.

The Summit document does not refer to preventive armed intervention and to these conditions.

As a *judiciary prevention measure,* the Panel had recommended that the Security Council use the powers set in the Rome Treaty to submit cases to the International Criminal Court. The Summit's final statement made no reference to the Court, in view of the aggressive opposition of the United States to the ICC.

Terrorism was rhetorically "condemned in all its forms and manifestations, committed by whomever, wherever and for whatever purpose," but terrorism could not be defined. A comprehensive convention on international terrorism should be concluded during the 60th session of the General Assembly, an unlikely prospect.

On the Security Council, the High-Level Panel put forward two options, both involving an expansion of the Security Council from 15 to 24: under Model A, six new permanent seats without veto power, two each for Africa and Asia and one each for Europe and the Americas, plus three new 2-year non-permanent seats. Model B provided for no new permanent seats. Instead it proposed the creation of a new category of eight 4-year renewable "semi-permanent" seats with one new non-permanent non-renewable seat.

Annan felt that the Council should be broadly representative of the realities of power in today's world. However, there was no agreement at the Summit on expansion and democratization of the Security Council.

Agreement by both the Security Council and the General Assembly to an expansion of the Council is unlikely soon. There is no agreement on the number of new permanent members, nor on the number of new non-permanent members. The United States has ruled out a veto for new permanent members. The five permanent members want to keep their status and the privilege of the veto power.

The G4, Germany, Japan, India, and Brazil, would agree to delay having veto power for 15 years, but the Africans want two African permanent members with full rights.

Argentina and Mexico oppose Brazil. Japan is opposed by China and the two Koreas. Italy opposes Germany, and Pakistan is against India's bid.

Early reform was supported, but the burden was passed on to the General Assembly to review progress later.

Technically, an amendment of the Charter would be needed to change the composition of the Security Council. An amendment needs the vote of two-thirds of the General Assembly's members and must be ratified by two-thirds of these members—including all the permanent members of the Security Council: a major obstacle indeed.

On the reform of the Secretariat, the Panel had asked that the Secretary General be given all necessary resources to manage the Organization. The Panel also proposed the appointment of a Vice-Secretary General in charge of peace and security issues. The Summit did not decide on any significant reform of the Secretariat. It mainly stressed the need for better and stricter oversight and auditing systems.

More positively, as an innovation long sought by humanitarians, the Summit affirmed that the international community has the *responsibility to help protect populations* from genocide, war crimes, ethnic cleansing, and crimes against humanity, a potential right to humanitarian intervention, long opposed by the developing countries as a breach of their sovereignty and as neo-colonialism. For Oxfam, this was a clear and historic commitment.

A *peace-building commission* was approved, a useful tool to help war-ravaged countries to help countries' transition from war to peace, backed by a support office and a standing fund.

The Summit approved the creation of a *Standing Police Capacity* as a component of peacekeeping missions.

A *Human Rights Council* replaces the ineffective Human Rights Commission, but it was left to the General Assembly to decide on its size and composition, accepting a reduction of the number of members, and screening of the members on the basis of democratic and human rights criteria.

The United Nations is made up of sovereign countries. Its members are not required by the Charter to have democratic credentials, unlike states members of the European Union and the Council of Europe. Hence a built-in conflict between declarations of adhesion to human rights treaties, while the practice of many governments shows no respect for their obligations.

The budget of the High Commissioner for Human Rights was doubled. A new Democracy Fund received pledges of $32 million from 13 countries.

16.2 Why These difficulties?

The 191 member states of the United Nations are deeply divided between North and South countries, between rich and poor countries.

North countries are themselves divided—the European Union and the United States do not have the same views of development.

South countries have different levels of development, different types of governance. They want more money for their development. Western countries want to spread good governance and human rights, as a condition for development aid. Their main security concern is the fight against terrorism. The European Union and other countries are for the Kyoto treaty on global warming and for the International Criminal Court, both of which are opposed by the United States.

There is a fundamental disagreement between Western countries and the South as to what the United Nations is and what the United Nations should do. The small, weak, and poor countries want a bigger role for the United Nations, the powerful want to limit its authority and keep it under their control.

16.3 Many Unsolved Problems

There is so much to do with such limited resources, with progress in parts of the world and decline in others, mostly in sub-Saharan Africa and Southern Asia.

According to the United Nations Statistics Division, in 1990, more than 1.2 billion people (28% of the developing world's population) lived in extreme poverty. The target of the first MDG is to halve this proportion and the proportion of those suffering from hunger by 2015. This is not likely to happen. By 2001, the proportion fell to 21%, due to progress in a few highly populated countries. In sub-Saharan Africa, which has the highest poverty rates in the world, millions more became poorer. The causes and consequences of poverty are many: among them, socio-economic stagnation or decline, poor governance, military conflicts, political instability, lack of resources, over-population, lack of adequate health services, epidemics, natural disasters, lack of education, and others.

The number of people suffering from hunger increased between 1997 and 2002.

Most developing regions have made progress towards universal primary education, but some 115 million children are still out of school (more than half are girls). Women's access to paid employment is still lower than men's in most developing countries.

Women's share of seats in parliaments has increased, but their share is only 16% worldwide.

16.4 In the Health Sector

Nearly 11 million children under the age of five die every year, mostly from diseases which could be prevented or treated with adequate means. Advances slowed in the 1990s.

More than half a million women die of complications during pregnancy and childbirth: maternal death rates are 1,000 times higher in sub-Saharan Africa than in high-income countries.

In the 25 years since it was first reported, AIDS has become the fourth largest killer worldwide. At the end of 2004, an estimated 39.4 million people were living with HIV, of whom nearly half are women.

Current health spending in most low-income countries is insufficient for the achievement of the health MDG. A fivefold increase in donor spending on health is needed.

According to the United Nations, the outlook for ensuring environmental sustainability is grim.

In Africa, massacres still occur in the Congo, Ivory Coast is on the verge of renewed civil war, and Iraq is in bloody chaos. The Palestine–Israel conflict is far from being settled. The United Nations is needed to help countries recover from civil wars or national disasters.

16.5 What can the United Nations do?

On the positive side, the United Nations is still an indispensable diplomatic forum. It is the only global institution where all nations have a voice.

The United Nations has "invented" peacekeeping, as an unwritten Chapter VI and a half of the U.N. Charter. It now has peacekeeping missions composed of 70,000 Blue Helmets in 18 countries.

It has promoted decolonization, fought apartheid, and sent missions to supervise elections and meet humanitarian emergencies. Its World Summits, the 1990 World Summit for Children in New York (1990), the 1991 Earth Summit in Rio, the Social Summit in Copenhagen (1995), the World Summit on Sustainable Development in

Johannesburg (2002), and the first phase of the World Summit on the Information Society in Geneva (2003) have opened new horizons, challenges, and hopes to the United Nations and to the world.

The United Nations has initiated a human rights regime with the 1948 Universal Declaration of Human Rights, the Covenants, other treaties, and the 1989 Convention on the Rights of the Child. It sets standards and monitors results through the new Human Rights Council.

It has created the International Criminal Tribunals for ex-Yugoslavia and for Rwanda, the Special Court for Sierra Leone, and the Tribunal for Cambodia; it has supported the creation of the International Criminal Court, a major achievement.

The United Nations assesses and sets goals for economic and human development. It has just established an ambitious programme of MDGs, to be achieved by the year 2015 (Reg. 4).

UN funds and specialized agencies fight against poverty and for development in their own areas; UNDP helps countries through its 134 country offices; it focuses on poverty elimination, environmental protection, and equal rights for women; WHO has launched campaigns against malaria and polio; it co-ordinates research and prevention of SARS; UNAIDS fights against HIV/AIDS; UNICEF promotes the equal education of girls and boys and monitors the implementation of the Convention of the Rights of the Child; UNHCR protects refugees; and the World Food Programme provides food in natural and manmade disasters.

In a controversial but beneficial initiative, Kofi Annan has opened the United Nations to the world of business through the Global Compact, thus adding the private sector to NGOs as legitimate partners (under certain conditions) and promoting the creation of many public/private partnerships, in particular in the public health field.

16.6 Conclusion

The proposals of the High-level Panel and of Annan were ambitious; were they over-ambitious? They were intended to jolt governments into action and restore the credibility of the United Nations. Unfortunately, the occasion of the 60th anniversary of the United Nations failed to produce a new climate of hope and innovation for the United Nations and for world solidarity and co-operation.

Heads of state and government and diplomats need to compromise. They all want the United Nations to continue for different reasons: belief in international co-operation, feelings of solidarity, prestige, advocacy for their own schemes, presence on the world stage, and financing. The world body, in spite of its obvious weaknesses, is still indispensable.

Internationalist countries, national associations for the United Nations, human rights, humanitarian, medical, and other professional associations, NGOs, civil society, and individuals should join hands with regional organizations and national parliaments and push their governments into promoting an effective reform of the United Nations and the UN system.

It is not too late: the survival of the United Nations is not at stake, its credibility is at stake, and without credibility, the imperfect but indispensable organization would lose all its influence.

The United Nations needs reform—the world needs a stronger and more effective United Nations.

Bibliography

A useful compendium is in the "International Symposium—Prospects for Reform of the United Nations System, 15–17 May 2002". Italian Society for International Organization, CEDAM, Padua, 1993.

Also "Rethinking International Organizations, Pathology and Promise", Dennis Dijkzeul and Yves Beigbeder, Berghahn Books, UK, 2003.

See "Progress towards the Millennium Development Goals, 1990–2005—Summary", U.N. Statistics Division. http://unstats.un.org/unsd/mi/mi-coverfinal.htm, 13 June 2005.

See also "The Humanitarian Force of the U.N. Millennium Development Goals", H. Mezoui, Journal of Humanitarian Medicine, 6: 1–4, 2006.

The Report of the High-level Panel on Threats, Challenges and Change is entitled: "A more secure world: Our shared responsibility," United Nations, 2004.

Kofi Annan submitted his report, "In larger freedom: Towards development, security and human rights for all" on 20 March 2005: U.N. Doc. A/59/2005, www.un.org/larger freedom

The full text of the 2005 World Summit Outcome is in U.N. General Assembly Doc. A/60/L. 1, 15 September 2005: www.un.org/summit2005.

Chapter 17
The Critical News Stories You Never Read*

Shashi Tharoor

While in Addis Ababa for the African Union summit meeting, UN Secretary General Kofi Annan had dozens of conversations and meetings with the region's leaders. He observed a strange thing: "Iraq didn't come up, terrorism didn't come up, weapons of mass destruction didn't come up. There were subjects on people's minds other than the ones dominating the media's attention."

"Iraq," Annan noted ruefully, "has sucked out all the oxygen and distorted the international agenda." This has been true, of course, for some time—at least since January 2003, when Annan held a press conference to cover 16 different issues on his global agenda, and every question addressed to him was about Iraq.

In response to the gap between what we at the United Nations thought the world should care about and what the media covering our work preferred to focus on, my colleagues and I came up with a list last May of the top 10 stories we felt were not getting enough media attention. The objective was not to point a finger at the reporters. We understood the pressures that drove the world's news agenda, and we didn't deny that Iraq was an important story.

We felt, however, that there were other important stories that were falling off the radar screen because the media didn't have the space or time for them. And what the world had not heard about, it would not be willing to do anything about. So we wanted to say to our friends in the press: "Would you please consider reporting these stories too?"

My team consulted every UN department and agency to find out what they thought the world needed to know more about. A list of over 60 issues emerged, which we whittled down to a more media-friendly 10.

For a while, the crisis in Darfur led the list, but as our deadline approached the media woke up to the sufferings of the people there. Other tragedies bubbled up to the top, but we were alert to the risk of crisis-fatigue. So we also tried to choose human interest stories and good-news stories, offbeat stories, and early warning stories.

The result was a mix of stories no one could plausibly claim were yawn-inducing: the brutal lives of child soldiers in northwestern Uganda, where kids are killers

* Reproduced from the *International Herald Tribune*, 14 July 2004, by kind permission Other United Nations features can be accessed on the web site www.un.org/events/tenstories.

131

(often of other kids); the tragedy of the AIDS orphans of southern Africa, where children are being brought up by grandparents, and sometimes by other children because their parents' generation has been wiped out by AIDS; the simmering cauldron of the Central African Republic, where an explosive combination of rich resources, acute poverty (95 per cent of the people live on less than $2 a day), political tension, population displacement, and widespread insecurity cries out for outside help. We knew the old cliché must be stood on its head: all too often, good news is no news. So we came up with positive stories that had been neglected: the steady building of a viable peace in Tajikistan on the ruins of a long civil war; the war that never happened as Nigeria and Cameroon peacefully worked out their differences over the resource-rich Bakassi Peninsula; the role of women in Rwanda—as 49 per cent of the Parliament—in leading their society away from the ashes of genocide.

There were more (for the full list, see www.un.org/events/tenstories). But why go on? None of the top-flight international journalists who turned up at my press conference to launch the list actually wrote about our list. I got a lot of airtime on the US public broadcasting system and one interview on CNN International (not domestic), and a lot of silence. We are persisting, though: in recent weeks, newspapers as far afield as Egypt and Hong Kong have carried the list.

We know we are making the smallest of dents in the public consciousness, but we could not forgive ourselves if we didn't try.

Four decades ago, the newsman Edward Behr came across a TV cameraman in a camp of violated Belgian nuns in the Congo calling out, "anybody here been raped and speak English?"

It's never enough to have suffered; you must be able to convey your suffering in the language the media wants to hear. That's where we at the United Nations will try to help—to give a voice to those who remain voiceless in the world media. Next year, on World Press Freedom Day 2005, we will launch another Top 10 list. Maybe this paper, at least, will cover it.

Chapter 18
United Nations Humanitarian Action and the Role of Non-governmental Organizations

Hanifa Mezoui, PhD

It seems that not a year goes by without some corner of the globe being devastated by nature or man in the form of floods, famine, chemical leaks, or, increasingly, armed conflict. Faced with the growing incidence of large-scale disasters, whether classed as natural, technological, or complex humanitarian emergencies, the international community has learned the value of working together to address today's multi-faceted emergencies through coordinated response mechanisms. Typically, complex humanitarian emergency situations will mobilize a myriad of bilateral agencies, international organisations, and relief workers from all over the world, including the hundreds of national and international Non-Governmental Organizations (NGOs) to act as implementing agents for others or to pursue independent programmes of their own. Needless to say, the multiple lines of responsibility, overlapping mandates and sometimes-divergent programmes of so many actors make effective coordination crucial to the success of the humanitarian effort. More often than not, this task will fall to the United Nations with its extensive presence in the field and network of humanitarian and development agencies.

The UN emergency management apparatus itself comprises humanitarian, development, political, and security components and falls under the UN Office for the Coordination of Humanitarian Affairs (OCHA). This Office is responsible for mobilizing and coordinating the collective efforts of the international community (particularly the UN System) to meet human needs in disasters and emergencies in a coherent and timely manner and to facilitate the smooth transition from relief to development.

The primary responsibility for delivery of humanitarian assistance is shared by four agencies: the *United Nations High Commissioner for Refugees (UNHCR);* the *World Food Program (WFP);* the *United Nations International Children's Emergency Fund (UNICEF);* and the *United Nations Development Program (UNDP).* As the majority of those affected by disasters tend to live in the rural areas of developing countries, the UN Food and Agriculture Organization (FAO) monitors the food situation and collaborates with the World Food Programme on emergency operations for food aid. In addition to its emergency health interventions, the World Health Organization (WHO) is increasingly concerned with clarifying the role of the health sector in conflict prevention and peace building. In order to provide early warning of impending conflicts and analyse possibilities for preventive action, the UN

Department of Political Affairs follows political developments worldwide; while the UN Department of Peacekeeping Operations (UNDPKO) provides monitoring, planning, and support of peacekeeping operations and is also responsible for the military, civilian police, and electoral components of complex missions that extend to rehabilitation and reconstruction.

Although the need has never been greater for the elaborate and admittedly quite impressive international emergency response machinery, there is a growing feeling among relief workers that this is not enough. Certainly, in the face of an immediate crisis, the first concern must be to provide the best, most effective humanitarian assistance to the victims. However, it does seem that if the same level of concerted effort were to be focused on preventing humanitarian emergencies from arising in the first place, we should be able to devise proactive measures that would be at least as effective as those now in place for reacting to emergency situations. With the alarming rise in the number and scale of the complex humanitarian emergencies all over the world, finding effective conflict prevention and peace-building strategies have become an imperative. In the health sector, one of the most definitive global directives came from the 1981 World Health Resolution 34.38, which asserted that "The role of physicians and other health workers in the preservation of peace is the most significant factor for the attainment of health for all." A decade later, the proliferation of complex emergency situations created by the escalating violence of armed conflict and civil strife led the World Health Organization to re-examine its humanitarian response mechanism. Humanitarian interventions could no longer focus on mitigating efforts, as had been the case in the past when WHO was dealing primarily with the victims of epidemics and natural disasters. Relief from acts of war could only be achieved by establishing a lasting peace. In this context, the concept of Health As A Bridge To Peace was formulated to provide a policy and planning framework for activities that would integrate peace building into relief and development initiatives primarily directed towards health.

Physicians and health workers, by virtue of their profession as caregivers, enjoy the trust of the community. Their training as diagnosticians has made them particularly observant and sensitive to seemingly insignificant signs. Even before hostilities break out, health care providers are in the position to use the comparative advantage of their profession to pick up subtle early warning signals. Moreover, by employing the same skills that make it possible to discover the causes of a particular symptom presented by a patient, the health professional can identify the root causes of brewing conflict. It is not beyond the bounds of possibility that placing this kind of information in the right hands might avert developing crises.

Further along the continuum, when hostilities have already broken out, medical NGOs can play an even more active role. I must stress at this point that first and foremost NGOs in conflict situations must maintain a strict neutrality. This does not mean that NGOs should work in ignorance; in order to be effective relief workers must have an understanding of and sensitivity to the political, legal, and socio-economic environment of the population in which they work and be able to assess the impact of the crises on their area of concern.

WHO has identified the major public health problems caused by war. First, there is a breakdown of supportive structure health care systems and normal preventative actions. This includes the destruction of the infrastructure, such as hospitals, other health institutions, and the lack of medical essentials and medicines. Young children, the aged, and the chronically ill, who need specialized care, are hit particularly hard.

Rehabilitation programmes directly suffer and in turn affect physically and mentally disabled peoples. Mental health problems are also a direct result of conflict situations, and include trauma, alcoholism, and drug abuse. Violence, suicides, and psychosomatic diseases increase, in turn further straining the already weakened health system.

As roughly the same levels of social, economic, and political breakdown are used to declare an area in a state of emergency, it would seem reasonable to assume that to a greater or lesser extent, the public health problems identified by WHO would be found in any country reduced to emergency status by armed conflict. In this case, an NGO willing to pursue the primary health objective in the context of peace building would do well to follow the lead of WHO by addressing the identified health problems through its humanitarian programme. Once into the implementation stage, NGOs can seek creative ways of using their health initiatives to foster the spirit of peace.

Certain strategies have been established as successful examples of the health-to-peace concept. One that I am sure that you are all familiar with is the health brokered humanitarian ceasefire, which not only brings opposing parties together to negotiate but also demonstrates that cooperation is possible in pursuit of a common goal. Cessation of hostilities can be valuable on many levels. First, it supports the health initiative by making health services available. Secondly, it opens the way for deliveries of food and other necessities and, finally, it contributes to the overall mental health of both combatants and civilians by providing a period free of the stresses of life in a war zone. These humanitarian ceasefires have been introduced into armed conflicts in the Philippines, Central America, Sudan, and even Afghanistan for periods of up to 2 months. It is important to bear in mind, however, that although the periods of peace were universally successful, they only provided a brief hiatus in the on-going violence. Nevertheless, in light of the effectiveness of this short-term peace-building activity, it would prove a worthy challenge for the NGO community to explore ways to extend the time frame of the present model of humanitarian ceasefires.

As an invariable result, violent, armed conflict is the widespread effect on the mental health of the population, another form of intervention that lends itself to innovation is the mental health programme. Several programmes have built upon the connection between the individual's physical and mental health and the overall health and peace of his or her society, and have integrated peace building into mental health initiatives.

Even the end of operation process can be used creatively. You are all aware, I am sure, of the importance of terminating activities. One of the most difficult problems for international NGOs is to know when and how to remove themselves while leaving something of value behind. For the humanitarian NGO, mastering this is essential, since emergency relief is by nature short-term. There are several ways for an NGO to contribute to peace and development on a continuing basis. The United Nations in general and my office in particular firmly believe in the value of forming strategic partnerships. I would encourage international NGOs to seek out a local counterpart who could turn their time-limited project into a sustainable activity. For example, some form of community development project could be designed as a follow-up to trauma healing and reconciliation interventions. On another level, sharing your expertise with local NGOs and other civil society organizations serves to empower the NGO sector and contributes to social development. This brief overview gives a glimpse of some of the ways that NGOs can diversify their field of action, while promoting their primary professional concerns. Even more, I hope that some of you will be inspired to take your valuable generosity of spirit and professional expertise to share with others in the field.

Chapter 19
The UN Founding Fathers and Dr Chisholm*

Sir Robert Jackson, KCVO [†]

I am honoured by this invitation to deliver the Brock Chisholm Memorial Lecture. This has come about following a conversation I had with Dr Gunn when we talked about the origins of the present United Nations system and "The Founding Fathers" who did so much to create it.

We have come here today to pay tribute to the work of a great man, Brock Chisholm. I can only describe that part of his distinguished career which reached its climax in the creation of the World Health Organization, and in order to relate my own experience to his achievements, I shall divide my talk into four parts.

For me, the story begins in the siege of Malta, which lasted from June 1940 until November 1942. Before and during that siege, we had racked our brains in devising ways to defend the island fortress with a minimum of supplies, for every replenishment demanded a full-scale fleet operation . . . . It was at that time (as far as I know) that the expression "optimum use of resources" was coined, and I was therefore interested to observe Dr Mahler using it, some 43 years later in his memorandum of 23 January 1985 about WHO's resources!

The Defence of Malta attracted worldwide attention, and at the end of 1941, I was told to go to the Middle East theatre and apply the same principles there. Pearl Harbor occurred just after I arrived in Cairo, and we were able very quickly to develop the first Anglo-American paramilitary organization of the World War II, the Middle East Supply Centre (MESC), which ultimately extended from Turkey to South Africa and from Cyrenaica to India, a population of about 100 million people.

By that combination of imagination, basic control procedures, and management by objective, it was generally agreed that MESC achieved the optimum use of resources in the region and, in so doing, was able to secure a remarkable degree of co-operation from the many governments concerned. It dealt with literally everything in the region: agriculture, industry, the infrastructure, education, currency, inflation, and so on, and, of course, health, including safe drinking water and sewerage disposal. The results were spectacular.

It was in MESC that a few of WHO's bricks were moulded, and in saying this, I appreciate that there were very many much older bricks, for example,

---

* Historical lecture delivered at the Medical Society of the World Health Organization. (published from the Archives)

[†] 1911–1991

the Lazarettos, the 14 International Sanitary Conferences, the Office International d'Hygiène Publique, and the Pan-American Sanitary Bureau (1902).

Shortly after the Centre was established, we set up the Middle East Medical Advisory Committee, which was composed of outstanding physicians, surgeons, and public health experts, drawn from the British and American Armies, as well as talented medical and health officials drawn from the Middle East countries themselves.

At the end of the war, it was acknowledged on all sides that the health of those 100 million people was better than before the war, and that was an accomplishment of which all concerned were understandably proud.

From the end of 1942, the Mediterranean opened up and, *inter alia* we were able to deal with epidemics in several countries and, in particular, start to attack malaria in Greece. As I shall explain shortly, those operations were picked up quite naturally by UNRRA. MESC was a major, if not *the* major, influence in determining the formation of the five Regional Economic Commissions which are now part of the United Nations itself. It also influenced thinking about the organization of WHO, a process reinforced by the fact that a basic regional organization for the Western Hemisphere called the Pan-American Sanitary Bureau already existed in Washington.

Other aspects of MESC's organization had also been noted: the continuous management by objective which demanded maximum decentralization and maximum delegation of power to our country Directors. Today the organizational legacy can be seen in the United Nations Development Programme (UNDP) Resident Representatives, but the decentralization and delegation of authority which I advocated in the UN Capacity Study (written in WHO's Annex where we were Dr Candau's guests in 1968–1969) have not yet come about.

Thus, in that stage of our brick-making, I think it can be said that MESC had a very direct influence on the organization of WHO, and was able to initiate operations which, in a modest way, would, in due course, assist WHO's own work when it came into being.

At the end of 1944, I was told to go to Washington, DC, as Senior Deputy Director-General of the United Nations Relief and Rehabilitation Administration, since UNRRA's operations would have many similarities to MESC. Now, in this day and age when the UN system seems to be called upon almost continuously to deal with various disasters, it must be remembered that UNRRA was unique in at least two respects and remains so to this day. First of all, it is the only organization that has ever been designed to deal with a vast disaster, the broad outlines of which could be seen in advance. Its second enormous advantage—in contrast to other disasters with which I have had to deal subsequently—was that it had substantial and ongoing funds at its disposal from the very beginning.

During the 4 years of its existence, UNRRA provided essential relief and rehabilitation supplies to about 25 countries in Europe, Asia, and Africa—directly contributing to the maintenance and preservation of the lives of several hundreds of millions of people.

In addition, as the war ended in Europe, it co-operated with the Allied Forces in dealing with about 8,500,000 displaced persons, plus the tragic survivors of the concentration camps. About six million of those people were returned to their home-lands, and UNRRA was able to persuade governments to accept another million or so of them in new homelands.

By 1947, it was clear that UNRRA would become a victim of the Cold War and action was taken quickly to arrange for its essential functions to be transferred to other organizations. From the moment they came into existence, UNRRA, with its very large resources of manpower and money, was able to provide invaluable assis-tance to the United Nations itself, to FAO, and to UNESCO in the early formative stages of their development, and to WHO.

From the outset, health (including water and sewerage disposal) and welfare, generally, occupied a vitally important part of UNRRA's work. The UNRRA Agree-ment provided that the new organization should take over virtually all of the ear-lier responsibilities enshrined in the League of Nations and, bearing in mind the tragedies that occurred after the World War I, had to prepare, as soon as staff could be assembled, for the endless challenges which would arise as hostilities began to end. The first winter after the end of the war in Europe was a harsh one, but by the time spring arrived in 1946, there had been no serious loss of life, thank God; a dramatic contrast to the 30 million people who died from influenza alone in the winter of 1918–1919, quite apart from the terrible toll of typhus and typhoid in Poland and Yugoslavia at that time.

By now, I hope that I have told you enough about the operations and organization both of MESC and UNRRA to illustrate their influence on the formation of WHO. Before I proceed, I suppose I should admit here that WHO has always had a very special place in my thinking and work within the UN system.

At this point, I need to reverse engines in order to place history in its proper perspective. At the San Francisco Conference, it became possible for three men whose names are well known to all of you—Dr De Paula Souza, Dr Szeming Sze, and Dr Karl Evang—to secure the all-important article in the UN Charter that made it possible for the World Health Organization to become a reality. Those three men and Lord Bruce were certainly brick-makers of the highest order!

And here, of course, our Architect and chief brickmaker enters the scene. Dr Brock Chisholm was Chairman of the Technical Preparatory Committee that met in Paris from 18 March to 5 April 1946, together with 17 other very distinguished medical men. Immediately, the breadth of his views commanded attention and had a decisive influence on the future of the organization. I am sure you will remember his prophetic words which were incorporated in the Preamble to the WHO Constitu-tion: "Health is a state of complete physical, mental and social well-being, and not merely the absence of disease or infirmity." I was pleased to see that in a record of a conversation with him in 1968, he observed that UNRRA had had great influence on his thinking because it was "an action organization" and was "made up of people who were in a hurry." I know that I was!

Then the International Health Conference followed on, meeting in New York from 19 June to 22 July 1946. Once more, Brock played a role of crucial importance, and it was not surprising that he was selected as Executive Secretary of the Interim Commission of WHO (IC-WHO), which could be regarded as the nucleus of WHO itself. Functions were steadily transferred in a regular and orderly manner from one organization to the other, and in most cases, key staff went with them.

UNRRA provided IC-WHO with two grants of $1,500,000 each, and UN extended two loans of $1.3 million and $1.2 million, respectively. They may seem small sums today, but they proved to be a classic example of tall oaks growing out of small acorns, for WHO today is certainly a very large and healthy tree.

We naturally worked very closely with Brock and his team during the 2 years when the Interim Commission was building the essential foundations of WHO; and Dr Chisholm impressed all who knew him by the clarity with which he defined his objectives for WHO, and by the managerial and diplomatic skill with which he steadfastly pursued those objectives. In the political field, he faced real difficulties as a result of the initial reluctance of the US Congress fully to support the new organization. But he persevered, and won.

I have already talked of the broad vision with which Brock Chisholm approached the task of creating WHO from the very outset, and throughout his professional career his deep humanitarianism was displayed again and again.

His physical courage was reflected in his outstanding record in the First World War, and his moral courage was reflected throughout the entire UN system when he flatly refused to permit the US Government authorities to trespass within his headquarters or intervene in his operations.

Brock had many admirable qualities, and modesty was one of them. He was well content for the record of his service—both in war and peace—to speak for itself, and no man could ask for better testimony.

He was one of the true "Founding Fathers" of the modern UN system. As a result of my own appointment in UNRRA, I was at that time working with all the Heads of the then existing UN organizations, and amongst the distinguished men who at that time were in charge, I would select John Boyd-Orr, who made FAO, Julian Huxley, who provided the intellectual stimulus for UNESCO, and Brock, who inspired the concept of WHO, as the three most outstanding leaders. All of them had first-class intellects; all had that priceless quality of imagination, and all were modest men.

In Thomas Hardy's *The Woodlanders*, one of the characters remarks: "You was a good man, and did good things." I am sure we would all agree with that judgement of Brock.

Chapter 20
Brock Chisholm—Doctor to the World

by Allan Irving, Markham, ON, Fitzhenry and Whiteside, Canada, ISBN I-55041-1845, 149 pages

Book Review by S.W.A. Gunn, MD

In 1954, the University of British Columbia bestowed the honorary degree of Doctor of Science on a Canadian doctor of medicine much honoured internationally as a world physician, but one who tends to be remembered in his country as a reforming iconoclast: Dr Brock Chisholm.

The Hannah Institute for the History of Medicine in Toronto is to be congratulated on publishing the "Canadian Medical Lives" series, of which volume 22 is about Dr George Brock Chisholm.

Brock Chisholm—Doctor to the World traces quite chronologically the life of this Canadian, who was born in Oakville, Ontario, in 1896, and died in Victoria in 1971.

It describes his growth and maturation, his brave soldiering in the First World War, his general practice and later specialization in psychiatry until the Second World War, his distinguished career and rapid military ascension to the rank of major general, his introduction of the PULHEMS test and military health reform, and thence to high civil service as deputy minister of health.

Except in the higher spheres of Health and Welfare, the popular memory of Chisholm within Canada remains quite hazy, indeed distorted. A capsule judgement of "the man who destroyed Santa Claus" somehow prevails, and Irving falls into the trap by constantly repeating it, presenting Chisholm as somehow obsessed by that Christmas figure, yet one wonders if it is not Irving himself who has the *idée fixe*, mentioning him no less than 32 times in the first half of the book alone. Chisholm, of course, was using the example as a metaphor for a legend that children know how to handle and that adults are mature enough to understand. Irving's overemphasis of this myth may be due to his heavy reference to the popular media. No mention of such myths exists in the scientific press or medical journals.

The second part of Irving's book is devoted to the man of WHO, the "Doctor to the World," the man with noble yet practical ideas of service and ethics, who insisted that even more than clinical prowess and technology, the future of mankind and its health was in the hands of the dedicated and enlightened younger generation. Chisholm served only one term as the first Director-General of WHO (1948–53); yet within this short period, he firmly anchored the organization as the most respected among the UN agencies. Representing Canada at the United Nations as from the embryonic days of the organization (1945, San Francisco Conference), through the Technical Preparatory Committee (1946), the Interim Committee (1946 to 1948), and finally the World Health Assembly (1948) when he was elected director-general, Chisholm toiled tirelessly to establish, ensure, and strengthen the mission and work of the new organization. Before joining WHO, I paid him a courtesy call at his peaceful retirement home in Sooke; his modesty gave no hint at all of his having been invested, that very day, with the country's highest accolade, Companion of the Order of Canada.

Just under half the book is given to Chisholm's medical international work. The facts are mentioned, but considering the special importance of this sector of the man's life and contributions, a more analytical study would have been welcome. One is left with the desire to know more on his far-sighted position against biological weapons and nuclear madness, as Pugwash was later (1995) to receive the Nobel Peace Prize; his vision for an international peace maintaining force, that is now being advocated by the United Nations; his ideas on world federalism, which are now in part being answered by the European Union. These are grouped rather hurriedly toward the end and keep the reader in the expectancy.

It is difficult to appraise this book. It gives a good, concise, chronological account, but one feels that this has been brought to a close rather hastily, and it falls short of a deeper study of a superior man. Doctors, health ministries, and medical libraries should have this slim volume, pending more extensive research.

The International Association for Humanitarian Medicine Brock Chisholm has been named as a tribute to his vision and action.

Chapter 21
The Language of International Humanitarian Action: A Brief Terminology*

S. W. A. Gunn, MD, FRCSC, DSC (Hon), Drhc

> *Not all humanitarian situations are emergencies. But all humanitarian failures should be treated as emergencies. For any such failure is a human disaster.*

If the Tower of Babel was a language disaster, disaster itself has a language. Whether act of God or act of man, disaster often calls for multinational assistance. The many governments, agencies, professions, and individuals from different parts of the world, representing different languages, specialties, religions, and cultures, yet all imbued with a humanitarian spirit of providing succour to the helpless, converge on the stricken land to help the victims, who are themselves of different language and background.

Communication among these diverse people and a certain understanding of the technical, administrative, and operational terminology of the many disciplines involved become paramount if the inherent difficulties of the disaster are not to be compounded by an overlay of communications disaster. In what often is a multidisciplinary operation, the physician has to understand the transport engineer, the meteorologist must be able to converse with the administrator, the volunteer with the EMS nurse, the planner with the journalist, the sanitarian with the nutritionist, the expatriate donor with the local government official, and the multitude of individuals whose normal life has been suddenly shattered by the earthquake, war, flood, refugee exodus, or the reactor accident.

If such understanding is essential in the field, it is becoming equally necessary away from the site of action: in planning boardrooms, lecture halls, statistical tables, press centres, and medical schools where disaster preparedness and humanitarian response increasingly are receiving attention. Indeed, it is heartening to notice that after many years of unplanned, ad hoc responses, disaster planning is becoming more and more conceptual and systematized and, with this trend, disaster medicine gradually is becoming a specialized field, within a broader humanitarian vision, humanitarian medicine.

All professions, techniques, and organized activities generate their own language, their specific terminology, and disastrology is no exception. Because it is relatively new and multisectoral in nature, its language is broadly based and evolving. In this

---

* First published in *Basics of International Humanitarian Missions,* and reproduced courtesy of Fordham University Press. The author is President of IAHM.

chapter, I shall offer a small selection of terms to show its concepts, scope, organization, and operation. I have intentionally chosen terms that are predominantly outside the medical field, but which the emergency practitioner or prehospital nurse will encounter in the course of his or her disaster mission and will use in humanitarian work.

21.1 Disasters: A Classification

Disaster: The result of a vast ecological breakdown in the relations between man and his environment; a serious and sudden event (or slow, as in drought) on such a scale that demands exceed available resources and the stricken community needs extraordinary efforts to cope with the situation, often with outside help or international aid.

Natural disaster: A sudden major upheaval of nature, causing extensive destruction, death, and suffering among the stricken community, and which is not due to man's action. However, *(a)* some natural disasters can be of slow origin, for example drought; and *(b)* a seemingly natural disaster can be caused or aggravated by man's action, for example, desertification through excessive land use and deforestation.

Man-made disaster: A disaster caused not by natural phenomena but by man's or society's action, involuntary or voluntary, sudden or slow, directly or indirectly, with grave consequences to the population and the environment. Examples: technological disaster, toxicological disaster, environmental pollution, desertification, conflict, refugees, epidemics, and fires.

Complex disaster/Complex emergency: A major disaster or complicated emergency situation affecting large civilian populations, which is further aggravated by intense political and/or military interference, including war and civil strife, resulting in serious food shortages, epidemics, population displacements, pauperization, loss of human liberties, and significant increase in mortality, rendering the management of the situation very complex.

Man-conceived disaster: Distinct from man-made disaster, man-conceived refers to disastrous actions like genocide, death camps, ethnic cleansing, forced disappearance, pauperization, torture, and other acts against humanity that are obscenely conceived, cold-bloodedly planned, and indecently perpetrated with impunity by evil rulers, dictators, terrorists, or kleptocrats with the aim of inflicting maximum suffering, death, and destruction, in full violation of personal, social, and cultural rights of humanity. While the response to man-made disasters is scientific, humanitarian, and managerial, the response to man-conceived disasters must be through the International Criminal Court.

Disaster preparedness: The aggregate of measures to be taken in view of disasters, consisting of plans and action programs designed to minimize the loss of life and damage, to organize and facilitate effective rescue and relief, and to rehabilitate after disaster. Preparedness requires the necessary legislation and means to cope with disaster or similar emergency situations. It also is concerned with forecasting and warning, the education and training of the public, organization, and management—including plans, training of personnel, the stockpiling of supplies, and ensuring the needed funds and other resources.

Disaster management: The study and collaborative application by the various pertinent disciplines and governmental authorities of decision-making processes, management techniques, and resource utilization to the entire process and different phases of a disaster, from prevention and preparedness to planning, immediate response, damage reduction, rehabilitation, reconstruction, and development.

Health: The state of complete physical, mental, and social well-being, and not merely the absence of disease or infirmity. Also, the state of an individual or a community free from debilitating conditions, demonstrating a reasonable resistance to diseases, and living in a salubrious environment.

International health: The study and systematic comparison of the multiple and variable factors that influence the health of human populations in different countries and different environments, and the resulting measures that need to be taken for its improvement.

Disaster medicine: The study and collaborative application of various health specialties—for example, paediatrics, epidemiology, communicable diseases, nutrition, public health, emergency surgery, military medicine, community care, social medicine, international health—to the prevention, immediate response, humanitarian care, and rehabilitation of the health problems arising from disaster, in cooperation with other nonmedical disciplines involved in disaster management.

Catastrophe theory: A mathematical and philosophical theory to explain and define transitional continuity whereby a disaster represents a brutal dynamic change in the forces present in natural, physical, or social phenomena.

Hazard: The probability of the occurrence of a disaster caused by a natural phenomenon (earthquake, cyclone), by failure of man-made sources of energy (nuclear reactor, industrial explosion), or uncontrolled human activity (overgrazing, heavy traffic, conflict). Some authors use the term in a broader sense, including vulnerability, elements at risk, and the consequences of risk.

Risk: The lives lost, persons injured, damage to property, and disruption of economic activity due to a particular hazard. Risk is the product of hazard and vulnerability.

Assessment: Survey of a real or potential disaster to estimate the actual or expected damages and to make recommendations for preparedness, mitigation, and relief action.

Acceptable risk: The eventual loss and agreed conditions or degree of human, material, and economic damage that a country or community is willing to accept as tolerable rather than provide the necessary finances and resources to reduce such a risk.

Mitigation: Separate and aggregate measures taken prior to, during, or following a disaster with the view to reducing the severity of the human and material damage caused by it.

Vulnerability: In a physical object, the degree of loss from a potentially damaging phenomenon, expressed in a scale from zero to 100 per cent. In a person or community, the potential extent of fragility and harm suffered.

21.2 Human Rights: A Brief Glossary

Human Rights: The inalienable entitlement by all humans everywhere and without distinction whatsoever to all the fundamental rights and freedoms enunciated in the 30 Articles of the Universal Declaration of Human Rights (United Nations, 1948) and other international instruments.

Humanitarian medicine: While all medical intervention to reduce a person's sickness and suffering is in essence humanitarian, Humanitarian Medicine goes beyond the usual therapeutic act and promotes, provides, teaches, supports, and delivers people's health as a human right, in conformity with the ethics of Hippocratic teaching, the principles of the World Health Organization, the Charter of the United Nations, the Universal Declaration of Human Rights, the Red Cross Conventions, and other covenants and practices that ensure the most humane and best possible level of care, without any discrimination or consideration of material gain.

Bioterrorism: Planning, threatening, using, or spreading of contagious disease organisms or toxins, for example, botulism, anthrax, smallpox, or other viruses, as a terrorist tool or weapon.

Conventional arms: Arms or forces pertaining to a nation's nonnuclear, nonbiological, nonchemical weapons, such as guns, tanks, battleships, aircraft, troops, and so on. The opposite of arms/weapons of mass destruction.

Crimes against humanity: Crimes concerning the international community as a whole, committed in widespread and/or systematic manner, and/or on a massive scale, and/or on specified grounds, in war or peacetime. They include murder, genocide, extermination, enslavement, rape, sexual abuse, or forced prostitution; deportation; persecution on political, racial, national, ethnic, cultural, and religious grounds; enforced disappearances; other inhumane acts of physical or mental injury; detention, imprisonment, or deprivation of liberty in violation of international law. Such crimes are punishable by the International Criminal Court.

Deportation: The unlawful and forcible transfer of a person, group, or population from its normal habitat; the forced transfer of children of a group to another group. This is considered a crime against humanity.

Disappearance/Forced disappearance: The arrest, abduction, forced detention, and cutting off communication of persons against their will, by or without the approval of the state or of a political organization, accompanied by refusal of the latter to acknowledge that abduction has taken place and denial of information on the fate of those abducted, thereby placing them outside the protection of the law. This is considered a crime against humanity.

Disarmament: The process of and regulations concerning the reduction of a military establishment to levels defined by international agreement.

Disaster epidemiology: The medical discipline, now extended to other fields, that studies the influence of such factors as lifestyle, biological constitution, and other personal and social determinants on the incidence and distribution of disease, both under normal circumstances and in markedly changed disaster situations.

Embargo: An order forbidding certain activities, often accompanied with certain penalties or sanctions in case of noncompliance. Article 41, chapter 7 of the UN

Charter provides for embargoes on a country that may pose a threat to peace, a breakdown of peace, or an act of aggression. Humanitarian goods such as food and medicine may be exempted.

Environmental pollution: Unfavourable changes and degradation of one or more aspects or elements of the environment by noxious biological, industrial, chemical, or radioactive wastes, from debris of man-made, especially nonbiodegradable, products and from mismanagement and inconsiderate use of ecological resources.

Ethnic cleansing: New term for an age-old illegal and decidedly unclean policy with the aim of removing, through hatred, intimidation, deportation, killing, genocide, or any other form of force, certain groups or minorities within the country, in order to homogenize the national population, acquire land, pamper to extremist pride, and ensure control.

Genocide: Acts committed with intent to destroy, in whole or in part, a national, ethnic, racial, or religious group or identity.

Guerrilla warfare: Literally "small war," which takes on a different meaning or interpretation according to whether it is justified or unjustified, a struggle for independence, liberation, resistance, or insurrection, destruction, or subjugation. International humanitarian law, the Geneva Conventions, and UN instruments have difficulty in dealing with such situations.

Incident/Accident: Although different in meaning and consequences, these two terms are often used interchangeably in emergency management. Incident is a sudden, unexpected occurrence that happens by chance and is usually without very serious consequences. Accident is also a sudden, unforeseen event, but more serious, usually with some resulting damage, injury, or death.

Internally displaced person(s) (IDP): Persons or groups of persons who have been forced or obliged to flee or to leave their homes or places of habitual residence, in particular as a result of, or in order to avoid, the effects of armed conflict, situations of generalized violence of human rights, or natural or man-made disasters, and who have not crossed an internationally recognized state border. According to established principles, these persons have the right to seek safety in another part of the country, to leave their country, to seek asylum in another country, and the right to be protected against forcible return or unsafe resettlement. But these are not refugees in the juridical sense.

Measures of effectiveness: In assessment techniques, the qualitative and quantitative criteria used to predict or correlate the value or measure of an organization or a system, such as disaster management. Such measures must be appropriate, measurable, sensitive, timely, cost-effective, and meaningful.

North–South: A theoretical division of the globe into north, representing the developed, more affluent, technologically advanced, financially rich, healthy, educated, and stable countries; and south, with developing, poor, indebted, technologically retarded countries where mortality is high, health levels low, and education deficient.

Posttraumatic stress disorder: Delayed or protracted reaction to an exceptionally strong stressful event of catastrophic dimension, which can cause pervasive distress in almost any person, but more marked in some, following a natural or man-made disaster, combat, violent death, torture, rape, terrorism, and so on. The onset may follow the trauma within a few weeks or at most six months. Typical symptoms include "re-living" or "flashbacks" of the event, "numbness" and detachment, fearful reminiscences.

Prisoner of conscience: Person imprisoned solely because of his/her political or religious beliefs, gender, or racial ethnic origin who has neither used nor advocated violence.

Prisoner of war: A member of the armed forces of a party to conflict; all members of armed groups and units that are under a command responsible to that party, and who have been caught and made prisoner by the opposing party in the conflict. Prisoners of war have rights and responsibilities defined by the Geneva Conventions. Guerrillas also benefit from POW provisions.

Refugee: A person who is outside his country of origin and who, due to well-founded fear of persecution, is unable or unwilling to avail himself of that country's protection. Different official categories of refugees include Convention refugee, de facto refugee, de jure refugee, mandate refugee, Protocol refugee, recognized refugee, refugee sur place, statutory refugee, environmental refugee.

The condition of being a refugee and refugee camps constitute a disaster. The problem comes under the jurisdiction of the UN High Commissioner for Refugees.

Resettlement: Relocation and more or less orderly settlement, for temporary or permanent habitation, of refugees and other persons displaced from their usual places of residence.

Right to intervene: By international law, every state has absolute sovereignty over its national territory and its internal affairs, and no outside interference is tolerated. In view, however, of certain unacceptable injustices and totalitarian acts carried out by dictatorial regimes, in 1991, UN Resolution 688 introduced the concept of "right to intervene" on humanitarian grounds. Subsequent decisions have further codified the concept of the right to intervene, while some even extend this to a duty to intervene.

Sustainable development: Development based on decisions, processes, and actions that meet the present needs without creating undue burden on society or the environment, and without undermining the ability of coming generations to meet their own needs in the future. The UN has set Millennium Development Goals.

Terrorism/Terrorist: Term referring to various kinds of illegal acts of violence, such as bombing, setting fire, abducting, intimidating, killing, and other forms of actions in order to create fear terror, panic, or submission among the public, state, or individuals. (Intolerant regimes tend to accuse freedom fighters and opposition actions as terrorism.)

War crimes: During hostilities, crimes committed in breach of established customs and principles of international law or the laws of war. They include the following: (a) grave breaches of the four Geneva Conventions and their Additional Protocols, such as willful killing, unnecessarily excessive destruction; (b) other serious violations of the laws and customs applicable to international armed conflicts, such as targeting civilians, pillaging; (c) violation of laws concerning armed conflicts of not an international character, such as cruelty against those not taking part in the conflict; (d) other serious violations of laws in noninternational conflicts, such as attacks on peaceful buildings. War crimes are considered as crimes against humanity.

Weapons of mass destruction: Offensive weapons whose destructive capability is derived from nuclear, chemical, or biological sources. Sometimes referred to as WMD or ABC: atomic, biological, chemical. Their use is prohibited by the UN and other international conventions. They are the opposite of conventional weapons or arms.

21.3 Laws and Organizations

Bilateral Cooperation: Technical cooperation or assistance by a donor country to a recipient country, through direct agreement between the two governments, without the United Nations or any other intermediary.

Geneva Conventions: The body of international agreements consisting of four Conventions (1949) and two Additional Protocols (1977) concerning the humanitarian treatment of victims of armed conflict, and put under the responsibility of the International Committee of the Red Cross. The first Convention regulates the care of the wounded and sick soldiers on the battlefield. The second is about the care of the wounded, sick, and shipwrecked in naval warfare. The third regulates the treatment of prisoners of war. The fourth is about the protection of civilians in time of war. Additional Protocols 1 and 2 ensure more humane considerations not only in international conflicts but also in national strife, such as the treatment of guerrilla fighters.

World Health Organization (WHO): The health arm of the United Nations aiming at "the attainment by all peoples of the highest possible level of health." The WHO coordinates efforts to raise health levels worldwide and promotes the development of primary health. Besides multiple public health programmes and actions, it is engaged in disaster preparedness and relief both at its headquarters in Geneva, Switzerland, and at six regional offices, and it coordinates the health sector of the UN involvement in major emergencies. The organization has compiled the Emergency Health Kit.

United Nations: The Office for the Coordination of Humanitarian Affairs (OCHA) mobilizes, directs, and coordinates the emergency humanitarian activities of the various UN agencies and other organizations. It has established the International Disaster Management Information Network (UNIENET), operates the OCHA warehouse in Pisa (Italy), and publishes studies on disaster relief and preparedness. In disasters and emergencies, OCHA dispatches field officers to the stricken site.

(Office of the) High Commissioner for Human Rights: The United Nations's central point for all human rights questions. Leads and stimulates human rights issues, responds to serious violations of human rights, investigates reports on their breaches, promotes human rights and strengthens national action in their favour, ensures that UN decisions on human rights are implemented, and the articles of the Universal Declaration of Human Rights are respected.

Human Rights Council: Permanent United Nations body that studies all issues and denounces violations of human rights, under the High Commissioner for Human Rights.

Biological Weapons Convention: United Nations Convention on the Prohibition of the Development, Production, and Stockpiling of Bacteriological (Biological) and Toxin Weapons and their Destruction, signed in 1972.

Red Cross: Red Cross, or International Red Cross, general terms used for one or all the components of the worldwide organization active in humanitarian work. The official name is The International Red Cross Movement, which comprises three components: (1) International Committee of the Red Cross (ICRC), acts mainly in conflict disasters as neutral intermediary in hostilities and for the protection of war victims. Guardian of the Geneva Conventions; (2) International Federation of Red Cross and Red Crescent Societies (IFRC), worldwide federation of the National Societies, active in nonconflict disasters and natural calamities; (3) The individual National Red Cross or Red Crescent Society of every country.

21.3.1 International Association for Humanitarian Medicine Brock Chisholm (IAHM)

A professional, nonprofit, nongovernmental organization that promotes and delivers health care on the principles of humanitarian medicine, named after Dr Brock Chisholm, first Director-General of the World Health Organization. In particular it provides medical, surgical, nursing, and rehabilitation care to patients in or from developing countries deficient in the necessary specialized expertise; brings relief to victims of disasters where health aid is lacking; mobilizes hospitals and health specialists in developed countries to receive and treat such patients free of charge; promotes the concept of health as a human right and bridge to peace; and advocates humanitarian law and humanitarian principles in the practice of medicine.

21.4 Summary

These are a few of some 2,000 terms (see Gunn dictionaries of disaster medicine and humanitarian relief)[1,2,3] that have been tested over many years in the field, in training programmes, and briefing sessions, and are established as the standard terminology in disaster management and humanitarian service.

It is the author's conviction that in the difficult emergency situations of multilingual and multidisciplinary *humanitarian action*, use of a commonly agreed vocabulary transforms a potential disaster of language into a commonly understood language of disasters and lessens the Babelian confusion that often risks to hamper the most well-meaning, humanitarian, disaster response.

---

[1] Gunn S.W.A.: *Multilingual Dictionary of Disaster Medicine and International Relief*, Kluwer Academic, Dordrecht, Boston, London, 1990.

[2] Gunn S.W.A.: *Dictionary of Disaster Medicine and Humanitarian Action*, Springer Science, New York, 2008. (In press.)

[3] Gunn S.W.A. and Murcia C.: *Dictonnaire des Secours d'Urgence en Cas de Catastrophe*, Conseil International de la Langue Française, Paris, 1984.

Part IV
Disasters and Conflicts

Chapter 22
Humanitarian Action in Major Emergencies

Boutros Boutros-Ghali

It is a great pleasure as well as a great honour for me to be with you on the occasion of the International Conference on Emergency Medicine and Catastrophes, amongst the men and women on the ground who have made the choice to serve their fellow human beings.

Following the recent murders of six employees of the ICRC, I would like to begin by paying public tribute to your actions, your dedication, and your commitment, as eminent specialists in emergency medicine and dealing with catastrophes.

I must say that if you were looking for a completely detached view of this question, I would be entirely the wrong man for the job. I would therefore like, quite simply, to share with you some of the thoughts that your actions inspire in me. Let me stress five points:

1. *It is difficult to isolate the issue of humanitarian action, in the broadest sense of the term, from a global geopolitical perspective.* It is clear that, since the end of the Cold War, and advances in promoting human rights, the humanitarian issue has acted as a stimulus in the international political arena.

One only has to look at the increase in the number of Security Council resolutions devoted to humanitarian issues and at the increase in the number of peacekeeping operations, which are largely intended to come to the aid of populations in distress. One only has to look at the increase in the number of NGOs in the humanitarian field, and at the increased efforts and resources devoted by international organisations, as well as national governments, and private institutions, to bringing help to the victims of natural disasters or technological catastrophes; to the victims of famine or pandemics, and to the victims of dictatorship or war.

2. *Recent decades have also been characterised by the significant increase in the number of conflicts.*

Never, since the end of World War II, has the world seen so many conflicts. Moreover, these are a new kind of conflict: conflict within nations and conflicts about identity and disintegration. Conflicts that affect civilian populations above all and that lead to huge migrations of displaced persons or refugees!

Conflicts that are sometimes accompanied by the disappearance of government structures, making it very difficult to perform independent humanitarian actions, and sometimes impossible to intervene at all. Conflicts where the boundary between acts of war and outright crime, between civilians and combatants, disappear. Conflicts in which the value of symbols is no longer respected, transforming humanitarian workers into the preferred targets of those who prey on humanitarian action, and in which international humanitarian law itself is no longer in a position to provide an appropriate response. It means humanitarianism finds itself confronted with new situations, new difficulties, and new challenges, all at the same time.

3. *It means that beyond the controversies, humanitarian action is the subject of more and more ethical and political debates, and it deserves to be defined more precisely.*

Whether it is a question of cost or a question of organising relief to avoid what Bernard Kouchner calls—I believe—"a catastrophe within a catastrophe." With all that implies in terms of disputes and coordination problems between multiple NGOs, NGOs and the population, and NGOs and the national authorities.

Whether it is a question of the legitimacy of wanting to respond to suffering when the country itself is opposed to it. Whether it is a question of a duty to bear witness. Whether it is a question, faced with a saturation of resources, of the necessity of choosing who should be abandoned.

All of this pushes us to keep on re-evaluating and to take better account of the wide diversity of situations, to acquire a better understanding, also, of the necessary interdependence between humanitarian action and political power, even if political power, as represented by nation states, must continue to play its role. In particular when, in certain situations, the disappearance of organised authority makes any kind of humanitarian action almost impossible. It falls, then, to the international community to avoid this kind of drifting and to compensate, through concerted political action, within the framework of the United Nations or regional bodies, for the powerlessness of humanitarian organisations.

We must also take better account of the diversity of the players involved and, as part of this much-needed dialogue, draw the line between necessary compromise and compromising principle. We must also define how far to take certain risks, which are inevitable in the current context. But above all, in all circumstances, we must keep in mind that all conflicts, all suffering—whether or not it is covered in the media—deserve our attention.

4. *If we need to pin down the scope of emergency humanitarian action, we must, also and above all—make the connection between emergencies and prevention, and between rebuilding and development.* Emergency humanitarian intervention must be supported and then replaced by political action, before, during, and after the event! Let us help people to understand that humanitarian problems do not only need humanitarian solutions!

First of all, it is before catastrophe, strikes—upstream of the event—that the problems of poverty, harm to the environment, and overpopulation must be tackled. It is also prior to any disaster that real, preventive diplomacy needs to be developed. Most conflicts that break out can be predicted, and an early warning system remains the best way to help avoid delayed, improvised, or disorganised interventions.

Then, when a crisis does strike, emergency humanitarian action must not act as an alibi for indifference, a lack of engagement on the part of the international community, or a refusal to tackle the core of the problem. We need to remember that once the emergency operation is over, we still have to help with the convalescence. It means, for example, after a conflict, helping with demobilisation, demining, returning refugees to their homes, rebuilding infrastructure, and getting institutions back on their feet again. It means that once we've handed out emergency food aid, we need to help with reorganising production and getting agricultural back-up and running. If these essential links to the "before" and "after" are not made, emergency medical care may, in certain circumstances—quite involuntarily—actually destabilise the situation further. It means that instead of acting as a substitute—the prevailing attitude during the actual emergency—we must move into an advisory and support role during the rebuilding and development phases, to avoid the same situation arising again.

5. *Humanitarian action must not take the place of development aid.*

The figures speak for themselves! In the early 1990s, the budget of the UN High Commission for Refugees doubled. The ICRC's did the same. About a quarter of UNICEF's resources—some one billion dollars—is devoted to humanitarian relief. The World Food Programme, created in 1974 to support development activities, now devotes 80% of its resources to emergency aid.

At the same time, development aid has continued to decrease. Politicians and the international community seem to want to abandon any kind of long-term vision or action, apparently satisfied with the immediate and the spectacular. In fact, we need to give ourselves the means to act in ways that go to the heart of the causes of poverty, tyranny, and war.

In other words, let us have the will to apply the principles of international humanitarian law, everywhere in the world, here and now. It is our duty of humanity, of sympathy, and of compassion towards those who are suffering! It is our duty of impartiality, tolerance, and respect for the dignity of all! It is our duty of solidarity with all those who need our support.

Humanitarian action must continue to fulfil its aims! But at the same time, we must begin to rebel against inaction!

Those are the thoughts I wanted to share with you.

The Nobel Peace Prize, which was awarded to "Médecins Sans Frontières" in 1999, has won acceptance for this long and quite remarkable tradition.

But the spirit of humanitarian action also bears witness to another aspect: a spirit of openness, fraternity, and solidarity shared in a context of friendship and peace.

Chapter 23
The Humanitarian Postulate
in Disaster Management

Jean Marie Fonrouge, MD and S. W. A. Gunn, MD, FRCSC

Disasters, unfortunately, and help, fortunately, are as old as humanity. As long as man has had a heart, some adrenalin and a physiological reflex for protection, he has had compassion and an urge to bring succour to those in distress.

Distress is not in short supply today. In fact the frequency and magnitude of disasters and major emergencies are steadily increasing throughout the world, imposing a heavy strain on the essential services and much suffering in individual countries and the international community. There are, currently, in the world's "disaster belt" of earthquakes, cyclones, and desertification over 100 developing countries, few if any of which have the technical knowledge, planning capacity and necessary resources to cope with such onslaughts. Add to these the constant risk of major technological disasters and the current post-Cold War sociopolitical upheavals, and we have a spaceship Earth in a chronic state of emergency.

Historically, assistance in such emergencies has evolved from early wound dressing and pain relief to specialized techniques like Emergency and Disaster Medicine, to institutionalized mechanisms like the Red Cross, and to newer social and political concepts of aid, as humanitarian intervention.

Whatever the motivation, whatever the magnitude of the emergency, whatever the scale of relief, and however genuine the goodwill, disaster response must, if it is to be efficient and effective, have a proper scientific base and solid technical underpinning. However, today we will concentrate not on the organizational and physical but on the humanitarian postulate of disaster relief, committed to peace and humanitarian service not only as a concept but also as a reality, as a way of life.

During the past decade or so, our ways of thinking about disasters and our ways of tackling disasters have changed dramatically.

- Major emergencies and disasters are no more considered fatalistic phenomena, but rather foreseeable and preventable events;
- Disaster-stricken communities are claiming assistance not as a charity but as a right;
- Those who provide assistance are looking upon it not as a sympathy but as a duty based on mutual aid;

- Disaster aid is being seen not as an ad hoc emergency repair episode but as an essential factor in long-term development; and
- The world community is now perceiving emergency relief not as a magnanimous contribution but as a humanitarian obligation.

We contend that this is a quantum leap forward in human and international relations.

Let us examine this humanitarian postulate of our specialty. And we unreservedly rank emergency and disaster medicine as specialties, which have come of age but which are young enough to provide dream, action, and growth.

Humanitarian we say. It is paradoxical that wars have engendered peaceful organizations and that new kinds of conflict are now engendering new concepts of peaceful response and humanitarian action.

The International Commitee of the Red Cross was born out of the battlefield of Solferino (1859) and resulted in the Geneva Conventions on decency between belligerents. World War I produced the League (now Federation) of Red Cross and Red Crescent Societies, and, of course, the United Nations, and its medical arm, the World Health Organization, were born out of the ashes of World War II.

But the end of World War II also resulted in the Cold War, which, until some years ago, completely galvanized international politics, quasi-paralysed the United Nations, distorted country-to-country intercourse, polarized all national expenditures, and limited humanitarian action.

Suddenly, with the end of the Cold War, all this has changed. The world is faced with a new situation, with new problems, and new challenges.

The *new situation* is that thermonuclear competition between the two major nuclear powers is virtually over, and that war between the leading nations of the East and West is most unlikely. It is no longer disrespectable among serious analysts to consider the probability of a nuclear-free world, and in large measure, international peace is at hand.

The *new problems* are equally real, but of an entirely different nature, with a most destabilizing effect on peace and security. One problem is the continuing presence of nuclear weapons under more fragile circumstances than before, and the other is the explosion of ethnic conflicts and centrifugal movements in many parts of the world.

In contrast with the relative calm on the *inter*national scene, *intra*-country strife of varying origins is showing up the United Nations and the international community ill-prepared and undecided for such new situations. For all their horrors, these internal conflicts do not threaten international peace; the strife in Sudan will not plunge Europe into war, the fighting in Chechnia is not an international war, and no outside power is invading Somalia, which is torn among its local warlords.

States, the international community, the United Nations, the disaster management organizations, relief societies, and even the military doctors are having to adapt to these changing circumstances and changing needs.

The changes perhaps affect less the non-governmental organizations and practitioners of disaster medicine than the government-based and diplomatically tied institutions. For disaster medicine is a humanitarian, emergency help, and health providing activity, related to man's suffering and unrelated to any political ideology or governmental ties. Somewhat in like manner, liberated from the strait-jacketing political constraints of the ex-Cold War, the United Nations too is redefining its capacities: it is moving from peacekeeping to peace-building, and this is to its credit.

This evolution, perhaps revolution, is recent. On 5 April 1991, the Security Council took a historic decision that has established new rules in international relations and intra-national behaviour, rules which have a tremendous impact on emergency assistance. Resolution 688 now gives the international community the "right to intervene"—"le droit d'ingérence"—on humanitarian grounds or for urgent human rights protection. Will this lead to . . . "duty to intervene"?

Furthermore, and this concerns more the non-governmental, voluntary, and emergency medical services; General Assembly Resolution 4–131 formally recognizes the role of NGOs in providing humanitarian aid in ". . . food, medicines and health care for which access to victims is essential."

These are landmark decisions. It was on the strength of Resolution 688 that outside forces were able to intervene in Northern Iraq in favour of the suffering Kurds, that made it possible for United States and other forces to mount Operation Restore Hope in Somalia, and that allowed some help to be channelled to Bosnia-Herzegovina.

We note with some pride that this takes us full circle to the basic precept of the World Health Organization: that health and security are a human right. Indeed the right to health is enshrined in WHO's Constitution, which states the following:

- The enjoyment of the highest attainable standard of health is one of the fundamental rights of every being
- The health of all peoples is fundamental to the attainment of peace and security.

Other UN instruments expand on and strengthen these ideals: Article 25 of the Universal Declaration of Human Rights states that

- Everyone has the right to a standard of living adequate for the health and well-being of himself and of his family, including food, clothing, housing, medical care and necessary services, and the right to security . . . in circumstances beyond his control.

Principle 4 of the UN Declaration of the Rights of the Child states that

- The child shall enjoy the benefits of social security. He shall be entitled to grow and develop in health . . . [and] . . . have the right to adequate nutrition, housing, recreation and medical services.

And the Universal Declaration on the Eradication of Hunger and Malnutrition adds that

- Every child has the inalienable right to be free from hunger and malnutrition . . .

All these expressions of intent took more substance in December 1991 when General Assembly Resolution 46/182 created the UN Department of Humanitarian Affairs to combat more effectively the major emergencies. DHA supersedes UNDRO and officially establishes the humanitarian nature of international assistance.

These then are some of the bases—and to us doctors some of the necessary underpinnings—of the evolving doctrine of humanitarian intervention in disasters. Translated into medical terms, there is already a feeling that Disaster Medicine is a sector of Humanitarian Medicine.

Naturally these ideas will not be enthusiastically espoused everywhere. The right to intervene, in particular, cannot be expected to receive universal acclaim, and even at this moment at the International Conference on Human Rights it is being opposed by some, who perhaps fear for their seats. For the former Minister of Health of France, Dr Bernard Kouchner, ". . . It is a dream. It is a sort of utopia. But it is obviously the only way." Former national-security adviser to President Carter, Zbigniew Brzezinski, also welcomes the concept and considers that "intervention is the flip side of interdependence." And are we not living in an interdependent world?

To be productive, credible, and impartial, any intervention must be decided upon and carried out under the strictest vigilance and unbiased adherence to international precepts in order to avoid abuses or excesses and not invite excuses. For, as one observer from the Third World has put it, intervention, however well meaning, must not become "a new form of colonialism; we can only accept it as a short-term solution." This is in fact capital: an emergency intervention, whether medical, military, or political, must be seen as just that—an emergency, with strictly specified conditions and limits to it in scope, time, and place.

Where does our profession stand in all this? Obviously, the old problems due to nature's fury and man's folly will be with us on an ever-increasing scale. On the other hand, the new challenges of humanitarian service will at once open new vistas and bring new satisfactions in emergency relief. If we as health practitioners can meet the old and the new with honesty, competence, and humanism, we shall have made our small step on this planet Earth.

Bibliography

Belanger M.: Le Droit International de la Santé. Presses de France, Paris, 1997.

Berner P. Fonrouge J.M, Gunn S.W.A.: Legal, diplomatic and geopolitical concepts for physicians on international humanitarian missions. Prehosp. Disaster Med., 14: S, 87, 1999.

Boutros-Ghali B.: De l'action humanitaire. J. Humanitarian Med., 1: 17–18, 2000.

Fonrouge J.M.: Droit international des catastophes, Doctorate Thesis, Université de Bordeaux, 1997.

Gunn S.W.A.: La Médecine des catastrophes: une nouvelle discipline. Helvetica Chirurgica Acta, 52: 11, 1985.

Gunn S.W.A.: Disaster medicine and emergencies. The international community's response. J. Irish Coll. Phys. Surg., 17: 14, 1988.

Gunn S.W.A.: Multilingual Dictionary of Disaster Medicine and International Relief, Kluwer Academic Publishers, Dordrecht, London, 1990.

Gunn S.W.A.: The scientific basis of disaster management. Disaster Prevent Manage. J., 1: 16 16–21, 1992.

Gunn S.W.A.: The role of the military in non-military disasters. Prehosp. Disaster Med., 9 (S): 46–8, 1994.

Gunn S.W.A.: Disasters and conflicts, Encyclopedia of Life Support Systems, UNESCO, Eolss Publications, Oxford, 2001.

Gunn S.W.A.: The humanitarian imperative in major health crises. In, Understanding the Global
    Dimensions of Health. Springer, NY, 2005.
Mahler H.: Health for all, or hell for all? J. Humanitarian Med., 3: 43–5, 2003.
Masellis M., Gunn S.W.A.: Humanitarian medicine: a vision and action. J. Humanitarian Med., 22:
    33–9, 2003.
Sullivan S.: A right to intervene? Newsweek, 16: 1, 1963.
World Health Organization: Principles of the rights of patients in Europe. EUR/R44/T.D. Rev. 1,
    1994.

Chapter 24
Health and Social Issues of Migrants and Refugees

Manuel Carballo, MD

This is a study of the process of social insertion of migrants, refugees and asylum seekers in one country in the context of access to and use of health and social services.

Migration has become an integral and important part of social and economic development everywhere. Whether it is precipitated by economic or political factors, there is always the risk that it will result in social and health problems for those who migrate and those who are left behind, as well as for the societies and social services that absorb migrants. Today a number of questions remain to be answered with respect to the relationship that exists between the social insertion of migrants, which is crucial for society as a whole, and how they relate to the social and health services in the communities that host them.

24.1 Methodology

The study involved structured interviews with 714 clandestine migrants, asylum seekers, refugees, doctors, nurses, social workers and professionals drawn from the educational sector and from the police force. The study also included a detailed assessment of how associations that work with and for clandestine migrants, refugees and asylum seekers are structured and function in the Canton of Geneva. It also involved a review of the policies that help define migration and the reception of migrants to one country, in this case Switzerland.

24.2 Clandestine Migrants

The 235 clandestine migrants covered by the study primarily came from Latin America (67%), Asia (21%), Africa (7%) and Europe (4%). In the case of Latin America, the main countries of origin were Bolivia, Colombia, Ecuador and Peru; in the case of Asia, most migrants came from two countries, Mongolia and the Philippines. The average age of clandestine migrants was 20 and over half of them (56 per cent) were female. More than half of them had been living in Geneva for less than 2 years. In general, their education level was high; 50 per cent had completed grade school and a relatively high proportion of them had university degrees.

24.2.1 Housing

The survey highlighted the challenge presented by housing for clandestine migrants and the fact that serious overcrowding is a major problem. It was not uncommon to find nine or more people of all ages and gender, including children, living in three-room apartments. Residential instability is also a problem and a large proportion of the clandestine migrants said that they had been forced to move more than three times since their arrival, that is to say on average 2 years.

24.2.2 Economic situation

Most clandestine migrants were working as domestic workers or in the service sector as restaurant staff. Job security was meagre and more than half (62%) of them had changed jobs at least three times since arriving in Geneva. More than half (54%) were also of the opinion that they were overqualified for the work they were doing, and 81% believed they were far less well paid than local Swiss people. Salaries of around 500–600 CHF were reportedly not unusual and contractual protection was relatively unknown.

24.2.3 Health situation

Nearly a quarter (24%) of the clandestine migrants felt their health had got worse since leaving their countries of origin. Fewer than 22% said they felt happy, and 85% said they were depressed. Problems of a psychosomatic nature, such as ulcers, back pains, chronic headaches, loss of appetite and sleep disorders were frequently reported. Their levels of knowledge about certain health matters were also often low, and they were often poorly informed about contraception and family planning. About 40% of all pregnancies were unwanted, and the rate of abortion was high with as few as 27% of pregnancies being carried to term. More than 36% of the women who had become pregnant said they did not know where to go for counselling; 84% had never had a breast examination, and 63% had never visited a gynaecologist since coming to Geneva. Violence and sexual abuse figured among the problems encountered by clandestine migrants with 37% of female migrants saying that they knew another migrant woman who had been a victim of domestic abuse, and 14% said they knew a woman who had been sexually abused in the work place.

24.2.4 *Relationship with health services*

Most clandestine migrants were not covered by any health insurance. For many of them, the price of health insurance was too high, and they said that even when they sought insurance, insurance companies typically refused them. More than half only knew of one hospital, and 60% could not name one. They were equally unin- formed about what health services were available to them as clandestine migrants. For example, almost half were unaware of the existence of UMSCO, and 61% do not know about the Points d'Eaux, both of which have been set up to respond to the needs of clandestine migrants. Even if the emergency services at the cantonal hospital were known by many to be an option, self-medication with the advice of pharmacists was the first health care recourse for most. Dental and ophthalmologic problems were badly neglected because they were seen as too costly. More than a third of clandestine migrants felt they were well understood by doctors, but nearly half felt just the opposite, and 34% believed doctors did not like them; 35% also believed nurses did not understand them, and 27% were of the opinion that nurses did not like them.

24.2.5 *Relationship with social services*

Familiarity with the network of locally available social services varied consider- ably; 74% of the clandestine migrants were familiar with Caritas and 68% with the Salvation Army, but only 41% knew of the Square Hugo, 37% the Contact Centre for Swiss Immigrants and 27% the Collective of Workers Without Legal Status. As far as other services were concerned, the Geneva Red Cross and the Protestant Social Centre were the most often mentioned, but even then only by 22% and 17%, respectively. When clandestine migrants did seek help from social services, the principle causes were economic problems (35%), employment-related difficulties (27%), housing problems (23%) and health (17%). At the same time, 86% of them said they did not know where the most appropriate place to go was, and 78% said they were afraid of being denounced if they did seek help. For 74%, the lack of legal status in Geneva was seen as the main obstacle to benefiting from available social services.

24.3 Asylum Seekers and Refugees

Of the 106 asylum seekers and the 28 refugees who were surveyed, 63% were between the ages of 20 and 34 years. Over a third (38%) of asylum seekers and 64% of refugees were men; 27% of asylum seekers and 64% of refugees were married. More than half of the asylum seekers (64%) originated from Africa and 26% from Europe, primarily Bosnia. Almost half (43%) of the refugees came from Africa, 29% from Eastern Europe and 22% from Asia. On the whole, levels of education were high; 35% of asylum seekers and 29% of refugees had completed high school or trade and business school, and a significant proportion of refugees had a university education. More than half of the asylum seekers (68%) had been in Geneva for less than 2 years, and 71% of refugees had been here for more than 5 years.

24.3.1 Housing

Most asylum seekers (84%) were accommodated in shelters where they said the living conditions were often difficult with serious problems of overcrowding, poor hygiene and lack of privacy. Nearly half of them shared bedrooms with three or four other people, often of different ages and backgrounds. The lack of privacy weighed especially heavy on elderly asylum seekers, even more so where there was overcrowding and poor hygiene.

24.3.2 Socio-economic situation

The rate of employment among asylum seekers was low, not only because of laws that limited their access to remunerated work but also because the jobs open to them were poorly paid and did not correspond to their qualifications. More than a half of the asylum seekers interviewed had not worked since arriving in Geneva, and there was a generalised feeling this was contributing to a loss of self-esteem.

24.3.3 Health situation

Almost half of asylum seekers and refugees rated their health as poor, and almost a third were of the opinion that their health had deteriorated since leaving their country of origin. Half of the asylum seekers and refugees said their psychosocial condition had worsened since arriving; nearly 70% of asylum seekers referred to frequent sensations of isolation, anxiety, nightmares, fear and difficulties making decisions. Asylum seekers in particular said they suffered from anxiety, often associated with waiting for their asylum requests to be processed. As far as reproductive health was concerned, 15% of the asylum seekers appeared to be unfamiliar with modern contraception, and 18% of them did not respond at all to questions on contraception. Over half (61%) of the female asylum seekers and 90% of female refugees had nevertheless consulted a gynaecologist since arriving in Geneva.

24.3.4 Relationship with health services

Most refugees and asylum seekers had experienced health problems since arriving in Geneva and more that 87% had received some type of medical care. In 50 per cent of cases, they had consulted a medical practitioner, but asylum seekers were more likely to have sought help from the Cantonal Hospital than refugees who were more likely to have resorted to self-medication with the help of pharmacists. Unlike clandestine migrants, asylum seekers and refugees had more access to ophthalmologic and dental care. A third of the asylum seekers thought that doctors did not understand them, and 28% were of the opinion that doctors and nurses were insensitive to their migratory experience. Both groups had a tendency to believe that nurses "understood" them better than doctors did.

24.3.5 Relationship with social services

Despite the high proportion of asylum seekers with psychological problems, only 7% said they knew about associations such as Appartenances, and only 3% knew Pluriels, both of which are organisations set up to provide psychosocial support services. The Centre Social Protestant, Caritas, the Red Cross and the EPER were the best known of the specialized associations followed by Camarada and AGORA, and the Hospice General was mentioned by 26% as the place they would go in case they needed help. In the case of asylum seekers, the main reasons for seeking help were administrative difficulties (34%), problems of training (20%) and job seeking. In the case of refugees, housing was the most important source of problems. Difficulties in making themselves understood, feeling that some services were not being made available to them, not knowing whom to go to and the feeling that the local community was unwilling to share its services with them were some of the reasons cited for the under-utilization of social services.

24.4 Health Workers

In all, 57 physicians and 24 nurses from surgery, obstetrics and gynaecology, paediatrics, psychiatry, clinical neuroscience, dermatology, community medicine and emergency medicine were interviewed; 54% of the physicians were men and 46% women. Among the nurses, 83% were women and 17% men.

24.4.1 Perception of migrants, refugees and asylum seekers

Most health care personnel felt their contact with clandestine migrants, refugees and asylum seekers had made them discover a new socio-cultural dimension of medicine, and most said it made them want to take a course in multicultural medicine and improve their foreign language abilities to better respond to the needs of foreign patients. They were nevertheless of the opinion that translators and cultural mediators should be made more available and they pointed out that in the current situation the children of migrants, refugees and asylum seekers are often called on to serve as mediators and translators for their parents.

Most health care personnel believed asylum seekers and refugees know where to go to get medical attention and do so effectively. Clandestine migrants, on the other hand, were seen as waiting too long before they sought medical attention. More than half (55%) of the physicians and 80% of the nurses thought this was partly because migrants had a tendency to underestimate their health problems. Most physicians (90%) also felt that once clandestine migrants knew how to use the system they had a tendency to over-use it; 30% of nurses were of the same opinion. They were also of the opinion that clandestine migrants often sought attention for problems that are not purely medical, but were often more of a social and economic nature.

In general health care personnel thought, the medical system had been well conceived to respond to the needs of clandestine migrants, asylum seekers and refugees, but 54% of the physicians felt that they lacked necessary information about the health care system, and almost all of them were of the opinion that the lack of legal status impeded the access of clandestine migrants to health care services.

24.5 Social Workers

In all, 47 social workers were interviewed; 62% of them were men and 38% women. More than a third (38%) of them worked for non-profit organizations; 30% worked for the Cantonal Hospital and 26% for the Hospice General.

24.5.1 Perception of migrants, refugees and asylum seekers

A majority of social workers (85%) thought that after a year in Geneva asylum seekers were on the whole capable of using the services available to them, but 50% doubted that they had the capacity to do so before that. Nearly half of them were of the opinion that the information available to clandestine migrants was not well adapted to their needs, and 40% thought the social services were not conceived in a way that allowed them to respond to the needs that are now emerging in the context of migration.

In general, they were of the opinion that cultural factors tended to be more problematic for asylum seekers and refugees than they were for clandestine migrants, but they also thought that one of the most significant problems was the overestimation of what social workers could actually do for them. Housing, health insurance and medical problems were felt to be the reasons most asylum seekers, refugees and clandestine migrants sought assistance.

There was also a sense among some social workers that they had to "fight" to ensure that migrants were well treated and looked after. In the case of the reproductive health of clandestine migrants, they frequently said becoming pregnant had become "a curse" for clandestine migrant women. Just as with health care personnel, social workers tended to think that contact with clandestine migrants had expanded their horizons and most of them said they would like to learn a new language in order to better intervene on their behalf.

24.6 Educators

In the educational sector, a number of professionals, including teachers, social workers, psychologists and administrators working with children of clandestine migrants, asylum seekers and refugees were interviewed.

24.6.1 Perception of migrants, refugees and asylum seekers

Most of the educators interviewed felt the educational sector in Geneva had become a model of what the state could do to support the social insertion of children of migrants, asylum seekers and refugees. They nevertheless believed that many migrants tended to mistrust the system for cultural reasons not fully understanding what it had to offer and afraid for their situation in Geneva. They generally shared the opinion that the academic performance of the children of clandestine migrants was often impeded by the conditions they lived in, and particularly referred to the impact overcrowding was having on the space needed for them to do their homework. They felt many children were also suffering from lack of sleep and mentioned the number of people sharing apartments as a cause of this. There were also frequent references to poor nutrition among children of clandestine migrants and the impact it was having on their academic performance.

Another problem that was cited was that children of clandestine migrants often felt they were "betraying" their parents because they saw themselves benefiting from conditions their parents could not take advantage of. At the same time, children were often afraid their parents might be identified by the authorities because they were enrolled in school.

People in the educational sector were also sensitive to the fact that children often had to serve as translators and mediators between their parents and the health and administrative systems, and feared this could have serious psychological implications for the children. They also highlighted the problems that adolescents encountered at the end of their schooling, suddenly finding themselves thrust back into the role of clandestine migrants without access to any further training or apprenticeships.

24.7 Police

Key representatives of the gendarmerie and officers of international security were interviewed at the suggestion and with the help of the Chief of Police.

24.7.1 Perception of migrants, refugees and asylum seekers

The police sector has created small "islands" in high-density migrant neighbour-hoods in order to better respond to the needs of migrants and help their social insertion. There was great sensitivity to the problems of clandestine migration and its contradictions, and this was felt to be a source of the difficulties between police and clandestine migrants. There was also a feeling that they were lacking in the type of training and support that might help them deal with difficult situations and complex decision-making. The living conditions of clandestine migrants and in par-ticular problems related to overcrowding and their precarious psychological and physical health were frequently referred to and there was a sensitivity to the fact that migrants, despite their clandestine character, were nevertheless contributing to the local economy and were often exploited. Police were also very aware of the growing industry of trafficking and smuggling of people into Switzerland and other parts of Europe and of the way in which clandestine migrants were being exploited financially by traffickers and smugglers.

24.8 Conclusions and Recommendations

Migration precipitated by both economic and political factors is changing the social, demographic and cultural character of Geneva and other large European cities and has also become an integral part of their economic development. The risk of social exclusion of these new arrivals nevertheless weighs heavy and with time could become a source of social and health problems for everyone concerned. Although much is already being done in Geneva for clandestine migrants, asylum seekers and refugees, a number of actions can be recommended with the objective of: (a) responding to the needs that have been identified in this study, (b) facilitating the social insertion of clandestine migrants, asylum seekers and refugees, (c) promoting and protecting their health and well-being, (d) rationalizing the use-effectiveness and costs of health and social services in the context of this migration.

24.8.1 Training

Given the multicultural nature of contemporary migration, continuous training of those who work with migrants, asylum seekers and refugees should be made avail-able, including for health care personnel, pharmacists, social workers, educators and others in the education sector and the police.

24.8.2 *Information and education*

Given that many clandestine migrants will continue to risk being marginalized from the health care system, ways should be found of giving them the tools to promote and protect their health. Information and education is called for in areas such as nutrition, reproductive and sexual health, work-related accidents and stress-related psychological problems.

24.8.3 *Pharmacists*

Given that many migrants and refugees go to pharmacists as a first resort when they need care, more should be done to create referral links between pharmacists and the health care services that clandestine migrants can have access to.

24.8.4 *Translators and mediators*

Given the many cultural and linguistic challenges faced in the health care system and by health care personnel, the number of translators and cultural mediators should be increased and more people should be trained in this field.

24.8.5 *Psychosocial personnel*

Given the high prevalence of psychosocial problems among clandestine migrants, refugees and asylum seekers, and given the implications of this for health, the number of staff with training in psychology should be increased in medical facilities.

24.8.6 *Screening*

Given that many migrants, asylum seekers and refugees present at medical facilities with problems whose underlying causes are psychosocial, more attention should be given to redirecting these people to relevant services and avoid overloading doctors and nurses with problems that are not purely biomedical.

24.8.7 *Medical insurance*

Because many migrants are willing to invest in medical insurance, more should be done to explore possibilities for making medical insurance available to them.

24.8.8 Working conditions of clandestine migrants

Given the very low wages being paid to clandestine migrants, more should be done to sensitize employers and the community at large of the vital role played by clandestine migrants in the local economy as well as the necessity for more justice in employment conditions.

24.8.9 Working conditions of asylum seekers

Given that many asylum seekers suffer from psychosocial problems associated with low self-esteem linked to employment constraints, more should be done to explore ways of giving them more rapid access to employment opportunities that correspond to their training and capabilities.

24.8.10 Housing

Given the acute problem of housing amongst clandestine migrants and asylum seekers, and also keeping in mind the lack of housing in general in Geneva, more should be done to ensure the best hygiene and health education adapted to their situation.

24.8.11 Children

Given the potential psychological impact on children acting as translators and mediators between their parents and the health and social service system, more should be done to find ways of reducing the need for children to do this and ensuring that children have a more harmonious education and development.

Given that many children of clandestine migrants live in overcrowded living conditions that limit their private space and impact adversely on their schooling, more should be done to find ways of providing them with environments where they can study after school.

24.8.12 Adolescents

Given that adolescents of clandestine migrants are prevented from pursuing any further education and training once they finish basic high school, more should be done to allow them continue their training and, in so doing, avoid this waste of human resources and the negative social consequences that can result from sudden exclusion.

24.8.13 Coordination

Given the large number of associations and organizations in the canton of Geneva working for and with clandestine migrants, refugees and asylum seekers, more should be done to harmonize objectives and coordinate activities.

Given the range and variety of specialized organizations working for and with clandestine migrants, more should be done to ensure that referral systems available to them be better coordinated and made known to them.

Chapter 25
Man-Conceived Disasters

S.W.A. Gunn, MD, FRCSC, FRCSI, (Hon), DSc (Hon)

Disasters are being studied more scientifically now, and disaster management, from prevention to planning, response and reconstruction, is being tackled more professionally—albeit desperately inadequately. Major emergencies and disasters are now subjects of investigation and teaching, and as such undergo the organizational and didactic techniques of classification and simplification. Thus, without in any way minimizing their catastrophic impact and destructive havoc, disasters are generally categorized as natural or man-made, with subcategories and combinations in between.

Natural disasters have been extensively investigated, and in the majority of cases are more straightforward both to understand and to manage, for example, a volcanic eruption. But here too an El Niño can turn completely upside-down our understanding of ocean meteorological phenomena, as was the case in Central America recently.

Man-made disasters are more difficult to categorize, as they include such diverse calamities as a badly constructed apartment block, a massive railway collision, a chemical accident like Bhopal, nuclear explosion like Chernobyl, mass exodus, war, major fires, and technological and environmental disasters that threaten the ecological balance of a community.

Complex disasters are yet another emerging concept where natural and man-made forces meet and where "the cause of the disaster as well as the needed assistance to the afflicted are bound by intense levels of political considerations", such as in the current Sudan catastrophe.

My long involvement in disaster situations and emergency management has, however, led me to the realization that, besides the inadequacy of classifying them, there is yet another category of man-made disasters that, beyond being a human-designed error, is a more sinister, indeed evil, catastrophic, totally lawless, and obscene type of disaster born in man's mind that I have called *man-conceived disaster.*

Not just a failed Chernobyl, with its genetic defects for generations to come; not just a Bhopal, leaving thousands dead, blind, and anoxic; not just a war that gives itself excuses of national security or territorial defence; but something that goes far beyond these calamities: a disaster that man—or a group of men—has set down, designed cold-bloodedly, planned, thought out in its minutest dark detail, *conceived and deployed for its maximum evil effect*, and carried out with all the finesse of scientific planning, cool rationalization, and sardonic satisfaction at its inhumane, destructive success.

I refer to such barbaric acts as ethnic cleansing, genocide, deportation, mass disappearances, death camps, and other crimes against humanity. The list goes on: should one also forget forced pauperization of entire nations by such kleptocratic autocrats as Mobutu in Africa, Duvalier in the Caribbean, or Karazic in Europe? Note that there is no geographic monopoly, and that, tragically for our profession both the last named torturers are medical doctors.

In a deeply thought-provoking presentation on torture, elsewhere in this volume, Ambassador Jaap Walkate rightly states that "torture is a man-made disaster . . . and a symptom of a sick society."

It is this kind of sick man or society that with cool rationalization and morbid precision devises and carries out this kind of horror: not just a man-made but a man-conceived disaster.

Endorsed by the plenary of the World Association for Disaster and Emergency Medicine in 1997, by the International Workshop on Disasters of the World Health Organization Collaborating Centres in 2001, and entered in UNESCO's massive *Encyclopedia of Life Support Systems* the term is now in the expanded edition of the Gunn *Dictionary of Disaster Medicine and Humanitarian Action*, as follows:

> Man-conceived disaster: As distinct from man-made disaster, man-conceived disaster refers to disastrous actions like genocide, death camps, ethnic cleansing, forced disappearances, pauperization, torture, war crimes, and other crimes against humanity that are obscenely conceived, cold-bloodedly planned and indecently perpetrated with impunity by terrorists, evil rulers, dictators, or kleptocrats with the aim of inflicting maximum suffering, death, and destruction, in full violation of personal, social, and cultural rights of humanity. While the response to man-made disasters is scientific, humanitarian, and managerial, the response to man-conceived disasters must be through the International Criminal Court.

Bibliography

Gunn S.W.A.: Disaster medicine, humanitarian medicine. Prehosp.Disaster Med., 13: 82, 1998.
Gunn S.W.A.: Disaster and conflict. Encyclopedia of Life Support Systems. UNESCO, Paris, 2000.
Gunn S.W.A.: Dictionary of Disaster Medicine and Humanitarian Action. New ed. in press, Springer, New York, 2008.
Gunn S.W.A.: [Jin ki sai gai]: Man-conceived disasters. Japan J. Disaster Med., 6: 193–195, 2001.
Gunn S.W.A.: On man-conceived disasters. J. Humanitarian Med., 1: 7–9, 2001.
Gunn S.W.A.: Catastrophes – New term for old tragedies. Medizin Katastrof Moscow, 2(38) 64, 2002.

Chapter 26
The Nuclear Issue and Pugwash

Sir Joseph Rotblat[†], DSc, PhD, KCMG, CBE, FRS

> Against a great evil, a small remedy does not produce a small result, it produces no result at all.
>
> John Stuart Mill

It is now more than a year since the Secretary General initiated a review of the Pugwash nuclear agenda. In an article in the Pugwash Newsletter (June 2000), he draws attention to substantial differences of opinion on these issues:

> There is now much support for the view that abolition of nuclear weapons is a remote and, perhaps, receding and misleading or unrealistic goal; and that, accordingly, the primary focus as regards nuclear weapons should be on measures that might, in the short and medium term, be effective in reducing the likelihood of their use

I took part in all but one of the forums. In addition, I had numerous conversations with Pugwashites in Cambridge. I did not detect much support for the views expressed in this quotation. On the contrary, it is my impression that the great majority of Pugwashites want the abolition (or prohibition)[1] of nuclear weapons to continue to be the main focus for Pugwash.

In this article, I want to present my opinion that our policy should be based on the premise that the elimination of nuclear weapons remains our principal goal and that priority should be given to discussing measures which lead directly to that goal. In view of the suggestion that Pugwash should abandon, even if only temporarily, that goal, I believe that we should begin by revisiting some fundamental aspects of Pugwash.

[†] 1908–2005

[1] *Side note on terminology.* Various terms have been used in describing the ways towards a nuclear-weapon-free world (NWFW). In this article, I use the term elimination because this is the word used in official documents, for example, the Preamble to the NPT, or in the statement from the 2000 NPT Review Conference. I am aware of the difference between elimination and prohibition, but in the context of this article, the difference is semantic rather than substantive. Any attempt to present the difference as a major problem would be misleading.

26.1 Some Basic Notions About Pugwash

The main task for Pugwash is to provide a forum for learned debate, but this was never intended to be a purely academic exercise, solely for the purpose of acquiring knowledge. Michael Atiyah put it in a nutshell in his Schrödinger Lecture when he said: "Knowledge brings responsibility." Pugwash has a strong moralistic element. There is a motivation for our actions. We aim at specific goals.

This was so from the beginning. The Russell–Einstein Manifesto implores: "Remember Your Humanity." At the First Pugwash Conference, we discussed the social responsibility of scientists on a level with the political aspects. Later this became enshrined in the "by-laws" of our (unwritten) constitution, which we have debated and adopted at successive quinquennial conferences. The document "Principles, Structure and Activities of Pugwash" states:

> The Pugwash Movement is an expression of the awareness of the social and moral duty of scientists to help to prevent and overcome the actual and potential harmful effects of scientific and technical innovations, and to promote the use of science and technology for the purpose of peace.

At these quinquennial conferences, we also adopt a document entitled "Goals of Pugwash," which sets out the objective of Pugwash activities for the forthcoming 5 years (and thus are mandatory on the Council). The goals adopted at the last quinquennium (Lillehammer, 1997) specifically include the elimination of nuclear arsenals. I believe that the time has come to reaffirm this goal, not only because of our belief that this is necessary for the security of the world but also because of equity requirements and ethical considerations.

There are many organizations, institutes, and commissions, which study the nuclear issue in its various aspects. We are different from most of them through our expressed concern with ethical values, yet we are disinclined to highlight this distinguishing feature. Indeed, we seem to shy away from mentioning this aspect probably because we are afraid of the criticism this might evoke; we are afraid of being labelled as naive, amateurs, and not a serious group. The so-called realists, many of whom are hawks and some are simply cynics, view ethical arguments with contempt. Remember the question reportedly put by Stalin: "How many divisions does the Pope have?"

Another probable reason is related to the general problem of specialization. Those who study a specific topic in its minutiae, and become experts engrossed in it, do not like to be diverted by other concerns.

I do not think that we should be influenced by such considerations. Of course we should be pragmatic, but not at the cost of abandoning basic values. We should try to put some idealism into realism; we should study topics in depth but be motivated by worthy ideals. We should not lose sight of the wood for the trees.

The fact that Pugwash has a good reputation in the world—evidenced by the award of the Nobel Prize—should encourage us not to be affected by negative reactions. Far from being ashamed of raising ethical issues, we should be proud of it. It is the cynics who should be made to feel ashamed, and we can do this by exposing the hypocrisy of their policies.

26.2 Moral and Legal Aspects

I make the above points in direct reference to our policy on the nuclear issue. Our ultimate aim is to create conditions for lasting peace in the world. Such a world would have to be based on moral principles, on equity and justice, on respect for the law both as individuals and as a society. The integrity of international treaties is of particular importance to Pugwash.

From the very beginning, nuclear weapons were abhorrent to people everywhere, and attempts were made to eliminate them by international agreements (e.g. the Acheson–Lilienthal Report).

The potential use of these weapons was generally described as a crime against humanity. It was in response to such feelings that the NPT came into being in 1970, and now counts among its members 98 per cent of the nations of the world. I am sure that even in the four countries that have not signed the NPT, the people have the same sentiments about nuclear weapons.

The NPT has been criticized as being discriminatory, which indeed it is. But the underlying concept was laudable: to get rid of *all* nuclear arsenals and thus end the discrimination. There was an apparent difficulty relating to the ambiguous wording of the all-important Article VI, in which the pursuit of nuclear disarmament is called for in the same sentence (though separated by a comma) as a treaty on general and complete disarmament. The hawks in the nuclear-weapon states deliberately interpreted this as meaning that nuclear disarmament can proceed only together with—and as part of—general and complete disarmament. Until the latter has been achieved, the nuclear-weapon states are legally entitled to retain their nuclear arsenals, they claimed. This ambiguity has now been removed.

In the General Assembly of the United Nations, there has always been strong pressure on the nuclear-weapon states to proceed with nuclear disarmament. This pressure has been steadily increasing since the indefinite extension of the NPT in 1995. A new group of seven nations, the New Agenda Coalition, was very vocal in this respect, and its efforts seem to have been successful. The NPT Review Conference in April/May 2000, in New York, came out with a long and comprehensive statement, signed by all five official nuclear-weapon states. It makes the issue quite clear. The section related to Article VI of the NPT includes inter alia: "An unequivocal undertaking by the nuclear-weapon states to accomplish the total elimination of their nuclear arsenals leading to nuclear disarmament to which all state parties are committed under Article VI." The previous description of nuclear disarmament as being an "ultimate goal" has also been dropped. The objective of ". . . general and complete disarmament under effective international control" is still mentioned in the statement, but in a separate paragraph, much further down in the document. The link between the two objectives is unambiguously broken. There is no longer any excuse not to fulfil the objectives of the NPT. This is where the hypocrisy comes in. The solemn declaration is belied by the actual policies pursued by the nuclear-weapon states (or at least by four of them). The pursuit of the policy of extended deterrence, whereby nuclear weapons would be used—if necessary—against attacks with chemical, biological, or even conventional weapons, implies the indefinite retention (or retention at least until general and complete disarmament) of nuclear weapons.

This is the actual policy of the United States; it is enshrined in the 1997 Presidential Decision Directive (PDD-60 document) which sets out the US nuclear posture, and clearly implies the first use of nuclear weapons.

If, at this stage, Pugwash were to give up the elimination of nuclear weapons as the primary focus, this would imply our connivance with the United States and the others in the violation of an international treaty. I do not think that this would be acceptable.

On the contrary, we must strongly oppose such an attitude; we must use every opportunity to expose the hypocrisy of the nuclear-weapons states in proclaiming one policy and pursuing just the opposite.

We should keep hammering home the fundamental thesis that compliance with international commitments is an essential requirement of a civilized state. We should keep on reminding people that world peace cannot be achieved without respect for international law. We should encourage other NGOs working towards nuclear dis-armament to make the call for the adherence to international treaties an important part of their campaigns. I suggest that we make this issue the subject of a Pugwash Workshop. We need to study the various aspects of international treaties; their role in national and international policies; and the ways and means of dealing with their violation. Some of the study would be concerned with legal issues, but this should not put us off (we are, e.g. dealing with legal issues in the Pugwash study group on Intervention, Sovereignty, and International Security).

26.3 The Ethical Dimensions of Deterrence

In reviewing the nuclear issues with which Pugwash should concern itself, as a group with moral responsibilities, we should—in my opinion—take up explicitly the ethical aspect of deterrence.

The concept of nuclear deterrence is historically and substantively at the heart of the whole nuclear issue. I used it way back in 1939 as the rationale for starting the work on the atom bomb (but soon realized its fallacy); it was the rationale for nearly all the scientists in the pre-Manhattan years. Deterrence—in its various forms—was the reason for the build-up of huge arsenals during the Cold War period, and it is being used now to justify the retention of nuclear weapons.

The problem of deterrence has of course been frequently debated in Pugwash, as well as in numerous other forums. But the arguments have usually been on the political, strategic, or military aspects; little attention has been paid to the ethical aspect. The reason for this is the one mentioned earlier: ethical issues have no place on the agenda of the cynics. But for Pugwash, the ethical dimension of deterrence should be of prime importance. If the use of nuclear weapons is a crime against humanity, how can the threat of their use ever be justified?

In discussing the problem of deterrence, I am primarily concerned with the doc-trine of extended deterrence, although the ethical element applies of course to all aspects of deterrence. The argument that nuclear weapons are needed to prevent any aggression is the chief reason for policies of indefinite retention of nuclear weapons. I believe that if this argument were shown, and accepted, to be invalid, it would open the way to the total elimination of nuclear weapons. The extended deterrence argument lacks credibility, largely arising from the general abhorrence of nuclear weapons. The existence of these weapons has not prevented the several hundred wars that have taken place since 1945. Nor has the possession of them prevented the United States and the Soviet Union from being defeated (in Vietnam and Afghanistan). No doubt, there were political and military reasons for the non-use in these cases, but the opprobrium associated with such use must have played a significant role.

The taboo against the use of nuclear weapons is still strong, and this weakens the threat of deterrence. On the other hand, if the taboo is too strong, the deterrence argument would cease to be valid. The whole thing is based on a deliberate ambiguity. We have made our security hang on uncertainty: on whether or not a would-be aggressor will take the threat seriously.

The deterrent would be effective only if it is made absolutely clear that the threat will be converted into action; otherwise, it would have no value and the bluff would be called. This means that George W. Bush, or Tony Blair, have to show convincingly that they will push the button and unleash the most destructive and omnipotent weapon in a dispute which could otherwise be solved with much less destruction. The threat may work for a time, but eventually an aggressor will gamble on the uncertainty. In the meantime, the security of the world is based on a balance of terror, and as Francesco Calogero pointed out a long time ago: "The fact that the survival of human civilization is predicated on such a policy may, in the long run, result in the disintegration of the ethical basis of civilized society."

Although the ethical aspect of nuclear deterrence is as old as nuclear weapons themselves, there are valid reasons for raising it now as an item for our agenda. There is growing awareness in the world community about individual and collective responsibility for one's deeds. With the establishment of the International Criminal Court, people may be put on trial for offences against international law even if these are legal under national laws.

This raises the much wider issue of the personal responsibilities of scientists working on military projects. If the use of a given type of weapon is illegal under international law, should not research on such weapons also be illegal, and should not the scientists also be culpable? And if there is doubt even about the legal side, should not the ethical aspect become even more compelling?

In this connection, we should be reminded of the call issued in 1995, on the occasion of the 50th anniversary of Hiroshima, by Hans Bethe, the most senior scientist in this field:

I call on all scientists in all countries to cease and desist from work creating, developing, improving, and manufacturing further nuclear weapons and—for that matter—other weapons of potential mass destruction such as chemical and biological weapons.

It seems to me that there are enough items for investigation in connection with the ethical issues of nuclear weapons to justify at least one workshop.

26.4 Steps Towards a NWFW

Apart from the two suggested topics for Pugwash study, centred on the social responsibility of scientists, I want to recommend other projects on measures that would lead to the achievement of a NWFW.

A nuclear-weapon-free world will not be achieved in one go: it will require a series of steps. Some of these steps may be the same as suggested by the "realists." There is, however, a significant difference: the latter view each step as an endpoint in itself, while we see them as part of a comprehensive programme of disarmament. Among the many steps that can be taken, we should give priority to those which lead us directly to the objective.

26.5 No-First-Use Treaty

As I have stated several times already, I consider the doctrine of extended deterrence —which means the potential first use of nuclear weapons—to be the major obstacle to the achievement of a nuclear-weapon-free world. This is a fundamental issue. If we concede that nuclear weapons are needed to deter even non-nuclear attacks, then these weapons will have to stay for as long as disputes are settled by military confrontations. And if they are needed for that purpose by the United States, then they are needed even more by weak states. Hence, the proliferation of nuclear weapons is bound to happen, with the eventual near certainty that these weapons will be used in combat.

The doctrine of extended deterrence has been discussed and potent arguments against it were presented in several studies in the 1990s, notably in the Report of the Canberra Commission. The matter was also discussed in two relevant reports from the US National Academy of Sciences published in 1991 and 1997. In the first of these, the following is stated in the Executive Summary:

> We conclude that the principal objective of the U.S. nuclear policy should be to strengthen the emerging political consensus that nuclear weapons should serve no purpose beyond the deterrence of, and possible response to, nuclear attack by others.

The 1997 Report goes a step further when it recommends that

> To this end, the United States should announce that the only purpose of U.S. nuclear weapons is to deter nuclear attacks on the United States and its allies, adopting no first use for nuclear weapons as official declaratory policy.

The great importance of a no-first-use policy is that it would pave the way to an agreement on the total elimination of nuclear weapons.

The no-first-use policy is usually presented in the form of unilateral declarations, or pledges, by the individual nuclear-weapon states. While this could be achieved more quickly than the alternative (a treaty), it would not be satisfactory, in my opinion. There is nothing—legally—to stop a unilateral declaration from being unilaterally revoked. This has in fact happened: the Soviet no-first-use pledge, in existence since 1982, was withdrawn by Russia in 1993. In the United States, a new president may decide that he does not like the policies of his predecessor and scratch a pledge. This cannot be done easily with international treaties, signed and ratified. International treaties can also be terminated by states parties giving suitable notice of withdrawal, but this usually creates quite a commotion (witness the current situation of the ABM Treaty), and does not occur often. Treaties may of course be violated by cheating, but this too is an infrequent event. In general, there is a tendency to adhere to the terms of a treaty. Certainly, in the light of what I said earlier, we in Pugwash should promote international treaties and seek ways to ensure that they are conformed with, both in letter and in spirit.

In line with this, I believe that a no-first-use policy should be enshrined in a No-First-Use Treaty to be signed and ratified by all official and non-official nuclear-weapon states.

As far as I am aware, not much research has been done (certainly not in Pugwash) on the terms of such a treaty and its possibly far-reaching consequences for military doctrine and nuclear force postures. For example, the treaty would probably have to include a formal agreement to abolish tactical nuclear weapons, in place of the 1991–2 unilateral declarations by Bush (senior) and Gorbachev/Yeltsin, since these are weapons most likely to be used to counter a non-nuclear attack. De-alerting of nuclear warheads, necessary to reduce the probability of an accidental or unauthorized launch, would be an essential part of a No-First-Use Treaty.

These, and other types of measures to make first use less likely, as well as possible obstacles to a NFU treaty, need to be discussed in detail, and should be the subject of a Pugwash project.

26.6 Verification of Nuclear Disarmament

The Pugwash study on the desirability and feasibility of a nuclear-weapon-free world (published in the trilogy of Pugwash monographs on this subject) makes out a consistent case for a programme of nuclear disarmament leading to the abolition of nuclear weapons. In the last of these books (A Nuclear-Weapon-Free World—Steps Along the Way), John Holdren makes a penetrating analysis of the pros and cons of going to zero, coming to the conclusion that "... prohibition is *clearly* desirable under appropriate conditions...." It is to these conditions, discussed in the last part of Holdren's work, that we must apply ourselves.

The argument used by those who would like to retain nuclear weapons indefinitely is that even if a NWFW were desirable, it would not be feasible because there are no means to guarantee that a treaty to eliminate nuclear weapons would not be violated, either by some nuclear-weapon state hiding away a small nuclear arsenal (the bombs in the basement argument) or by some rogue state acquiring such weapons clandestinely at a time in the future (the breakout argument).

In a work by Tom Milne and myself in the second book (*Nuclear Weapons—the Road to Zero*), it is argued that the probability of such events occurring, once a treaty to eliminate nuclear weapons has been agreed to, is very small, although not zero. One hundred per cent security can never be achieved. Our main proposition is that a world without nuclear weapons would be safer than a world with them (quite apart from being a better world for moral reasons as outlined above). All the same, we have to substantiate this proposition by showing that it is possible to realize a safeguard regime, with a verification system—both technological and societal—robust enough to reduce the probability of breakout to a vanishingly small value.

Although the topic has been studied by Pugwash sporadically, a new systematic study is warranted, to take into account the changes that have occurred as a result of the development of new technologies and the greater opportunities provided by the advances in information technology, such as the Internet.

Methods of technical surveillance are improving all the time. Although the advanced technology may also be used by those who contemplate illegal schemes, the overall balance probably makes feasible enhanced verification (the relative advantage should be part of the study). Similarly, reliance on societal verification is becoming stronger with the much greater openness and better facilities for transmitting information through the Internet. In general, the current tendency to greater openness makes verification easier.

The various agreements between the United States and Russia to improve strategic stability, for example, the decision to set up a Joint Data Exchange Centre, should also be helpful in this respect. A workshop devoted to these issues seems to me to be highly desirable.

26.7 Nuclear-Weapon-Free Zones (NWFZs)

The second method of achieving a nuclear-weapon-free world by gradually reducing the area of the globe where nuclear weapons are allowed—is making steady progress. More than half of the surface of the earth is now officially a nuclear-weapon-free zone, although in terms of the world population more than half live in the eight countries with nuclear weapons (plus NATO), this number having gone up considerably since 1998.

There is an urgent need for instituting NWFZs in at least three more areas, in Central/Eastern Europe, in Northeast Asia, and in the Middle East. Efforts to establish these seem to have evaporated recently, and there is a need to revive them, in view of the heightened tension in Eastern Europe following the expansion of NATO, the concern about the nuclear policy of North Korea (described again as a "rogue" state by the administration of George W. Bush, and the chief excuse for national missile defence), and the extremely volatile and dangerous situation in Israel/Palestine. All three potential NWFZs present special problems since they would border directly on official nuclear weapon states, or include an unofficial nuclear weapon state.

The controversial issue of transit and deployment of nuclear weapons in the waters of all the nuclear-weapon-free zones also requires more study, as does the formal recognition of the status of NWFZs with appropriate verification systems.

Chapter 27
Quantifiable Effects of Nuclear Conflict on Health and Society*

S. W. A. Gunn, MD, FRCSI(Hon), DSc(Hon), Dr h c

27.1 Introduction

On 6 August 1945, an atom bomb shattered the then enemy and heralded new hopes for mankind. Sixty years later, in this new century, those hopes remain mainly shattered.

The end of the Cold War in the early 1990s again introduced a glimmer of hope. But that too was shattered, and today the risk of nuclear conflict remains real, though less obvious.

The much-heralded Non-Proliferation Treaty is now taking hard knocks—sadly and paradoxically from its initial proponents, and governments are glibly talking of the possibilities of nuclear accident, nucleo-terrorism and nuclear threats, as if it were hurricane Katrina, the London tube or the Twin Towers. With deference to our Pugwash friends, even some of them were tempted at one time (2000) to think mainly of reducing the likelihood of the use of nuclear weapons, until that wise peace-monger, Joseph Rotblat, reminded us all that nothing but *total* elimination of weapons should be our main focus, echoing the Russell–Einstein Manifesto: "Remember your Humanity." This paper, which is based on some work we did together, is respectfully dedicated to the memory of Sir Joseph Rotblat.

To the credit of society, during the past few decades this Humanity *has* been remembered. At least insofar as no nuclear device has been dropped on people since Nagasaki.

But we have neither stopped producing them, nor testing them, nor threatening to use them. And at the side of bristling new warheads, the old rusting stockpiles, the melting chemicals, the rising culture of violence, the easy availability of black market ingredients and the general international indifference have all rendered the risk of nuclear hazards very real today. Pakistan, Israel and North Korea are not mirages.

Indifference, I was saying, and perhaps this explains why, of late, there have been few serious, objective studies on the short- and long-term effects of nuclear war on man, society and the environment. For objective calculations and independent

---

* The inaugural Sir Joseph Rotblat Lecture of the International Association for Humanitarian Medicine.

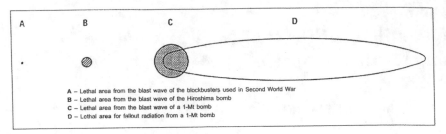

A – Lethal area from the blast wave of the blockbusters used in Second World War
B – Lethal area from the blast wave of the Hiroshima bomb
C – Lethal area from the blast wave of a 1-Mt bomb
D – Lethal area for fallout radiation from a 1-Mt bomb

Fig. 27.1 Comparison of the effects of bombs

opinions, we have to go back some 20 years to the studies based on scientific integrity carried out at the World Health Organization in 1987 and 1993, on the Greater London War Risk Study in 1986, the US National Academy of Sciences investigation of 1985 and a few others.

Although these studies go back some two decades, their results remain very much valid, even though their effects have not had to be tested in actual war. Thank goodness.

Having been personally involved in the WHO and London investigations, I shall draw my examples and conclusions from them. And if I may add a personal note, having carried out some of these studies with Professor Rotblat, particularly the health effects of nuclear attack on London, I should like to acknowledge his valuable help and gentle friendship.

The Second World War is behind us by 60 years, and the peace-promoting United Nations is celebrating a similar anniversary. Yet conflicts have not ended, and new conventional weapons have made their destructive capacity cruelly evident. The visible spectre of nuclear conflict appears receding, and we all hope that it is more than appearance. For today, a single thermonuclear bomb has the explosive power of a million times the largest conventional device, with not only devastatingly immediate effects but also extremely harmful long-term consequences, at the site of the attack and far away, in time and space, on man, society and the environment (Figure 27.1). Health will be the principal casualty.

To avert the risk of subjective exaggerations and value judgements, I have chosen to present in this survey certain quantifiable parameters on the immediate health needs and availability of health personnel, supplies and medical equipment following nuclear conflict. I shall also briefly touch upon some health-related problems of society that man will face.

These are based on scientific research, mathematical modelling, statistical techniques and socio-economic analyses by some 49 investigators and experts in their respective fields, who included Professor Rotblat.

27.2 The Health Consequences

Within the overall damage to all services, to the built environment, the means of communication and the technological armamentarium, health personnel will be killed or injured, and hospitals, medical services, pharmaceutical supplies, food and technical equipment will naturally be destroyed. These will, in fact, suffer proportionately greater damage as they are usually situated in urban centres and prime target areas. In the United States, approximately 80 % of all medical resources are located in such vulnerable areas. Moreover, following an attack, greater demand will be made on those that have survived or escaped damage, to a degree that available manpower and facilities, such as remaining drugs, X-ray films, beds, blood or ambulances, will be rapidly depleted, and replacement will become extremely problematic.

27.3 Physicians and Other Health Manpower

In line with material health facilities, doctors, nurses and other health professionals tend to be congregated in central, vulnerable areas. In the United States, 87 % of physicians live in cities, and in England, the Greater London area alone has a concentration of 13,454 medical practitioners and 67,330 nurses. As cities are priority targets, deaths and casualties will be proportionately higher among the medical personnel than among the rest of the population.

In Hiroshima, most of the hospitals were centrally located and all within 1 km of the hypocentre were totally destroyed, with a mortality rate of 100 % of the occupants, including all the health personnel.

Following an attack over the United States, there would remain only one doctor for 663 casualties, and the ratio for London would be 1/550. Table 27.1 from our GLAWARS study gives the casualties among the health personnel in metropolitan London according to different magnitudes of attack.[1]

Even if patients could find and reach a doctor, it would be an enormous logistical problem to arrange for all the injured and sick to be seen, were it only once, for just a few minutes. The few available doctors and nurses would need to work round the clock under most impossible conditions.

Table 27.1 Casualties among medical and auxiliary staff [a]

Type of personnel	Pre-war numbers	Numbers left uninjured in scenario			
		2	3	4	5
Hospital doctors	9,400	7,940	7,240	1,420	280
General practitioners	4,054	3,430	3,120	610	120
Dental practitioners	2,790	2,360	2,150	420	80
Nurses	67,330	56,900	51,800	10,200	2,000
Ambulance personnel	3,525	3,000	2,710	530	100

[a] Calculated from casualty rates to the general population according to Steadman, Greene and Openshaw (1986); similar calculations based on casualty rates provided by Rotblat, Haines and Lindop (1986) indicate even fewer surviving medical personnel.

---

[1] Most figures and statistics refer to the period of our GLAWARS study, 1986 (Clarke et al., 1986). The paucity of independent scientific investigations since then indicates the decline of general concern despite the persisting risks.

Clearly, in such circumstances, medical care could only be elementary at best. In the above calculations, information about dental practitioners is included as their experience in administering anaesthetics might be of value, although it is most likely that surgery would have to be performed without anaesthesia and at a most rudimentary level.

27.4 Hospitals and Hospital Beds

Hospitals situated in the blast and fire area would be totally or extensively destroyed. Those in the fallout zone would become inoperative and the remaining peripheral supporting hospitals would be entirely overwhelmed.

In Nagasaki, 75 % of all hospital beds were in the University Hospital, which was extensively damaged, with a mortality rate of 80 % of its occupants. Against this destruction, among those who survived 65 % of them needed treatment of more than 3 months' duration.

H.L. Abrams in the United States and our Greater London Area War Risk Study Commission in the United Kingdom have extensively investigated the problem of medical supply and demand following nuclear attack. Excluding psychiatric beds, the United States in 1978 had 1,137,666 hospital beds. Of these, 76 % were located in urban areas and can be assumed to be destroyed in war, leaving 273,000 beds available after an attack. Disregarding those with radiation syndrome, some 55 % of the multitrauma and burn cases would require hospitalization.

According to the estimates of the Federal Emergency Management Agency and other scenarios, in the United States there would be 93 million survivors, with 32 million injured. As 55 % of them would need beds, there would be only one bed per 64 candidates. Presuming that 20 % of the beds were already occupied at the outbreak of hostilities, there would remain one bed for every 81 patients. In the Greater London area, it is assumed that some 25 % of beds would have been already occupied at the time of attack.

Burns are a major problem, yet even in most developed countries burn care facilities fall far short of needs. In the United States, there are some 135 burn centres with a total of 1,400 beds. Considering only burn casualties—estimated at 5.3 million—2.12 million beds would be needed for burns alone, almost eight times the total number of all beds remaining for all other conditions. And it must be stressed that burn patients stay an average of 60.8 days and require some 40 operations.

The situation is even more dramatic for intensive care beds. After an attack, there would be 563 extensively injured and sick candidates for each available bed.

In the most thorough investigation carried out by any non-political, scientific commission, the effects of five scenarios of nuclear attack on London were studied from every conceivable angle, including all aspects of health. It becomes evident from this that the health facilities would be totally insufficient. Greater London has 270 hospitals with a bed capacity of 57,620. After a major nuclear attack, only one

Table 27.2 Percentage damage to hospitals and hospital beds in the GLC area

Damage	Scenario 2 Hospital	Beds	Scenario 3 Hospital	Beds	Scenario 4 Hospital	Beds	Scenario 5 Hospital	Beds
Severe to moderate	3	3	9	9	69	67	79	81
Light	3	3	12	12	16	15	14	13
Undamaged	94	94	79	79	15	18	7	6

Totals: hospitals, 270; hospital beds, 57,620.
Source: Rotblat, Haines and Lindop (1986).

out of seven hospitals would be serviceable. There might remain 7,500 beds against a demand of 1.1 million casualties, or 150 candidates for each bed.

Table 27.2 gives further details.

27.5 Pharmaceutical Supplies

Retail pharmacists depend on manufacturers and suppliers for their inventory. Hospital pharmacies usually hold about 8 weeks' supply of drugs. In Greater London, there are some 1800 chemists' shops. Following an attack, only between 7 and 15 % would remain undamaged, and their supplies would become rapidly depleted. They would also be vulnerable to looting.

In the United States, it is estimated that 90 % of the pharmaceutical industry would be destroyed. Thus, an estimated national inventory of 34,000 kg of tetracycline would be reduced to 8,600 kg, while the needs would rise to 314,000 kg. The same disproportions would apply to most of the other essential drugs (Abrams).

The multiplicity and great variety of pharmaceutical preparations can become a liability in disasters. The WHO Emergency Health Kit, with drugs specially chosen for disaster situations and quantified for the needs of 10,000 persons over 3 months, would be more useful. However, here again, supplies would be liable to destruction.

27.6 Equipment, Bandages, Needles

Besides pharmaceuticals, medical supplies include a wide variety of products, ranging from simple gauze bandages and scissors to surgical instruments, sophisticated diagnostic machines, computers and electronic equipment.

For a US population of 226.5 million (1980 census), the normal stocks of absorbent gauze would be 25 million square metres: hypodermic needles, 32 million; and general operating scissors 426,000. Following an attack the demands and needs would be entirely different. Thus, against 161 million square metres of absorbent gauze needed, there would be 6 million available; for 76 million needles needed, only 4–6 million available, and against a need for 5.2 million scissors, there would be only 85,000 pairs (Table 27.3).

Table 27.3 Some basic surgical supplies in the United States

	Normally available stocks	After attack	
		Remaining stocks	Amount needed
Absorbent gauze	25 mln. m^2	6 mln. m^2	161 mln. m^2
Hypodermic needles	32 million	4–6 million	76 million
Operating scissors	426.000	85.000	5.2 million

After Abrams:
    The Medical Implications of Nuclear War
    © 1986 by the National Academy of Sciences

27.7 Blood and Replacement Fluids

In normal times, the Greater London area has three regional transfusion headquarters which receive 588,000 blood donations annually, or 2,550 daily. In an attack, two centres would be put out of action and the third made almost inoperable. The same applies to the blood products laboratory of the metropolis.

In 1979, in the United States, 11.1 million units of blood were collected, representing 16.7 million units of blood and blood products. A total of 213 blood centres, representing 88 % of the nation's blood supplies, are situated near hospitals and, like hospitals, 76 % are likely to be destroyed, leaving only 13,985 units for daily use, totally inadequate for the overwhelmingly increased needs.

Albumin as a volume expander has a longer shelf life and would normally be available in sufficient quantities. But 80 % of the albumin supplies are likely to be destroyed. After an attack, only 680,000 units would be available for a total need of 3.4 million units daily.

Intravenous solutions—dextrose, sodium chloride, Ringer's lactate—represent a daily inventory of 7 million litres in the United States. After an attack, 1.4 million litres would be available. The demands would be enormous, as follows: 33.9 million litres of 5 % dextrose solution; 27.6 million litres of electrolyte solutions; 1913 million litres of Ringer's lactate (Abrams).

27.8 Ambulances and Transport

London has the highest concentration of ambulances in the world. A total of 1,070 vehicles, operating out of 74 stations, answer some 2,000 emergency calls a day and additionally provide transport for 10,000 outpatients. According to estimates, the main headquarters, 4 district headquarters and 66 stations would be destroyed in an attack. The remaining ambulances would be totally inadequate for the greatly increased demands.

Furthermore, undamaged medical transport would have great difficulty in moving about rubble-blocked streets, and disorganization, lack of gasoline and electromagnetic pulse (EMP) interference would virtually bring all communications and traffic to a halt.

27.9 Power Supplies

Health services are heavily dependent on the supply of power. From telephone communications to sterilizing facilities, refrigerators, light, X-ray machines, lifts, hospital kitchens, warning signals, cardiograms, computers and electronic equipment, electric power is indispensable. Power sources and distribution lines are very likely to be destroyed. EMP would disrupt radio communications and electronic equipment even in the few buildings that might have escaped structural damage.

Medical technology as known today would simply cease.

27.10 The Social Consequences

This brief examination of the quantifiable health consequences of nuclear war shows sufficiently clearly how woefully inadequate the medical services would be. But an extensive examination must also take account of the less obvious and less easily measured effects. These include the consequences of attack on the complex organization of an advanced urbanized society and the ability of such a system to survive. If the social, economic and political factors are ignored—and all these play an important role in a nation's health—the costs of a nuclear attack will be severely underestimated. With one exception (Katz, 1982), the GLAWARS investigation is the only major study to have explored these issues.

From this investigation, let me take but two elements affecting a changed society.

Among the studies our Commission carried out was a sociological assessment of the perception of Londoners of the threat of nuclear war and of the effects of war.

Normally, Londoners, you will agree, form quite a disciplined and socially conscientious citizenry. They gave ample proof of this by their self-sacrifice and mutual solidarity during the harassing bomb attacks they endured throughout the war and in recent terror bombs.

If this was so in World War II, it does not seem that it will be so in World War III. Faced with the threat of nuclear war, the Londoner, according to the GLAWARS survey, will have a different sense of social responsibility, an altered work ethic.

It is likely that the majority of those who work, in whatever category, will not report for duty. Table 27.4 shows that 69 % in the public sector and 82 % in the private sector would stay away from work, however essential that might be for society. A disturbing finding, and this applies not only to waiters, shopkeepers or clerks but also to teachers, doctors, nurses, ambulancemen and fire-fighters who are normally committed to their tasks (Table 27.4).

This is a very significant social reversal and one that tells much on the fear of nuclear war. One's principal obligation becomes one's own immediate family; social

Table 27.4 Whether those in work would go to work during the emergency

	Go to work?		
	Yes	No	
Public sector			
Stay in London	27	41 ⎱	=100%
Try to leave	8	28 ⎰	Base = 157
Private sector			
Stay in London	12	40 ⎱	=100%
Try to leave	6	42 ⎰	Base = 199

GLAWARS

ties do not count. The very fabric of society becomes frayed and torn; indeed, it collapses.

In the same order of social disintegration, the Commission also noted a certain readiness to disobey consciously rules and governmental precepts—if, that is, any government survived, and to take matters into one's own hands. And all this, for a normally orderly, advanced, civic-minded population as Londoners. Yet, it is perhaps not an unexpected reaction when one considers that in a nuclear debacle 90% of the metropolis is expected to be totally destroyed, governance to be in shambles and out of control, and all known medical and social methods of treatment and survival to be totally inadequate.

It would take 185 years to rebuild the semblance of an organized city, if, that is, that were possible.

27.11 Conclusions

This is the 60th "anniversary" of the tragic use of the atom bomb. Since then humankind has had the common sense and decency of averting such madness. But the danger is not altogether gone. The earlier, wiser measures of an international Non-Proliferation Treaty are being eroded, governments are lightly talking of nuclear accidents, nuclear terrorism is becoming increasingly cheaper and possible and old rusting facilities and warheads are sitting there as a constant source of catastrophe.

If such catastrophe happened, if there was nuclear war, wreckage would be incalculable, society would be disintegrated and disease and suffering would be rampant. No amount of help or response would meet the enormous needs in all fields, in health and in societal order. It would be somewhat academic to distinguish between the uninjured and the injured, from disorder to total social breakdown. After nuclear conflict, all systems and all survivors would be casualties in a final epidemic.

It can still happen. To avoid such misery and irreparable collapse, the World Health Organization has concluded that the only way is to avoid nuclear conflict. The International Association for Humanitarian Medicine totally agrees and, with Professors Russell, Einstein and Rotblat implores, "Remember your Humanity."

Bibliography

Abrams H.L.: Medical supply and demand in a post-nuclear world. In: The Medical Implications of Nuclear War, Solomon F. and Marston R.Q., eds. National Academy Press, Washington, 1986.

Bruce M., Milne T., eds: Ending the War: The Force of Reason, MacMillan Press, London, 1999.

Clarke R., Ehrlich A., Gunn S.W., et al.: London Under Attack: Report of the GLAWARS Commission, Blackwell, Oxford, 1986.

Clarke R., Gunn S.W.: Attacco alla Città, Guida, Palermo, 1987.

Gunn S.W.A.: Effects of nuclear war on health. Ann. Burn Fire Disasters, 1: 175–180, 1988.

Gunn S.W.A.: The inaugural Sir Joseph Rotblat Lecture. J. Humanitarian Med., 5:43–47, 2005.

Hinde R., Rotblat J.: War No More: Eliminating Conflict in the Nuclear Age, Pluto Press, London, 2003.

Rotblat J.: Pugwash and the nuclear issue. Pugwash Newsletter, 38: 46–51, 2001.

Rotblat J.: Scientists, doctors and nuclear war. J. Humanitarian Med., 5: 29–31, 2005.

Wittner L.S.: Towards Nuclear Abolition: A History of the World Nuclear Disarmament Movement, 1971 to the Present, Stanford University Press, Stanford, 2003.

United Nations: Attack on the city (Review). UNDRO News, 3: 23, 1988.

World Health Organization: Effects of Nuclear War on Health and Health Services, 2nd ed., WHO, Geneva, 1987.

World Health Organization: Health and environmental aspects of nuclear weapons. Report of the Director-General to the 46th World Health Assembly, WHO, Geneva, 1993.

World Health Organization: WHO Emergency Health Kit, 1984. New edition 1998. WHO, Geneva.

Chapter 28
Avoidable Tragedy Post-Chernobyl—A Critical Analysis

Rosalie Bertell, PhD, GNSH

28.1 Introduction

Journalists and mathematicians have a way of focusing on one aspect of a complex situation in order to give a snapshot view of its magnitude. For example, one might read in the newspaper that a "six alarm fire" had occurred in some neighbourhood. This immediately conjures up the image of a very large fire requiring six fire stations to send trucks to the scene. It gives one no clue as to the magnitude of loss of life or property, the water or smoke damage, the impact on human lives and health, ecological impact, and so on. Another example is that of a television show rating scale. If you see an estimate of five million viewers of some special event on television, you immediately understand that this is a "rounded number" meant for comparison only and which does not reveal how many people actually watched the show. Certainly, some televisions played to an empty room and some to a large number of people watching the display in the local pub. It gives no indication of whether the watchers reacted positively or negatively to the programme. If the event is important, we expect professionals to fill in the details later.

Another misleading human custom is presenting an event as "small" when there exist more traumatic forms of the event. For example, the radiation exposure to depleted uranium in the Gulf War is presented as "small" in the face of a nuclear holocaust. Such exposure is not "small" for the victims.

Unfortunately, many government officials, physicists, engineers, and others have used this tactic to deliberately minimize the health effects of radiation and, in particular, the immense suffering after the 1986 Chernobyl disaster. For example, some people actually believe that the magnitude of a nuclear accident can be gauged by the potential number of cancer deaths it will cause and, further, that cancer death is the only consequence! Minimalist reporting occurred after the Three Mile Island (TMI) accident, downwind of nuclear weapon testing, and at serious military accidents like the one which spread plutonium in farmland in Spain. Most recently, it has attempted to deny that exposure to depleted uranium weapons has caused severe health damage to the military veterans and the civilians in Iraq, Kosovo, and, most likely, in Afghanistan.

The minimalist reporting went even further with Chernobyl. The IAEA (International Atomic Energy Agency) and UNSCEAR (United Nations Scientific

Committee on the Effects of Atomic Radiation) recent statement that "only 32 deaths occurred, 200 were heavily irradiated and 2000 avoidable thyroid cancers" resulted from the Chernobyl disaster goes well beyond a mathematical short hand which gives an immediate sketch about a disaster. This 15-years-later report about a complex painful situation should be much more precise and believable! It rather tries to obliterate from people's minds and concerns the suffering of millions of persons in rural and unevacuated areas who were exposed, and hundreds of thousands evacuated but not medically examined victims. When one probes a little more deeply, one finds that the honest scientists and physicians, trying to explain the widespread injuries and long-term effects of nuclear exposure, have been silenced.

In fact, immediately after the disaster of 26 April 1986 due to IAEA policy, unless a person had been declared "overexposed" at the medical tent set up for the "liquidators" of the disaster, he or she was officially considered to be a "radio-phobia" case, a purely psychological phenomenon. Local physicians told people that there would be no medical effects of exposure, until, perhaps in 10 or 20 years, they might happen to develop cancer. But not to worry! These future radio-genic cancers would be indistinguishable from "natural" cancers. The physicians soon learned from direct evidence of pathological injuries that this information from the physicists was less than candid. It was not surprising to learn that those who tried to minimize the disaster were the same people charged with promoting nuclear industries, for example, marketing nuclear reactors to the developing nations.

The experience of Chernobyl is not unique but follows the secrecy pattern used at many lesser accidents which were mishandled in the same way. This has occurred both in the developed and the developing world. In particular, I would note the radioactive pollution of the Mitsubishi Asian Rare Earth facility in Bukit Merah, Malaysia, the radioactive waste dumped in Nigeria, and the contaminated food distributed to Egypt, Papua New Guinea, India, and other countries during the Chernobyl disaster clean-up.

However, the health problems due to Chernobyl continue to be very acute right now and demand international attention and action. Scientists and physicians are deprived of their freedom, and people, especially children, are suffering. This crisis can serve to point out the serious secrecy, vested interest, and collusion of international agencies protecting nuclear technologies. The public face of the nuclear industry has been "clean and safe." It is important and fair to unmask this public face, serving as a warning to economically developing countries deciding on energy technologies and bringing needed humanitarian aid to the victims. Preserving the false image of nuclear technology keeps the industry and nuclear agencies in business.

28.2 Lessons from Hiroshima and Nagasaki

Unlike the general study of toxic materials, handled by toxicologists, the field of radiation and health has been dominated by physicists, engineers, and mathematicians since the dawn of the nuclear era in 1943. Their health-related communications differ radically in content from similar communications of health professionals in toxicology, occupational health, or public health.

This field or radiation health was, with a few exceptions, taken over by the physicists of the Manhattan Project after World War II in their effort to contain the secrets of the nuclear age. Radiation was an effect of the atomic bomb. Secrecy caused these "hard scientists" to fail to consider the broad range of responses and varieties of vulnerabilities possessed by a living population exposed to this hazard. Such variation in biological responses would have been expected by health professionals.

Because of Hiroshima and Nagasaki, most people now know about acute radiation exposure syndrome, with vomiting, hair falling out, alterations in blood cells, and so on, and this bit of information has been translated into a naive belief on the part of the public that unless acute radiation sickness has been documented (often by the government physicists) any subsequent severe illness observed in radiation-exposed persons is due to something, anything, but not radiation exposure. This has some historical validity, but at Chernobyl, with millions of exposed persons in rural unevacuated areas, with hundreds of thousands evacuated but not medically examined, and with the population's continuous ingestion of contaminated foods for the past 15 years, demanding documentation of radiation sickness is ridiculous. Even in the Japanese cities, radiation sickness went undocumented for many victims. Radiation injury is not predicated on documentation of acute radiation sickness, but rather on the alteration of a cell leading to a fatal cancer. It is well documented that these cellular level events can occur well below the level of exposure which causes overt sickness. The amount of energy released by just one nuclear transformation of one atom of a radioactive material is measured in thousands or millions of electron volts. It requires only 6–10 eV to break the molecular bounds in the cellular DNA and RNA which carry the genes for life.

In Hiroshima and Nagasaki (1945), exposure and subsequent health records were not complete. The research stations did not begin to select a study population until after the 1950 Japanese census identified survivors and a 1967 dose estimate was derived by the scientists at Oak Ridge National Laboratory in the US deaths prior to 1950 were ignored. Death certificates, which were at times incomplete, were used to determine the first cause of death of the study population. Cancers that were not fatal were not reported until 1994. Most survivors are still alive so their "cause of death" has not yet been studied. Other non-cancer health problems were considered to be "not of concern" and have not been systematically reported.

There were persons who entered the contaminated territories of Hiroshima and Nagasaki after the fire died down, or who consumed radioactive food and water and experienced radiation sickness, but were not officially recognized as "exposed." They are in the radiation exposure control group. This is easily explained to the mathematician, who is told that the Hiroshima and Nagasaki studies looked for the effects of the immediate penetrating radiation from the exploding bomb on the persons who were within 3 km of the hypocentre at that moment. For the military person looking for information on the health effects of radiation due to the bomb, this artificial limitation made some sense.

However, if a civil society is seeking information on the effects of man-made radiation on the human body, then all sources of that man-made radiation, including that from nuclear fallout, food and water contamination, residual radioactive debris at the bomb site, are important. Changing the definition of "exposed to man-made radiation" to mean "exposed to the bomb" and then using this research to back public and occupational health policy is problematic, to say the least! Because of this concentration on the first flash of the atomic bomb, serious mistakes have been made by the radiation physicists in estimating the biological damage done by ingested or inhaled radioactive particles, many of which remain in the body for a long time and even enter into biochemical reactions of the cell's genetic material.

It is this atomic bomb study which appears to be dictating much of the inappropriate behaviour of officials with respect to the medical treatment of survivors of Chernobyl and other nuclear accidents. It has also caused harsh treatment of the honest scientists and physicians who spoke directly for the needs of the exposed suffering people. Many of these scientists and physicians, now in prison or effectively silenced, have conducted well-designed and well-executed scientific studies.

Due to the complications generated by the study of external irradiation by a bomb being used to evaluate civilian exposures to inhaled or ingested radioactivity and the use of this research to educate young physicists and nuclear engineers, many scientific blunders and administrative problems were generated. The failure to deal with the whole breadth of radiation problems became entrenched in the very agencies which were created in the 1950s to protect the public at risk from atmospheric nuclear testing. I will try to unravel the problems with the IAEA, the UNSCEAR, the International Commission on Radiological Protection (ICRP), the US National Academy of Science Biological Effects of Ionizing Radiation Committee (BEIR), and the World Health Organization (WHO). All of these organizations except WHO, which was relegated to treating the victims rather than understanding the problem, play key parts with respect to current radiation and public health policies and understandings. Ironically, the WHO, created by the United Nations in 1948, was not given any role in the health assessment of this global threat to human and ecological health.

28.3 United Nations Initiatives

Nuclear bombs were first used in war in 1945, when the United States used them against Japan in Hiroshima and Nagasaki. As early as 1946, the United States began atmospheric testing of nuclear bombs in the Marshall Islands in the Pacific Ocean. The former Soviet Union demonstrated that it had the nuclear bomb in 1949, and there was tangible fear of a nuclear exchange during the Korean War. The United Kingdom began nuclear weapon testing off the coast of Australia in the 1950s and then on the continent itself and in the Pacific Islands. The first atomic bombs were based on fission, and because of this, they were limited in their destructive power. The force of the explosion blew apart the fissioning materials, terminating the explosive energy release. In 1954, the United States tested a thermonuclear device (hydrogen bomb), called Bravo, at Bikini Atoll in the Marshall Islands, demonstrating that a nuclear device with unlimited power could be built. This one was about one thousand times more powerful than the Hiroshima bomb. It was this military accomplishment which prompted the "Peaceful Atom" speech of President Dwight Eisenhower before the United Nations in 1954.

The speech followed a shift in US military policy to dependence on nuclear bombs and a rush towards production of uranium and the technology necessary to carry out a major weapon replacement programme: uranium mining and milling, uranium-processing facilities, nuclear fuel fabrication facilities, nuclear production reactors, reprocessing facilities, and the hazardous transportation and waste associated with each of these industries. In order to obtain American and global co-operation during peacetime, there was a perceived need for commercial or the so-called peaceful uses of nuclear technologies which would justify everyone's co-operation in the nation and the international community. Nuclear electrical production was billed as capable of fulfilling all of the energy needs of the developing world, and being "too cheap to meter." It was promoted as the hope of preventing future wars since no country would be in need!

The United Nations responded by creating, in 1955, UNSCEAR (Res. 913(X) 1955) to "assess and report levels and effects of exposure to ionizing radiation." According to the UNSCEAR website, "governments and organizations throughout the world rely on the Committee's estimates as the scientific basis for evaluating radiation risk, establishing radiation protection and safety standards, and regulating radiation exposure." UNSCEAR was envisioned as an organization of physicists, who at that time were the only ones who could measure radiation since it escapes our senses and requires specialized instruments for detection.

They were the experts on the hazard of ionizing radiation, but failed to have the expertise to predict the varied human response to exposure to this hazard. In an odd way, perhaps because of their training in physics, they managed to average all exposures over the entire population of the world, some six billion people. Natural background, because it is ubiquitous, rather homogeneously exposes everyone. However, a localized accident or relatively small work force's exposure, when averaged over the whole population, can be made to seem trivial. It is not trivial to those who receive the exposure!

UNSCEAR became primarily a reporting agency, detailing the measurement of radioactive fallout, worker exposures, and eventually emissions from nuclear power plants. I would assume that legislators saw this agency as providing independent monitoring of nuclear activities as a check on predicted pollution and theoretical estimates of harm. Unfortunately, UNSCEAR incorporated into its midst those same scientists who were making the predications and estimating "no harm from low-level radiation." No other industry is allowed to monitor itself. We do not ask the tobacco companies to tell us about tobacco's harm or the pesticide companies to tell us the effects of their products on children. More on this point later.

In 1957, in response to the "Peaceful Atom" speech, the United Nations also established IAEA, which is described as "an independent intergovernmental, science- and technology-based organization, in the U.N. family, that serves as the global focus point for nuclear corporation." Its mandate is described as follows: "to promote peaceful uses of nuclear technology, develop safety standards, and verify that

nuclear weapon technology did not spread horizontally to the non-nuclear Nations."
They had no mandate with respect to the nuclear weapons of the five nuclear states.
Because of their nuclear watch-dog task, IAEA reports directly to the UN Security
Council.

28.4 Response of the World Health Organization

In 1957, the WHO, which had been founded by the United Nations in 1948, became
alarmed about the atmospheric nuclear testing and the proposed expansion of this
technology for "peaceful uses." It called together eminent geneticists to consider
the threat this exposure would pose to the human and ecological gene pool. Prof.
Hermann Muller, the geneticist who received a Nobel Prize for his work on genetic
mutations of the fruit fly, using ionizing radiation, in 1944, was a participant at this
conference. Although the United States had not sent him as its delegate, he received
a standing ovation at the conference for his work, and he consistently opposed extension of nuclear technology into civilian uses. The conclusion of this expert group
was that there was not enough information available in the scientific community to
assure the integrity of future generations, should the burden of ionizing radiation
exposure be increased. They called for extreme caution and further genetic investigations, especially in Kerala, India, where there is a high natural background level
of radiation, and people have lived in this environment for hundreds of years. These
recommendations were never implemented by governments anxious to get on with
nuclear activities.

Later, an independent NGO in India studied genetic damage in the high-radiation
background area and found it indeed significantly increased. An article by B.A.
Bridges in *Radiation Research* (vol. 156, 631–641, 2001) suggests that genetic
mutations due to radiation imply that "the nature of the radiation dose response
cannot be assumed." There is more complexity than was expected in the health consequences of changed DNA sequences. The serious implications of nuclear pollution
for future generations are still an area of research demanding more than ordinary
caution. One can guess at the politics behind a second WHO conference, called later
in 1957, of psychiatrists to consider the public health impact of peaceful nuclear
activities. These professionals concluded that such activities could cause undue
stress to the population because of the association with atomic bombs. One finds
that this has become a mantra for the physicists who have subsequently controlled
all information relative to the health impact of nuclear technologies. Most recently,
when UNSCEAR released its 15-year assessment of the Chernobyl disaster, one
of its spokespersons, Dr Neil Wald, Professor of Occupational and Environmental
Health at the University of Pittsburgh School of Public Health, stated, "It is important that public misperceptions be reduced as much as possible in this area, because
unwarranted perception and fear of harm can itself produce avoidable health problems, as well as erroneous societal benefit vs risk judgements." Loosely translated,
Dr Wald appears to be saying, "if the public gets upset we will not be able to make
our money with this nuclear technology."

After the TMI accident in 1979, in response to the people's demand for a health study, the government organized a study headed by a psychiatrist from the Annapolis Naval Academy. He drew concentric circles around the failed nuclear reactor and compared the cancer rates and also the levels of fear and tension of those living within these layers. A sensible study would have looked downwind for airborne radionuclide effects and downstream for the waterborne effects. This official study found only fear, which was positively correlated with distance from the plant.

There were about 2,000 injury cases from the TMI population taken to court for compensation of health damage due to the radiation exposure. The nuclear company fought all the way to the US Supreme Court against the courts even hearing these cases, and lost. Then the industry found an old law stating that an expert witness must use the methodology used by other professionals in their field, and using this, the nuclear company managed to disqualify every expert witness (physicians, epidemiologists, botanists, biologists) brought in by the victims. The physicists and engineers claimed sole expertise in the area of radiation health effects. All cases were dismissed by the court without one being heard.

28.5 A 1959 Deal Between WHO and IAEA

This potential conflict between those who wished to exploit the new nuclear technology for both profit and military power and the custodians of public health was superficially resolved.

28.5.1 III—Disasters

Agreement (Res.WHA 12–40, 28 May 1959) stating that the IAEA and the WHO recognize that "the IAEA has the primary responsibility for encouraging, assisting, and co-ordinating research on, and development and practical applications of, atomic energy for peaceful uses throughout the world without prejudice to the right of the WHO to concern itself with promoting, developing, assisting, and co-ordinating international health work, including research, in all its aspects." If the reader is confused, so is the writer. To understand this, one needs to know that the health effects of radiation were classified as secret under the US Atomic Energy Act for national security. The "international health work" assigned to the WHO was taking care of the victims. While technically IAEA and WHO are "equal" in the UN family, those agencies which report directly to the Security Council, as does IAEA, have more status.

In Article I (3) of theWHO/IAEA agreement, it is stated that "Whenever either organization proposes to initiate a programme or activity on a subject in which the other organization has or may have a substantial interest, the first party shall consult with the other with a view to adjusting the matter by mutual consent." This clause seems to have weakened the WHO from investigating the Chernobyl disaster and gave the IAEA a green light to bring in physicists and medical radiologists to assess the damage relative to their limited knowledge of the health effects of radiation. (Note: while radiologists use ionizing radiation in their work, they deal with health damage only after the patient receives therapy levels of radiation.) This first evaluation used a different epidemiological protocol in each geographical area and with different age groups, eliminated all concern for cancers as not having sufficient latency periods, and failed to note the extraordinary epidemic of thyroid diseases and cancers. From the point of view of medical epidemiology, they failed miserably to deal with the reality. The director of this 1991 epidemiological study, Dr Fred Mettler, is a medical radiologist. There were no epidemiologists, public health professionals, or toxicologists on the IAEA team.

28.6 The Self-established ICRP

UNSCEAR has continued to be the measurement agency, which verifies that all planned releases of ionizing radiation to the environment and all exposures of workers are "acceptable." It fell to the IAEA to "establish or adopt, in collaboration with other competent international bodies, standards of safety for the protection of health and to provide for the application of these standards."

Neither the IAEA nor UNSCEAR turned to the WHO to develop such protective health standards. Instead, they both turned to a self-appointed non-governmental organization formed by the physicists of the Manhattan Project together with the medical radiologists, who had organized themselves in 1928 to protect themselves and their colleagues from the severe consequences of exposure to medical X-ray. This new organization, called the ICRP, has a Main Committee of 13 persons who make all decisions. Members of this Main Committee were originally self-appointed and have been perpetuated by being proposed by current members and accepted by the current executive committee. No outside agency can place a member on the ICRP, not even the WHO.

The UNSCEAR 2000 Report was prepared by a Committee including seven persons who also serve on the 13-person Main Committee of ICRP. It is the ICRP that makes recommendations for the protection of human health for workers and the general public. By their own admission, they are not a public or environmental health organization. They have given themselves the task of recommending a trade-off of predictable health effects of exposure to radiation for the benefits of nuclear activities (including the production and testing of nuclear weapons). Their recommendations were first set in 1957, when the medical radiologists accepted the proposal which had been hammered out by the British, Canadian, and American physicists after World War II.

The original recommendation that workers be allowed 15 rad (150 mSv) per year was opposed by the British and an independent committee called the BEAR (Biological Effects of Atomic Radiation) funded in the United States by the Rockefeller Foundation. This forced the nuclear workers to 5 rad (50 mSv) per year. Maximum permissible doses for members of the public were ten times lower. This recommendation remained in effect until 1990, when under pressure from more than 700 scientists and physicians and after a reassignment of doses at the atomic bomb research centres, the worker exposure was reduced to 2 rad (20 mSv) per year, while exposures to the public were reduced by another factor of 5 to 0.1 rad (1 mSv) per year.

28.7 Who Takes Responsibility?

It is important to note that no agency takes responsibility for these recommendations, and the WHO is excluded from professional collaboration or comment on them. ICRP recommends, and the Nations are free to implement or not these recommendations. The Nations generally accept ICRP recommendations claiming that they do not have the expertise or money to derive their own standards. The recommendations are for a risk benefit trade-off and do not pretend to be based solely (or primarily) on protecting the public or worker health.

The IAEA states, "The underlying biological basis of the standards over the last several decades has rested primarily on UNSCEAR. This Committee was originally formed during the period of atmospheric weapon testing to assess the physical processes and health effects of fallout, but has since broadened its remit considerably."

UNSCEAR contains and depends on the leaders of the Main Committee of ICRP. Those who set the standards also judge them to be adequate! Usually scientific theory is tested against reality and rejected if it fails to conform. Radiation health predictions are tested against the reality of the victims, and if reality fails to conform to theory, reality is rejected. The suffering is blamed on some unknown cause! Another body that also assesses radiation risk is the BEIR Committee of the US National Academy of Science. The Committee was established in the United States around 1978 to counter accusations that the Nevada atmospheric nuclear tests had caused the deaths of thousands of American babies. BEIR is essentially a report and interpretation of the Hiroshima and Nagasaki studies of the effects of the atomic bomb, as previously discussed. These atomic bomb studies do not underpin the radiation standards, which actually were established some 17 years before the 1967 dose assessment for atomic bomb survivors on which the atomic bomb studies are based was completed.

IAEA radiation standards for nuclear waste were made "on the basis of recommendations by a number of international bodies, principally ICRP," and estimations of radiation risks made by UNSCEAR. IAEA Safety Requirements for radioactive waste, including standards, codes of practice, regulations, "may be adopted by Member States at their own discretion for use nationally." These IAEA requirements are mandatory *only* for the IAEA itself.

28.8 What Happened to the People of Chernobyl?

One can easily imagine that there were civilian victims of radiation sickness in the midst of the chaos during and after the Chernobyl disaster who were never seen at Hospital Six in Moscow! However, the IAEA continues, even in 2002, to insist that only 32 persons died of radiation exposure at Chernobyl! These "counted" deaths were all men from the firefighting brigade identified as seriously exposed and sick by the heroic physicians and other health personnel at the emergency medical tent near the crippled reactor. This type of counting goes even further than the usual mathematical and journalistic approach—it deliberately and maliciously minimizes the scale of this disaster and leaves the public vulnerable. Those who were exposed suffer without appropriate medical recognition and help, while those at a distance remain unprepared for another, perhaps worse, disaster.

Moreover, since the land contaminated by the failed reactor was poisoned, the fruits and vegetables grown on it, and the domestic animals that feed on it, and their milk and meat are also contaminated. Russia, Ukraine, and Belarus have taken this contaminated food and, with the advice of the IAEA, have mixed it with uncontaminated food from other parts of the former Soviet Union. This diluted (or adulterated) food has been given to the people to eat, subjecting them to continuous low doses of internal contamination with radionuclides for the last 20 years. In Belarus, people actually received money from the government for moving back onto the badly contaminated areas and setting up new farms.

The false claims of the IAEA have also failed to rally the international community to help the victims of this disaster. People have not responded internationally, with their characteristic generosity, to the tremendous needs of the people whose health and lives were cruelly disrupted.

The IAEA and its companion body, UNSCEAR, have gone even further, in the spring of 2002, by recommending that Chechen and Central Asian refugees re-populate the still contaminated area around the failed reactor. This raises some very serious questions about the mismanagement of information and communication around this serious disaster.

These two UN bodies, namely IAEA and UNSCEAR (and their partner the ICRP), have apparently supplanted the WHO in speaking to the health risks of this nuclear technology, and in particular, to the post-Chernobyl contamination of the people and the land. Whether or not this land is fit for inhabitation or for food production requires health assessment, not a promotional OK from two agencies which have financial ties to the polluting industry!

The WHO tried to take some initiative on behalf of the suffering people, and in 1996, its director-general, Dr Hiroshi Nakajima, organized in Geneva an international conference with 700 scientific experts and physicians, many of whom came from Russia, Belarus, and Ukraine. The IAEA, which to its dismay was not invited to jointly sponsor this international conference, nevertheless blocked publication of the proceedings.

The physicians of Chernobyl then organized a conference in Kiev, Ukraine, in June 2001, and invited Dr Nakajima (who was no longer director-general of WHO) to be their Honorary President. He was asked about the proceedings of the 1996 WHO Conference about the health of the Chernobyl victims which had never been published. He answered as follows, "I was the Director-General and I was responsible. But it is mainly my legal department... Because the IAEA reports directly to the Security Council of the United Nations. And we, all specialized organizations, report to the Economic and Social Development Council. The organization which reports to the Security Council—not hierarchically, we are all equal—but for atomic affairs . . . military use . . . and peaceful or civil use . . . they have the authority."

Because of the internal UN structure on Chernobyl, which is grossly out of date, the voices of the physicians and scientists actually dealing with the situation were not heard. It is outrageous to measure the radiation and then present a theory that no one has been hurt! It is imperative to look at the victims and assess their injury. Internationally, the theoretical voice of the ICRP, an NGO, which speaks through the IAEA and UNSCEAR, has prevailed! All three agencies have a vested interest in maintaining the reputation of nuclear industries as "clean and cheap," even if they are not! The representative of the UN Office for Humanitarian Affairs, D. Zupka, was present at the Kiev Conference, and he shared with participants the view of Kofi Annan, who estimated that the number of victims of Chernobyl is nine million! They are predicting that this number will increase. However, their voice is overpowered by the "scientific" voice of the ICRP speaking through the IAEA and UNSCEAR. This seems incredible, but it is the heavy burden which we suffer as a legacy of nuclear secrecy.

Because of the self-serving theoretical predictions and safety recommendations of the ICRP which colour the expectations of these radiologists, physicists, and engineers, even when they are confronted with the reality of the suffering of the Chernobyl victims, these scientists strongly declare that the observed health problems could not be due to the radiation exposure. Health problems are instead assigned to an unidentified factor in the environment or lifestyle. The director of the IAEA at the time of the Chernobyl disaster went so far as to say, "The atomic industry can take catastrophes like Chernobyl every year." There is an obvious conflict of interest for this agency mandated to promote nuclear technologies!

At the Kiev Conference, Alexey Yablokov, president of the Centre for Political Ecology of the Russian Federation, pointed out that the data used by UNSCEAR had been falsified by the State Committee for Statistics, and the officials were arrested in 1999 for this crime. He charged that UNSCEAR continued to use these falsified data to support its minimization of harm.

The medical research of Prof. Y. Bandazhevsky, a medical pathologist, Rector of the Medical Institute of Gomel, in Belarus, had to be presented by a colleague, Prof. Michel Fernex, as Prof. Bandazhevsky was under house arrest. Belarus received the heaviest fallout from the Chernobyl disaster. After 9 years of research in Chernobyl-contaminated territories, he had discovered that caesium 137 incorporated in food leads to destruction of those vital organs where the caesium 137 concentrates at higher than average body levels. With his wife, a paediatric cardiologist, Bandazhevsky described what he called "caesium cardiomyopathy," which others say is a syndrome which will eventually be named after him. The cardiac damage becomes irreversible at a certain level and duration of the caesium intoxication. Sudden death may occur at any age, even in children. After publishing this finding, denouncing government non-intervention policy, and arguing against the lack of resources given to the medical investigation of the disaster, Bandazhevsky was arrested, tried, and condemned to prison for 8 years.

The trial of Prof. Bandazhevsky was observed by lawyers from the Organization for Security and Co-operation in Europe (OSCE), from the French Embassy in

Minsk, and from Amnesty International. These observers documented irregularities and legal errors from the time of his arrest. In the middle of the night of 13 July 1999, Prof. Bandazhevsky was arrested by a group of police officers, who informed him that the arrest was by presidential decree aimed at fighting terrorism. This was never charged in court. In fact, it was not until 4 weeks after his arrest, August 1999, that he finally charged with taking bribes. These proved to be trumped-up charges by two defendants who later recanted their testimony saying it was forced under duress and threats. Prof. Bandazhevsky was denied access to a lawyer for the entire duration of his detention, and during the trial, there were serious breaches of Belarussian and international law. Amnesty International has listed Prof. Bandazhevsky as a prisoner of conscience. He is not well, and his important research is being kept from his scientific and medical colleagues.

Professor Bandazhevsky is not alone. The Russian, Belarussian, and Ukrainian medical communities, though silenced in international circles, were still present and active in alleviating the suffering and noting the causes of their people's pain. Many have carried out detailed high-quality scientific studies on the genetic, teratogenic, and somatic damage done by radiation exposure. They have confirmed their analyses by demonstrating the effects in animal experiments. The rest of the world is being deprived of this research through heavy-handed silencing of the scientists by their national authorities, acting on the recommendations of the IAEA and UNSCEAR (and especially ICRP).

28.9 Recommendations as Conclusions

While many individuals have been trying to make known this disaster and major UN problem, it has been difficult to get this complex situation across to the public in "sound bites." Serious study on the part of the United Nations will be needed to undo all of the damage caused. However, it seems possible to make the following recommendations to the United Nations.

1. WHO should be mandated to review all radiation research and to recommend health-based safety regulations. This mandate should be carried out by health professionals, including epidemiologists, oncologists, occupational and public health specialists, geneticists, and paediatricians (not linked with the nuclear industries or nuclear medicine) rather than other scientists.
2. The IAEA mandate to promote "peaceful nuclear technologies" should be withdrawn.
3. The IAEA mandate to safeguard the spread of nuclear weapons should be expanded to include monitoring the reduction and abolition of all nuclear weapons in the nuclear nations.
4. The UNSCEAR mandate needs to include the monitoring of increasing levels of background radiation and nuclear emissions from reactors and nuclear accidents. They should not be entrusted with estimating risk, which is the prerogative of the WHO.

5. Decisions relative to the safety of farmland, food and water ingestion, and refugee relocation should be entrusted to the WHO.
6. Investigation into the imprisonment of scientists and physicians who have spoken out on behalf of public health relative to radiation exposure should be undertaken by a special rapporteur of the UN Human Rights Council in Geneva.

Part V
Science, Research and Perspectives

Chapter 29
The Role of Science to Improve the Quality of Life: Reflections on the Post-Genomic Era

Anthony Piel, LLD

As we consider the role of science in the 21st century, let me start with a quotation from the 19th century ascribed to that great scientist, Alexander von Humboldt (1769–1859), who encouraged "that scientific conspiracy of nations which is one of the noblest fruits of modern civilization."

Humboldt worked at the boundaries of the science of his day, in pursuit of an ever-moving frontier of knowledge at the cutting-edge and state-of-the-art science, with innovation and commitment to progress.

In this perspective, I hope to bring a view from the World Health Organization (WHO), which I have served for a quarter century in various functions, from law, planning, and administration. I am neither a scientist nor a medical doctor, but I have worked with and admired many. So, I will address the general context of progress, not the technical specifics.

I will divide my remarks into roughly five parts: (1) the origins of WHO and the "Health for All" movement, with emphasis on Primary Health Care and research; (2) the pioneering role of countries in that movement and the challenge of harnessing the power of science, technology and medicine for the attainment of "Health for All"; (3) the WHO/Advisory Committee on Health Research (ACHR) "Research Policy Agenda for Science and Technology to Support Global Health Development; (4) the geopolitical and economic environment of research in the post-genomic era"; and (5) some scientific promises and opportunities at the sub-cellular level for accurate diagnosis and effective treatment of certain major conditions of ill health, which are of increasing global importance.

WHO was established on the heels of World War II, as a "specialized agency" related to but legally independent of the United Nations. The Constitutional idea was that WHO should be "the directing and co-ordinating authority on international health work," but maintaining a degree of independence from the United Nations would avoid the previous strategic mistake of tying the fate of the health arm of the League of Nations too closely to the main political body. The central idea was to depoliticize science and medicine. Almost as a direct result of this, WHO's governing body, the World Health Assembly, has always had more Member States (as many as 193) than has the UN General Assembly.

However, "health" has turned out to be one of the more politicized issues in our time. The first three directors-general of WHO (Drs Brock Chisholm of Canada,

Marcolino Candau of Brazil, and Halfdan Mahler of Denmark) built WHO into a major technical co-operation agency in international health work, with six Regional Offices, WHO Representative Offices in 110 countries, health programmes with all countries, a biennial budget of $1.7 billion, a staff of 5,500 including some 1,500 medical doctors and scientists, plus several thousand experts and consultants working with WHO worldwide each year. In co-operation with Member countries, WHO carries out a wide range of operational programmes in disease control, health systems development, and health promotion. WHO operates as the medical science agency of the UN system. WHO's keystone responsibility within that system is the transmission of knowledge necessary to health protection and development.

Research has become increasingly important in the work of WHO—consistent with its constitutional function "to promote and conduct research in the field of health." Two "Special" research programmes were launched in the 1970s: Human Reproduction Research (HRP) and Tropical Disease Research (TDR), because these were two areas of great importance that were likely to be overlooked by industry. Since then, there has been increasing emphasis on research, and this trend has continued under Directors-General Nakajima, Brundtland, and Lee, so that today there is an important research component integral to every major WHO programme.

In the 1970s, Director-General Dr Halfdan Mahler set WHO's sights on the ambitious global goal or target of attaining "Health for All." This expresses an equity principle, with the emphasis on "all"—given that "Health" is constantly moving target. The WHO Constitution states that "The objective of the World Health Organization shall be the attainment by all peoples of the highest possible level of health"—at any point in historical time. In 1978, a major international conference at Alma-Ata, attended by all Member States and major international organizations, confirmed the target of "Health for All" and declared that "Primary Health Care is the key to attaining this target." There are many different variations and attributes of "Primary Health Care," but if I had to boil it down to just five words, I would say, "PHC is democracy in health." With the setting of this operational goal of HFA/PHC, it became fully evident that the highest immediate priority of WHO and Member States alike had to be given to health system research and development in countries. All of us, in almost all nations of the world, have been beneficiaries of that strategic, global decision. This has been particularly true in developing countries, as the example of Thailand will show.

It is most impressive that in Thailand most major decisions about scientific and health system research and development have been taken openly, with full participation of the citizens, scientists, and health providers most affected. In the mid-1980s, several hundred Thai communities, both urban and rural, took part with health officials and personnel from Mahidol University, in developing and defining their own "Basic Minimum Needs" with agreed indicators of attainment, and identification of key initiating steps. Gradually a national consensus emerged, covering everything from nutrition, water, and housing to basic medical and social services, security, and even spiritual and cultural opportunity and freedom. These are not the kinds of things a central bureaucracy or financial interest group is likely to imagine and promulgate.

What has been striking about this experience has been the Thai democratic control over the health planning process.

To give just one example of the specificity of some Thai BMNs, here is the element of water within environmental health: "Every Thai family should have safe drinking water, defined as a minimum of 2 litres per person per day (of rainwater, filtered water, piped water, or pond water)." Having defined this "Basic Minimum Need element" of safe drinking water, it became the task of community, district, and national personnel to sit down and begin to identify the more specific actions, activities, and programmes necessary for attainment of at least this minimum, and in consequence, the knowledge, technology, research, training, and resources required. Although starting at the basic or primary level, the approach addressed the entire secondary and tertiary support network of the national health "system." Thai planning integrated public and private initiatives, but there is no doubt in my mind that leaving the determination of the "public good" to the vagaries of the "free" market enterprise system could not possibly have achieved the spectacular health development results we have witnessed in Thailand in the last three decades. I am sure that Thailand has helped shape WHO as much as WHO has helped Thailand. WHO has pursued these kinds of experiences in well over 100 countries. In doing so, we have had to learn, or re-learn, some basic truths.

One primordial, obvious lesson is that the success of even the most basic health initiatives is dependent on the supporting productivity of basic and applied scientific research. Often, today's dramatic scientific breakthrough becomes tomorrow's almost banal, but vitally necessary, diagnostic or therapeutic intervention. We have to make it affordable, available and acceptable to our citizens.

One of the Alma-Ata Declaration statements defines PHC as "essential health care based on practical, scientifically sound and socially acceptable methods and technology made universally accessible." PHC is not primitive medicine for the poor.

Another basic, obvious lesson is that our sheer success in basic health development places higher and higher demands on science and changes the kind of science and technology required. In many typical so-called developing countries, such as Thailand or Tunisia for example, we have witnessed a health indicator, such as average life expectancy at birth (taken as a proxy for good health, more than as a goal in itself), rise in a couple of short decades from around 40 years of age to well over 75 years of age now. As infant mortality rates decline, as traditional communicable and tropical diseases are better controlled, people live longer, to the point where the health system and supporting science have to contend more and more with burdensome conditions of ageing, industrialization, pollution, population, and effects of modern "lifestyle." The scientific and health communities have to deal, for example, with greater incidence of cardiovascular diseases, cancers, metabolic abnormalities, mental stress, and genetic disorders. Thus, we are faced with Lewis Carroll's dilemma of the "Red Queen": the scientific and health communities have to run faster and faster just to keep up!

Fortunately, the post-genomic era places new weapons at our disposal. In 2003, we celebrated the 50th anniversary of the discovery by Watson and Crick of the DNA double helix. The Human Genome Project has announced its completion of the "final draft" of the DNA sequence mapping for *Homo sapiens*. Suddenly, problems of health and ill health can be addressed at the subcellular level. We are seeing a veritable explosion in medical and scientific breakthroughs and corresponding potential for technological application in support of global health development. And this is accompanied by a revolution in informatics and communications technology.

The problem is how to stimulate, co-ordinate and exploit all this potential in support of global health. It goes without saying that no single organization, and certainly not the WHO alone, can do it all. No single country has all the answers.

And no one can dictate to scientists, at least not for long. By nature, scientists are inherently unmanageable. Many businessmen, politicians, and laymen probably think that the money carrot is the key to influence. True, our scientists are largely underpaid.

Yes, we should pay them better. But most scientists are driven, more than anything else, by personal intellectual, scientific curiosity.

From the WHO perspective, we cannot dictate to scientists—but maybe we can entice them. We can entice them if we can suggest that their personal scientific interest lines up with the global public interest.

There's one undeniable strength of WHO: as Nobel Prize Laureate Joshua Lederberg has said, "WHO possesses unique 'convening power' to call on the best brains in the world to help address major scientific, medical, and health development questions."

Indeed, WHO does have a plethora of scientific expert panels, expert committees, scientific groups, study groups, and collaborating centres. The highest-level scientific advisory body is the ACHR. Why not exercise that WHO "convening power" and ask them, the experts, how to "promote and conduct research" needed for global health development?

Enter Professor Theodor M. Fliedner, a distinguished scientist at Ulm University in Germany, a haematologist by training, and a pioneer in blood stem cell research and radiation medicine, a member and then Chairman of the WHO Advisory Committee on Health (and Medical) Research. In the late 1990s, Professor Fliedner and the members of the ACHR set about the task of developing and publishing a comprehensive "Research Policy Agenda for Science and Technology to Support Global Health Development." (Although the main Research Policy Agenda document is many hundreds of pages in length, a shorter "Synopsis" brochure is available. See WHO/RPS/ACHR/97-3.)

Briefly, the Agenda announced a vision for global health and a determination to pursue a more rational approach to scientific cooperation, as we enter the 21st century. The Agenda explores evolving problems of critical significance to global health. Chapter 4 deals with harnessing the power of science and technology and medicine and it describes tasks and challenges for the scientific community. The basic argument here is that evolving problems in health arise from a multiplicity of contributing factors; therefore, problem solution requires the combined inputs of a multiplicity of scientific disciplines, and it highlights the responsibility of the scientific community and other partners.

Chapter 5 of the Agenda goes into considerable detail on Research Imperatives and Opportunities in "Substantive domains," meaning, for example, communicable

diseases, constitutional diseases, impairments, health systems, family and reproductive health, environmental health, food and nutrition, mental health, and healthy
behaviour, for convenience discussed under five "health domains."

The main background document of the Research Policy Agenda goes into "substantive domains" in considerable detail—more than 30 pages. By way of example, diagnostic, therapeutic, and rehabilitative technology mentions everything from
coagulation microbiology to positron emission tomography. Why so much detail?
I think ACHR had two reasons in mind. First, to simply emphasize the truth: the
scientific development requirements to support global health are myriad, varied, and
complex. The second, related reason is that ACHR wished to counter the simplistic
notion held in some circles that it is only necessary to make a concerted, planned
effort with a few centrally defined global health priorities and let all other needs be
met by the normal workings of the "free" market private enterprise system. ACHR
is saying that all these needs are too urgent to just "laissez-faire."

Chapter 6 describes "Methodological needs." These include ways of analysing,
presenting, and interpreting data, modeling and simulation, "knowledge-based"
expert systems, constraint logic programming, as well as priority-setting and planning methodologies. One interesting method of data presentation is the "Visual
Health Information Profile" of a community, country, region or the world. Obviously, there is nothing sacrosanct about this methodology, but it is an innovative
way of saying a lot with few words, and it sits on top of a huge, detailed database.

Chapter 7 discusses a strategic concept for Implementation of the Research
Agenda System—a dynamic process of continuous planning, monitoring, course
adjustment, and action. In my opinion, the key to making operational the Research
Agenda is the establishment and systematic use of "Intelligent Research Networks"
(for convenience referred to as "IRENEs" although, as the saying goes, "a rose by
any other name . . ."). There is nothing "proprietary" intended about an "IRENE."
Indeed, many already exist.

But there are certain characteristics that ACHR wishes to stress about an IRENE.
An IRENE is a form of partnership, based on common purpose, and intended to take
advantage of modern science as well as information and communication technology,
to address research imperatives and opportunities in a rational way in order to bring
scientific and technological results expeditiously and co-operatively to the point of
application beneficial to human health, locally, nationally, and globally. IRENEs
offer scope or a "Planning Network for Health Research," or "Planet HERES."

An IRENE seizes opportunities for interactive planning among scientists and
others, research co-operation, financing, peer review, training, monitoring, quality
control, and evaluation.

It represents participation and openness in science. The use by the IRENE
of Internet and telecommunications technologies, including teleconferencing and
transmission of digital, graphic, imaging, and other forms of data, makes it possible
for scientific and health institutions and individuals to interact more quickly and
closely, without the necessity of always having to travel. This is especially beneficial to enhance co-operation among scientists and other partners in industrial and
industrializing countries—so that each can tap the energies, brains, and resources of
the other.

Before a formal IRENE can be established, it may be desirable for potential future partners to get together on a more informal basis, where they begin to develop understanding and working relationships, in full confidence of each other, in what has been described as the informal "Club" stage, which sets the groundwork for successful co-operation, that is, Competence, Creativity, Confidence, and Continuity. A more formal IRENE is then developed, bringing together individuals, scientific institutions, health planners, donors, and other partners. In some cases, one or more institutions may be willing and able to carry on certain "leading" functions, or act as regional "hubs," "focal points," or data bank holders, serving the larger network.

One way (of many) to initiate such an IRENE is to identify key players and organize a colloquium or other forms of meeting of experts and interested parties focused on a particular scientific or health objective or technology, a "Club stage" informal arrangement among persons having mutual confidence and shared purpose.

This can be followed up by high-level scientific exchanges, interactive demonstration or training courses and by institutional arrangements of a more formal nature. Fliedner, for example, has taken this approach through an "International Centre for Advanced Studies in Health Sciences and Services," known for short as "ICAS." Recently, ICAS has been offering advanced training courses in such diverse subject matters as epidemiology, clinical trials, diagnosis of acute illness, laboratory medicine, blood stem cell transplantation, and radiation accident management. Each of these ICAS courses has the making of an informal "Club stage" association, with potential for an enduring formal IRENE network, built around common purposes and technologies.

It is almost axiomatic to the thinking of an ACHR, and indeed it is the observed experience of WHO, that there is an enormous, sometimes untapped, wealth of brains, ideas, and experience in the scientific and health communities of virtually all countries, developed and developing. There is compelling need to bring this potential to bear on global health. What we have to nurture and promote is open science and the free communication of knowledge within and between all countries. There is the contrary view held in some circles that most scientific progress is assignable to just a few countries and that the transmission of knowledge is essentially "a one-way street." In fact, the reality is rather different, and the street runs two ways.

If you will allow me to indulge in a little friendly nepotism, let me mention my uncle, Gerard Piel. You may know of him as the founder and publisher of the modern Scientific American magazine, as we know it today. (Gerard Piel, by the way, has recently written a most interesting book entitled *The Age of Science—What Scientists Learned in the Twentieth Century*, Perseus Press, 2001.)

The experience of Scientific American is rather instructive. To date, the magazine has published the work of 81 Nobel prize winners, and this publication was done—and here is the point—before they received their recognition from Stockholm. That is quite a feather in someone's cap. It is also a reminder that the scientific community can recognize good scientific work long before the lay community or "officialdom" can take due notice. Another item: at a dinner for "The Nobel Prize-Winners in North America." Gerard Piel told the US President's Press Secretary, however, that they could not very well have a dinner for the "American" Nobel prize winners "on account of not all of them spoke English so good." Let me translate: at the time of the Kennedy Administration something like 80 % of all "American" Nobel prize winners in science had been born outside America. So, if there is a "one-way street," it is more like a "brain drain" in-bound. More telling, it suggests that brains are, and should be, transportable.

In defence of "my" country, the United States, I would look to the bright side: the key to American success has been (1) open science, (2) freedom to do research, (3) good communication, (4) good research facilities, and (5) availability of research funding.

Can we keep this progress up? Can we foster this kind of success everywhere? What does it take to promote good science worldwide? And what are the pitfalls we have to avoid in this post-genomic era of the 21st century? It is one thing to discuss the potential within the scientific and health development community. But we also have to address the ambient environment outside the scientific and health development community.

I am going to pick two interrelated issues: the rise of deregulated "free" market capitalism and the emergence of international terrorism. What do these developments, these "facts of life" in the new era, have to do with the future of science and health?

Ever since the collapse of the Soviet system, circa 1991, we have witnessed the extraordinary rise of deregulated "free" market capitalism, sometimes referred to as "globalization." In principle this should be a good thing. Access to up-front capital should spur large-scale industrial and economic development, create new markets, and create new jobs. This should mean greater demands on science and, therefore, more funding for scientific research. But does it?

My own "anecdotal" experience in country after country is that the imposition of deregulated "free" market capitalism in recent years has been doing at least as much harm as it has done good. As the bigger fish swallow up the smaller ones, still smaller enterprises suffer, economic disparities increase, and people lose jobs— all too often. In one Latin American country I visited recently, where giant malls and shopping centres are the new look, I had the impression that for every single "new" job created, about seven "mom and pop" jobs were lost. Furthermore, while a segment of consumers undoubtedly benefited from more and more, the majority of the population nevertheless could afford less and less.

In other words, the ideology of the deregulated "free" market systems is "out of sync" with the observed facts. In science, when a theory is "out of sync" and does not match the observed facts, the theory fails.

Now, is it "un-American" to call attention to observed facts? I would suggest that the burden is on the apologists for deregulation. The apologists have to contend with the harsh fact that in "my" country, in the last 2 years alone, more than 200 major US corporations have had to "re-state" their earnings (a euphemism for papering over fraudulent accounting practices) and prepare their legal defences to cover the actions of high-ranking corporate executives who have stolen from their own companies, misinformed the public, cheated their shareholders, evaded taxes, gouged the consumer public, destroyed employee benefits and pension funds, created unemployment, and practically ruined the US economy. These are harsh words for harsh facts.

In "the country I know best," there has been a significant drop in funding for education, training and scientific research, especially basic research. The largest US electrical company, for example, has abolished its research departments entirely, preferring instead to acquire new products and patents, not by research but by corporate takeover. Decisions about what products and patents to acquire are based on year-end corporate return on investment—not on an assessment of priority for long-term human well-being. (Why would a pharmaceutical company enjoying a patent monopoly on an existing drug pay for research to find a better one?) Scientists themselves are barely consulted. Most decision-making is done behind closed doors by senior executives, the very ones who have been engaging in the kind of malpractices just mentioned.

Are these the people best qualified to be making decisions about the future course of scientific research? The research departments of virtually all American universities are suffering from deep budget cuts. Government funding priorities are increasingly diverted elsewhere. Yes, we need the resources industry can generate, but only if scientists, health providers, and citizens have a say in decision-making.

Unfortunately, the ideology of the deregulated "free" market is not restricted to "my" country. "Free" market ideology is actively promoted by transnational corporations and international organizations, such as the International Monetary Fund, the World Bank, and the World Trade Organization—bodies that represent corporate interests, not science. Again, the initial advantages are there: up-front capital, grants and loans, fuelling large-scale projects.

But in all too many developing countries, "structural adjustment policies," so-called poverty alleviation programmes, "free" trade agreements, and other deals, struck with elitist interest groups behind closed doors, have had disastrous results, building up insurmountable debt, and "privatizing," that is to say, taking away people's land, water, air quality, food and agriculture, oil, and other mineral resources and wrecking small farms and businesses.

The small print in many "free trade" agreements requires the "benefiting" counties to surrender their resources to transnational "privatization." The losers are the ordinary citizens. For example, recently thousands of citizens in one South American country literally had to march in the streets, to force their government to buy back public water supply systems that had been taken over by foreign "investors," thanks to a World Bank leveraged buyout. Is this democracy? Is this how major decisions should be made about research and development? I think not. Scientists and health planners can do it better, with the support and co-operation of the private sector. Self-interest is not going to solve the world's ills. Democratic decision-making will.

The deregulated "free" market private enterprise corporate system is on a collision course with the socially responsible democratic health planning approach long advocated and practised by WHO and Member countries like Thailand. Recently, I had occasion to read a report on the US "Health System of the Future," presented to the US National Academy of Science, and others.

The report is full of enthusiastic declarations, information, and graphic presentations. But underlying all this is the notion that in the health system of the future the decision whether to offer a medical service or intervention will be based on its relative "profit margin," and determined by "free" market forces, rather than its relevance to the priority needs of the population served. This is dangerous stuff. It is common knowledge that "my" country, with the largest domestic product in the world, has the least affordable and most inequitable health care system among all so-called developed or industrialized countries; "enterprise" is based on corporate self-interest—as distinguished from what motivates scientists and health providers, which is duty to others ("Non sibi, sed cunctis"—"Not for oneself alone, but for others").

The warning is clear: Scientists, health providers, planners, and citizens must not abdicate their responsibility to society. They must not lie down in front of the juggernaut of deregulated, self-interested global capitalism. Health does not have to justify itself in economic terms. Rather, it is the other way around: economic policy must justify itself in human health and social development terms. If, in actual practice, "globalization" fails to meet this test, then we, the citizens of this Planet, have to take back ownership of the public good and slam the lid of regulation down on corporate and investor malpractice.

The other big issue looming on the horizon of this post-genomic era is the emergence of international terrorism and the war against it. The observed effect, of course, is to divert funds, interest, and energy away from humanitarian scientific research and development purposes and channel them towards military and security purposes. We are seeing this on a grand scale in "my" country, the United States, at the present time.

Unfortunately, the emergence of international terrorism, the culture of violence, and the triumph of deregulated capitalism are not unrelated issues. There is a great reluctance to examine this issue in a serious manner. Basically, terrorism is a criminal reaction or response to perceived irresponsible behaviour and abuse of power. A century ago, it was the abuse of advantage by the industrial and banking "robber barons," and the governments they controlled, that gave rise to the extremes of communism, fascism, and anarchism—the "terrorism" of that day. Today, terrorism is not about jealousy of failed cultures wishing to have our wealth, our freedom or our pop culture. It is not about "us" being "good" and "them" being "evil." It is about historical as well as recent abuse of political, economic, and military power and the exploitation of other people at the expense of their democracy, freedom, human rights, and welfare. When we fail to address people's needs, rights, and concerns, we invite crazed, desperate people to commit unforgivable criminal acts of terrorism. This is a threat to civilization and global development, and it is also a threat to open science.

Barry R. Bloom, Dean of the School of Public Health at Harvard, has discussed this threat in a recent article on "Bioterrorism and the University—the Threats to Security—and to Openness" (Harvard Magazine, November 2003). Bloom points out that the combined effects of the US Patriot Act, the Bioterrorism Act, and the US Presidential Decision Directive 2 have been to discourage research work on over 80 "select agents" (such as "dual use" biological agents useful in medicine and agriculture), prevent certain international students from receiving research and training in "sensitive" areas and prohibit publication of findings on biological and chemical agents that could be deemed "sensitive," or used for acts of terrorism. Now, how can a publisher of a science journal (such as *Scientific American*) predict how any fundamental scientific discovery is likely to be used or misused? Bloom cites three examples remote from bioterrorism to make the point.

> *Recombinant DNA.* "Would it have been obvious a half century ago that a study of sex in bacteria, ridiculed at the time as a frivolous use of public funds, would become the basis for all recombinant DNA, the genetic revolution, and the biotechnology industry?"
> *Sequencing the genome.* "Would it have been suspected that studying why certain tiny viruses that infect only bacteria are able to grow in some strains and not in others would provide the tools to clone DNA and sequence the human genome?"
> *Monoclonal antibodies.* "Would most people have cared whether fusing a cancer cell to a white blood cell producing antibodies extinguished the blood cell's ability to produce its specialized product? That is the experiment that created monoclonal antibodies used every day in diagnostics, in tumor treatments, and in creating vaccines against HIV and other diseases."

No one could have foreseen these outcomes—which we owe to open science, the curiosity of scientists, the freedom to do basic and applied research, the ability to communicate freely, and the availability of research funding—based on rational decision-making, identification of research "imperatives and opportunities" and the pursuit of socially responsible aims and purposes.

As Bloom concludes, "We need to find the means to prevent bioterrorism without crippling biomedical research, essential for developing drugs and vaccines to protect not only our population but people everywhere."

A phenomenon related to this social instability and terrorism is the culture of violence. Already we witness the cultural impact of deregulated corporate globalization: displacement of local and individual self-reliance and self-determination, provoking and compounding unsocial behaviour and violence, practically everywhere in the world. In the United States today, there is a virtual corporate conspiracy of "supply-side" consumerism, and "dumbing down" of the citizenry through deliberate disinformation and a manufactured fascination with violence as "entertainment" and as expression of "reality." This is the new imperial "bread and circuses," designed to keep the populace apathetic, doped, obese, malleable—and violent. This culture of violence has become yet another export commodity—dehumanizing, insinuating, and destructive.

When more traditional, moral cultures in other countries resist this trend, they are described as "backward" and as "enemies" of freedom and free speech. Many countries that really do face long-standing problems of insecurity and that really do seek freedom from fear and want are faced with a juggernaut of corporate, commercial, and political pressures and influences that can only lead to further insecurity, social unrest, and violence. Thus, deregulated capitalism is giving birth to its own Frankenstein monster, a culture of violence that will return to plague us all.

As we enter this post-genomic era of the 21st century, I find, among the most intellectually fascinating and medically productive fields of science and technology, those dealing with

- gene expression and pattern analysis, to predict risk, developments, and outcomes and to tailor diagnosis and treatments of many diseases, including cancers;
- gene therapies and related techniques, to actually correct mutated, defective or missing genes, and thereby reverse certain genetic or hereditary diseases of constitution, including cancers;
- stem cell research and engineering and related technologies, including transplantation, which can prevent disability, save lives, restore healthy function.

As Fliedner has observed, "the great challenge and opportunity of the 'post-genomic era' in medicine is to go beyond the traditional organ system approach to system regulation at the subcellular level, understanding and modulating metabolic systems, their regulation, growth and development, resistance to disease, and contribution to overall human health. Much of the research at the sub-cellular level is being carried out by in vitro experiments outside the human body. What we have to do now is confirm the validity and effectiveness of these approaches at the level of the integrated human body." It is difficult to imagine a greater intellectual challenge, or opportunity, for international scientific co-operation.

Chapter 30
The Ethics of Research: The Responsibility of the Researcher

Ivan Wilhelm, PhD

The theme—the ethical aspect of the activity of the researcher—is one of the most fundamental issues in academic life and needs to be accorded due attention. Medicine is of course one of the scientific disciplines most closely connected with the human individual, affecting his or her life in the most fundamental ways, and especially at times when he or she faces health problems. The influence of medicine on the human population as a whole is also enormous, and I would like to come back to this aspect later on. All this means that medical ethics has been very much to the forefront practically throughout the entire history of medicine. Medical ethics are not only of great concern to practising doctors and ethical philosophers attached to medical departments, but also occupy considerable space in initial medical education. As the rector of a university that has five medical faculties, I have had a chance to get to know some of the issues involved quite closely. My own field of research as a physicist is quite different, however, and I can therefore report that relatively very little explicit attention is paid to ethical questions of research and scholarship in the academic community at large, and by extension in the preparation of young specialists during university studies. The reason for this is the surviving traditional concept of academic research as something pure, orientated above all to scholarship, and reserved for a tiny percentage of people, a select group wholly devoted to their discipline and loyal to their society. Right at the start, however, we need to stress that this concept is no longer applicable. More and more people are working in research and it can hardly be assumed that the motive behind the choice of each one of them is a pure desire for knowledge. Personal desire for success in a professional career and above all the influence of those who commission or fund research and their pragmatic interests are all factors that can encourage unethical behaviour. At the same time it is clear that the results of research are having an ever more obvious impact on practical life and are therefore affecting more and more of the population. Moreover the state apparatus, as the main "shareholder" in research, ever more obviously seeks to influence research programmes. Hence science plays an ever more important part in human life. The growing number of research workers and the ever faster translation of research into practical life—these are the two basic reasons why questions of the ethics of research work and the responsibility of the researcher are even more important today than they were until relatively recently.

The increasing influence of science on the development of society is obviously the main reason for putting forward the theme of the ethical behaviour of the research workers for broader public discussion. Let us remember that the scientist or scholar works on the border between the known and the hitherto unknown, and that his or her path leads into uncharted areas where it is often impossible to predict quite what the results will be even when they are more or less anticipated, let alone when they turn out to be unexpected. And the general public has no chance at all of keeping up with the research situation in detail, in a way that would allow it to understand these results just as they emerge. As far as research in public institutions is concerned, or in institutions that have public statutes or if otherwise established still have the same basic organization, such as universities, public and private, the democratic internal system of such institutions provides a certain level of guarantee that there will be relatively systematic control of research activity above all inside the academic community. The transparency of the structure of decision-making in these institutions, the way in which decisions are achieved through bodies involving a large number of members of the academic community, means that to keep the existence of a major research programme from the public would require a conspiracy of a kind that would hardly be practicable. In my view this is one of the main advantages of the cultivation of research in public rather than private institutions, where I am convinced it is relatively easy to conceal quite large parts of research programmes from the public at large. The public availability of detailed information on research activities on the one hand creates the conditions for ethical evaluation of research, including the possibility of public pressure to regulate the ambitions of researchers and on the other, allows research and its implications to be judged by specialists from other fields. Given the current trend to narrow specialization and minimum interdisciplinary interaction this last argument is particularly important.

The present conditions of research and academic activity have not, of course, arisen purely by chance or overnight. They are the result of historical development and our task is not just to accept them, but to try and influence their ongoing development. Here I should like to consider the development of scientific disciplines, using a pivotal example that also happens to be the example where I feel I am on home ground, that is, physics.

The last decade of the 19th century was an important period for the progress of the natural sciences, and above all physics. The successes of earlier 19th-century physicists had meant an overall ordering of fundamental physical ideas and comparison of notions of physical processes including their mathematical description: what is known as "classical" physics had acquired a coherent, apparently comprehensive theoretical form. It was generally believed that all the basic questions in physics had been answered and that further research would concentrate on improving the precision of experimental results and achieving a complete fit between empirical finds and theoretical calculations. Essentially therefore, both theory and practice were directed simply to making minor corrections to existing models and descriptions.

But in the last decade of the 19th century physics started to undergo a major upheaval. Many physicists were obtaining experimental results that could not be explained by the existing theories, whether what was at issue was the description of photo-effect, the existence and behaviour of X-rays, or, above all, the discovery of radioactivity and new types of radiation. With the discovery of the electron, detailed study of the structure of matter began, a whole field of new, entirely unanticipated questions opened up, and the first efforts were made to formulate the principles of quantum theory. Ernest Rutherford's experiments, published in 1911, led scientists to accept as unchallengeable the idea of the structure of the atom as a material force centre with orbiting electrons, but it was only later, with the results of quantum mechanics, that these atomic processes and phenomena could be explained and comprehended. While it arose from the practical needs of the physics of the microworld, quantum theory provided a new theoretical groundwork and system of mathematical abstraction comparable in its revolutionary effects to differential calculus and the Newtonian view of nature. The conclusions of what is known as the Copenhagen School, led by Niels Bohr, are today formulated in universal terms as classical quantum mechanics; they represent not just a remarkable description and explanation of a number of physical processes, but above all a new concept, a new paradigm with all the philosophical aspects that this implies, and so the beginning of a new era in physics.

The beginning of the last century also saw crucial work that brought a paradigm shift in views of the dynamics of material bodies. In this context the key figure was Albert Einstein, as the author of the complete formulation of the general theory of relativity, meaning the generalization of the Galilean–Euclidean description of space or space–time. It is worth noting that what motivated Einstein to this theoretical leap forward was not in fact the lack of fit between experimental results and theoretical description evident above all in astronomy. In his own words, the attempt to make theory and experiment agree by introducing more and more corrections was so aesthetically ugly that it simply could not represent the right approach to a solution. It should be added, of course, that the theory of relativity certainly meets aesthetic criteria, and not only in terms of its elegant mathematical formulation. Here we might note the importance of the work of Ernst Mach, Rector of Charles University in the academic year 1879–1880 and then in 1883; his theories, which preceded the work of Albert Einstein, represented an important contribution to the problem of time and space and strongly influenced Einstein's thinking.

Thus new horizons opened up for research in physics. New discoveries came thick and fast, and it is no exaggeration to say that the end of the 1920s was the start of the golden age of physics. Thomson, Dirac, Anderson, Nedermayer, von Laue, Mottelson, Heisenberg, Schroedinger, Raabi, Segre and especially Fermi and Chadwick and many others made unique discoveries, pushed forward the frontiers of knowledge, and also won Nobel Prizes for physics. James Chadwick's discovery of the neutron (1932) was the impetus for development of nuclear physics, a field that now looked so promising that it attracted more and more specialists.

I would now like to turn, however, from the actual intellectual content of physics to the very interesting social aspect of the question of the development of physics research. Until what we might call the take-off of nuclear physics, that is, roughly in the first three decades of the 20th century, only a very small number of teams, each with only a very small number of members, had been engaged in physics research. This becomes very obvious if we look, for example, at the number of people attending the conferences on the most recent results in modern physics that were organized annually during this period in Copenhagen: not even once did more than 60 people attend, even though the conference programme was by no means restricted to one theme. This was also a time when research costs were relatively modest and were normally covered from the budgets of individual universities. The centre of gravity of these activities was Europe, with an emphasis on Germany, but European conditions in the later 1930s, and the rise of fascism in Italy and then in Germany, meant a major exodus of physicists. The centre of gravity of physics research went with them to the USA. The discovery of the process of nuclear fission came just before the outbreak of the Second World War (Halm et al., 1938), and experimental study of nuclear fission soon uncovered the possibility of creating a chain reaction and the prospect of a source of enormous energy. Unfortunately, of course, international politics was in the process of a chain reaction; the critical point was reached and Europe erupted into war. Communication between scientists was either suspended altogether or very much curtailed. The physicists who studied nuclear properties and processes at the time immediately realized that the chain fission reaction could be exploited to construct weapons of unprecedented destructive power. The road to such weapons, however, was long and first a large number of theoretical and technical problems needed to be solved. Here it is worth mentioning that the development of nuclear weapons might easily have come earlier. As early as 1934 the group led by E. Fermi in Rome had conducted experiments with neutrons and observed the process of nuclear fission. The situation was the same at the same time in the laboratory of Marie Curie–Sklodowska in Paris, where the Joliot–Curie team conducted similar experiments. But the explanation of the observed effects in both laboratories was mistaken and so the process of fission of the atomic nucleus remained, for the time being, hidden from humankind.

Many scientists were extremely worried about the rapid development of research on nuclear weapons in Hitler's Germany and the prospect that the Wehrmacht might acquire these and so win the war. There was no doubt that physicists of the stature of W. Heisenberg or C. von Weizsäcker were capable of turning the nuclear weapons project in Germany into a reality. For this reason physicists, emigrants from Europe now living in the USA, turned to the government and President Roosevelt to warn them of the danger. The result was that intensive work on the development of nuclear weapons went ahead above all in the USA. The Soviet Union did not as yet have the resources for undertaking military nuclear research on the same scale as in Los Alamos, and the German physicists deliberately slowed down their work in an attempt to avoid responsibility for the results of the world war.

What we have here, of course, is a textbook example of scientists taking an ethical attitude to a state commission with a pragmatic purpose. The concrete form of the nuclear weapon and its destructive power were as yet matters of guesswork, but there was no doubt that it would be a weapon with unprecedented military potential. The effects of radiation on live organisms was a particularly uncharted and speculative area. Indeed, around 1939–1940 there existed fewer than 20 physicists, anywhere in the world, with the knowledge and ability to conduct developmental projects of this type, and it is noteworthy that none of them were fanatical followers of the national–socialist ideas that were fuelling political conflicts in Europe, but also in Asia and Africa.

In 1942 the state of war and the absence of reliable intelligence led Roosevelt and Churchill to a formal agreement to combine English and American resources to develop nuclear weapons, and then the launch of the "Manhattan" project in Los Alamos, New Mexico. This was a project that at the height of its activities employed 150,000 people, more than a quarter of them scientific workers, and cost sums unprecedented for research before that time. It was also the state of war that motivated everyone to work on their tasks with great commitment, without moral and ethical doubts. Most of the physicists who had contributed in any significant way to the realization of the Manhattan Project personally attended the first nuclear test explosion in the Nevada Desert (Jordana de Muerto, not far from the village of Oscuro, by the township of Alamogordo, USA) in July 1945. It is well known that E. Fermi, overwhelmed by the experience of watching the explosion, reacted with the words "God, how beautiful physics is!" It is a sentiment that illustrates the general attitude of these international scientific authorities not just to the way the problem of nuclear arms was tackled scientifically, but to the actual results of their efforts. Many physicists immediately contacted US political and governmental leaders including the President himself to point out that no one else in the world yet had such a weapon and the mere fact of holding it and readiness to use it against the enemy meant a military advantage that would force the enemy into rapid capitulation. They appealed to the fact that the destructive power of this weapon, at a time when the result of the Second World War was essentially already decided, could be merely demonstrated to great psychological effect on the enemy without major loss of life. It became apparent at this point, however, that scientists' ideas of political decisions are very naive, and if the results of research are handed over to politicians, their authors cease to have any influence on the way they are used. That is one of the lessons of the development of nuclear weapons, which could of course have been predicted, but could scarcely have been taken into account in the course of the developmental work itself.

The example of nuclear weapons is not just a typical example of the military exploitation of scientific research. Of course, science and military necessity have often gone hand in hand throughout human history, whether we are talking about the ingenuity of Archimedes in using his discoveries in the defence of Syracuse against the Roman ships, or the use of chemical weapons in the First World War. But the military importance of the nuclear arms project in the most destructive war in history, and the way the project was applied, brought about a qualitative shift in the meaning of scientific research and changed the social status of scientific researchers, not just for the period of the project but forever. It had been shown that incomparably larger teams than had ever been assembled before could successfully tackle complex scientific problems. Many important scientists had convinced themselves of their managerial and organizational capacities and gave scientific research an entirely new character. The state, above all through its pragmatic interest in the results of the research, but also by creating the material conditions for the research, had become deeply involved in the whole sector.

These were changes that could not be reversed. The academic community began to become accustomed to ever-greater funding and ever-greater needs for funding, to the ever more intensive influence of the state on scientific activity, and gradually to pragmatic links and bonds between academic and state structures. Of course, the great majority of research programmes are not focused on the development of destructive discoveries, but the reverse. Their constructive effect on the over-all growth of the economy, production, services, and culture can be documented quite precisely. At this assembly it is unnecessary to draw attention to the efforts of medicine to free humanity from fear of whole constellations of diseases or to take examples from the unending list of successes in this respect. The character of development as I have described it cannot be changed in any essential way, nor would it be desirable to change it. It means not only that the importance of science for everyday life has been increasing, but also that some aspects of the model, procedures, and mission of the exact sciences have increasingly been taken over in the fields of the humanities and social sciences. The pattern is being followed by other academic disciplines such as biology, chemistry and technical sciences, but also sociology, history, political studies, and of course economics. Research in the humanities is now being expected to contribute to the solution of the social problems of the modern world, such as co-existence between different communities, religious conflicts, the demographic boom in the developing countries, cultural aspects of the quality of life and so forth. And in these circumstances more and more people are deciding on an academic career. The influence of academic research and the application of the conclusions of research are ever more evident in the practical decisions of the management teams of companies, and above all of politicians. The rule of competition in a market environment is simple—victory goes to the person or organization who comes first and reacts fastest. The customers for the results of research are therefore insisting on a speeding up of the research–application–production–sale cycle. In this context there is little time for consideration of risks associated with a piece of research or of the influence of new knowledge on other fields. The demand that research should have direct outputs and the linkage of financial sponsorship to such outputs (to put the "rules of the game" rather schematically) have led to generally accepted criteria that mean a certain trivialization of the relationship between the academic community and the state, and are of course still a subject of wide-ranging debate today. Furthermore, the ever-growing competition and rivalry in the academic community and the personal ambitions of each individual member are tending to encourage a casual attitude to the ethical norms and moral barriers that ought always to take precedence over any kind of pragmatism.

This risk of moral deficit is certainly a major focus of interest in any research institution, but in university conditions it is a particularly urgent concern, because a university is not just a research but a teaching establishment. The task of the universities is not simply to train a qualified labour force for the needs of the job market. That is only one and, I would venture to say, the lesser part of educational activity. The mission of the university in the educational process is to equip students to live their own lives in the best way, in terms of their own expectations of themselves and in relation to the world around them. There is no doubt that, for every individual, education should have not just a price, but a value. Every university graduate ought to become a cultured, ethical, spiritual and professionally qualified person. It cannot be any other way, if universities are to continue to be regarded as the bearers of the cultural values of civilization. Ethical norms and moral barriers naturally depend on the overall cultural level of society, which in turn depend on the level of knowledge and understanding. The level of knowledge and understanding ought therefore to inform the ethical behaviour of every individual. Just as universities contribute through their research to the enlargement of knowledge, so they must also take care to ensure that the ethical side of life develops in harmony with this knowledge and understanding. Because the academic community is part of society, this is a crucial and essential task, and means that every member of the academic community should be aware of his or her responsibility, because his or her research is also helping to form new ethical norms of behaviour.

Allow me to conclude by quoting V.F. Weisskopf, one of the leading nuclear physicists of the 20th century (who also worked on the Manhattan Project), and wrote:

> All parts and all aspects of science depend on each other. Science cannot develop of itself, unless it is consciously cultivated for reasons of pure desire for knowledge and understanding. Yet science cannot survive unless it is passionately and wisely used to improve life and not as an instrument by which groups of people control another group. Human existence depends on two aspects – mutual compassion and knowledge. Knowledge without compassion is inhumane; compassion without knowledge is ineffective.

Chapter 31
The Cost of *Not* Doing Health Research

William C. Gibson OC, DPhil, FRCPC, LLD(Hon)

It is a pleasure to note the ties of the International Association for Humanitarian Medicine with Italy, the land of Galileo, Leonardo, Spallanzani, Fallopio, Aselli, Galvani and his wife, Malpighi, Bellini, Fabricius of Acquapendente (the teacher of William Harvey), Realdo Colombo, Domenico Cotugno, Golgi, Cerletti and Bignami and many more, never forgetting the two Nightingale sisters: Parthenope, born in Naples, and Florence, born in Florence.

Their beautiful garden still flourishes there, looking out over the Duomo. And in Palermo, there was Professor Leonardo Bianchi, who contributed so much to brain research.

When we speak of research, what do we mean? When President Roosevelt put that Socratic question to his ever-present advisor, Harry Hopkins, more than a half-century ago, Hopkins replied in his condensed and forceful way: "Research is spending to save." This definition, it seems to me, speaks volumes.

Historically, the cost of the research was negligible in some amazing investigations. For instance, in 1540, a medical student, Valerius Cordus, first synthesized ether by pouring inexpensive sulphuric acid over his family's Christmas wine. Besides adding to the festive cheer, he showed ether's anaesthetic effect on chickens, which went on a "binge" by eating grain moistened with the new liquid which he named *oleum dulci vitrioli*. They fell senseless to the ground but soon recovered and consumed even more of this new general anaesthetic. Four years later, alas, Cordus died in the malarial marshes of Italy's south coast where he was busy collecting 500 botanical species for study, and his pivotal experiments were forgotten.

Much later, 300 years later, the first major use of ether anaesthesia was demonstrated in Boston by a medical student, William Morton, on a surgical patient of the 68-year-old professor of surgery at Harvard University, John Collins Warren. Where had this 300-year-old discovery been hiding, and why?

The results of research in the medical sciences are sometimes lost to mankind for such lack of communication. In 1897, a medical student, Ernest Duchesne, at the University of Lyons where he was subsidized by the Army, carried out the experiment for which Florey and Chain received the Nobel Prize 45 years later. In his graduation thesis of 54 pages, Duchesne described the protection against *Bacillus typhosus*, which the mould *Penicillium glaucum* conferred on his test animals. His controls, without the protection of this mould, all died.

Why was this delay possible, and what were the costs of *not knowing* this landmark work? No one read Duchesne's little thesis, and on graduation he was required to take up his service duties with the Army. His expressed hope was that others would follow up his modest contribution. It is said that he died of tuberculosis, unremembered and unsung.

Discoverers themselves may have been attacked by the existing "establishment" in medicine. William Harvey's account of the circulation of the blood was ignorantly attacked by critics who said it was not true. When it was proved to be true, his critics said it was already known *before* Harvey! When the British general practitioner, George Bodington (1799–1882) wrote his slim but sound volume on the fresh-air treatment of tuberculosis, he was excoriated by noisy, ill-informed physicians. Thomas Lauder Brunton (1844–1916), an Edinburgh medical student, in his first paper on amyl nitrite, advocated its use in angina pectoris. Thirty-four years later, he dared to suggest that mitral stenosis in humans might be relieved by surgical means. *The Lancet* thrashed him in its columns, in which Brunton was accused of inciting others "to pursue a path into the unknown which must be beset with very grave difficulty and responsibility." Brunton replied that he had been thus operating on animals for the last 35 years. Also, no contemporary took up this challenge, so mitral stenosis went on.

The cost of doing medical research—the cost to the researcher—is further illustrated in the life of Edward Jenner (1749–1823), the discoverer of an effective method of vaccinating humans against smallpox. He was harried for much of his life by one part of the medical profession and praised by the other. It took leaders of the calibre of Dr Brock Chisholm to galvanize the World Health Organization to mount the eventual campaign which freed the entire world from any further danger of smallpox. It is fitting that the International Association for Humanitarian Medicine should be named after this visionary doctor.

Research is one thing, but its application is another. From Jenner's proof, in 1796, that vaccination could prevent smallpox, to the World Health Organization's embodiment of Brock Chisholm's army general's approach to a war on this massive enemy took 10 years, and only $100 million. I say "only" because this unique, scientifically based campaign against mankind's old and insidious enemy was finally stopped in its tracks through good science and even better application of it. Two things have to be shouted to the world from the top of every chimney pot—(a) the victory over this deep-rooted evil saved the world $2 billion *per year*; (b) this saving goes on *in perpetuity*—a yield rarely demonstrable in any other human endeavour. We are proud that Chisholm's successor, Dr Halfdan Mahler, who sealed the official eradication of smallpox, is here as an illustrious Regent of IAHM.

Let me be clear—the medical profession *has not been alone* in decrying the work of pioneer scientific researchers. As Britain's great neurosurgeon Wilfred Trotter, FRS, recorded, J.J. Waterston, an engineer, was at least a generation in advance of his contemporaries in his work on the molecular theory of gases. Unfortunately, the Royal Society's reviewer said his paper was "nothing but nonsense."

Exit Waterston, alas! This loss put back new engineering by 20 years. Flight Lieutenant Frank Whittle, an engineering graduate of Cambridge University in 1932, published his research on jet propulsion. Yet, by the end of World War II,

13 years later, only a relative handful of jet aircraft had been in combat. A wise Chancellor of the Exchequer in England, Sir Stafford Cripps, awarded the then Air Commodore Whittle 100,000 pounds tax free in 1945 for his invention and years of frustration in its application.

A century and more ago, the great researcher Paul Ehrlich said that there were four "G's" needed for the discovery of effective therapeutic agents. These were *Geld* (money), *Geduld* (patience), *Geschichte* (ability) and *Gluck* (luck). I should tell you what my teacher in pathology at Oxford, Howard Florey, told me about one of these requirements—that of luck. A member of his staff at the William Dunn School of Pathology was passing a fruit stand in London when she saw on a rotting melon a luxurious growth of a bright yellow mould. She was astounded that such deteriorating fruit should be on sale, but recognized the value—not of the fruit, but of the mould. Back in Oxford, she presented it to an exophthalmic Florey. It was the "golden penicillium" mould which was the most productive ever seen in the laboratory—and brought with it Ehrlich's fourth requirement, *Gluck*, luck, and untold blessing to humanity. Now that smallpox has been overcome worldwide, the guns of war can be turned similarly on poliomyelitis, that scourge whose name means "grey matter destruction in the spinal cord." In 1954, three American medical scientists, Enders, Weller and Robbins shared the Nobel prize for their work leading to a vaccine protecting humans, mainly children, against this paralysing disease. They had succeeded in growing the viral agent—known since Biblical times—in tissue culture, thus leading to a vaccine.

These workers were standing on the shoulders of Ross Granville Harrison (1877–1959), a biologist from John Hopkins and a medical graduate of Bonn University. Working at Yale in 1907, he gave the world one of the most powerful techniques in medical history—that of "tissue culture." This revolutionary method of studying growing cells and tissues in artificial conditions outside the body was the key that unlocked countless doors, closed since time began. Why Harrison was never awarded the Nobel prize even in 1954 for this fundamental advance has puzzled scientists for generations. He would be the first to cheer on Brock Chisholm's troops today.

At all events, the cost of the research which produced the polio vaccine was only $40 million, and its worldwide application now in progress, thanks to the World Health Organization and to Rotary International, will bring health to all children in the year of its global success and thereafter *in perpetuity*.

The world will ever be grateful to Louis Pasteur for his researches which conquered many diseases—and concomitantly for his encouragement of all researchers. Pasteur used to say that "fortune favours the prepared mind." He also wrote, "Men without laboratories are as soldiers without arms." He knew that while bricks were needed, brains were the essential, living ingredients in discovery. Without carefully nurtured brains, the bricks can be mocking monuments to folly.

Close to General Chisholm's heart would have been Dr John Shaw Billings, a Civil War veteran who found an inadequate library of 2,700 volumes in the Surgeon General's office in Washington, DC, to which he had been posted. When he died, full of military and civilian honours, he left us the world's largest medical library and the very tools needed by future researchers. When asked by Sir John Y.W. MacAlister how he accomplished so many useful things in one lifetime, Billings replied, "There is nothing really difficult if you only begin. Some people contemplate a task until it looms so big it seems impossible. There would be no coral islands if the first bug sat down and began to wonder how the job was to be done."

Mention of Billings brings me to a brief but necessary inclusion in this lecture of medical libraries as the touchstone of all would-be researchers. Whether conveyed by books or journals in one's hand or by the magical electronic devices of today, knowledge is the lifeblood of future ideas. We have already seen how ignorance of Ernest Duchesne's early work on penicillium had delayed the work of three Nobel prize winners, and how ignorance of the trials by Valerius Cordus on ether delayed its use as anaesthesia in surgery for three centuries.

When Dr Frederick Banting, like Brock Chisholm after World War I, was trying to establish a medical practice in his home province in Canada, he was dependent on a poorly paid post as a lecturer in the Physiology Department of the University of Western Ontario, under Professor F.R. Miller, who had trained with Sherrington at Oxford. Thus Banting, a struggling orthopaedic surgeon, was preparing for his next day's lecture on carbohydrate metabolism. On his way out of the medical library late one evening, his eye caught the title of an article in a surgical journal concerning the destruction of all but the islands of Langerhans in a stone-obstructed pancreas. Taking the journal home to read of the effect on the circulatory blood sugar, Banting could not sleep.

At 2 a.m. he wrote in his notebook, "Ligate pancreatic duct of dogs. Wait six or eight weeks. Remove residue and extract." Working through a torrid summer and with the help of a graduate student, Charles Best, and a new PhD biochemist, J.B. Collip, Banting produced insulin, which went on to change the world of diabetics. He never forgot the library's role in this success nor the author of the article, Dr Moses Barron of the University of Minnesota. The total cost of the research was $15,000 in 1921 dollars.

Before concluding, perhaps I may ask, "What disease ever cured itself?" Human beings have to plot against disease and sustain the gifted troops required to win. In the century just past, it was possible for elected leaders to proclaim that they had "nothing but praise for medical research" but "nothing" is no longer good enough.

Volunteers are in the vanguard in financing medical research, in whatever country, today. If I may be permitted a personal reference I would cite the Muscular Dystrophy Associations of the United States and Canada, where committed volunteers have collected, in the past half-century, more than one billion dollars for research and treatment and education in 40 neuromuscular diseases. They have supported 400 research projects around the world—including Italy.

General Brock Chisholm would have seen this and similar efforts everywhere as the "*internal defence*" components of an awakened world. Successful industries put at least 10 % of their funds into research. Surely great countries could put 10 % of the cost of diseases into research now, and until the diseases of this shrinking world are prevented or eliminated, as the World Health Organization has done in the case of smallpox. How is it that the shameful 10/90 Gap should have been allowed to develop, whereby only 10 % of current global research expenditure goes to 90 % of the diseases that afflict mankind, a disequilibrium that adds so much to the cost of ill-health? The cost of not doing health research is unacceptably high.

Years ago, two great medical researchers, Sir Charles Sherrington and his pupil Harvey Cushing, spoke at the opening of a new Biological Sciences Building at McGill University in Montreal.

Sherrington's final words there are as *à propos* today as they were then: "Do not, O my brothers, forget research. Science calls us all to it—and the call is from humanity as well."

If researchers are to produce useful discoveries, they need our support, morally and financially. I can hear, over the years, the supporting voice of the British poet, John Masefield, calling to all medical researchers:

> Adventure on, for from the tiniest clue has come whatever worth man ever knew; the next to lighten all men may be you.

Chapter 32
Reflections on the Past, Present and Future of Medicine

Radana Königová, MD, CSc

In 1850, Armand Trousseau spoke in Paris of the *fascination* which accompanies the study of medicine: "Literature, painting, and music do not yield an enjoyment more keen than that which is afforded by the study of medicine. Whoever does not find in it, from the commencement of his career, an almost irresistible attraction, ought to renounce the intention of following our profession."

In 1902, Sir William Osler defined the *task* of medicine:

> To wrest from nature the secrets which have perplexed philosophers in all ages, to track to their sources the causes of disease, to correlate the vast stores of knowledge, that they may be quickly available for the prevention and cure of disease—these are our ambitions. To observe the phenomena of life in all its phases, normal and perverted, to make perfect that most difficult of all the arts—the art of observation, to call to aid the science of experimentation, to cultivate the reasoning faculty, so as to be able to know the true from the false—these are our methods. To prevent disease, to relieve suffering and to heal the sick—this is our work.

Rudyard Kipling—10 years later—in his *Book of Words* set forth a portrait of the doctor:

> The world has long ago decided that you have no working hours which anybody is bound to respect, and nothing will excuse you in its eyes from refusing to help a man who thinks he may need your help at any hour of the day or night. In all time of flood, fire, famine, plague, battle, murder, it will be required of you that you go on duty at once, and that you stay on duty until your strength fails you or your conscience relieves you.

In 1928, Sir Robert Hutchinson published in the *British Medical Journal*:

> Every doctor must be a judge. He has to weigh the evidence of symptoms and signs, and allot to each its proper value in making the diagnosis. We can increase our powers of observation by training and practice, we can increase our knowledge by study and experience, but *judgement seems to be an inborn faculty*—the result of a union of mind and character which a man either has or has not. It may be improved only by general mental culture, and not by purely scientific training.

Historically, all health professionals have followed the powerful traditions of Hippocrates, whose thoughts may be summarized:

> . . . declare the past, diagnose the present, foretell the future; practise these acts. As to disease, make a habit of two things: to help or at least to do no harm.

The emphasis on doing no harm was justified at a time when most medical treatments were useless and frequently dangerous.

Once medical science began to develop effective treatment, physicians were forced to *balance burdens* and *benefits* as they decided what was in the best interest of the patient. Making moral choices is the basis of *medical decision-making* but the choice is often between two apparently "good options."

Traditionally, the physician's duty is to the patient, and this duty only extends to the family in a diluted fashion when the patient becomes incompetent. The strong point of entrusting the use of extremely complex life-support systems to physicians is that the physicians have the knowledge and judgement to use them in a teleologically effective manner. This premise also implies that they have the expertise to know when this technology has no benefit and should not be used.

Recently, the focus on *the patient's right to refuse treatment* has shifted to the *patient's right to demand treatment*, even if doctors believe that such treatment is futile. "Right to care" is the next step in defining the boundaries of patient autonomy. These situations involve a conflict of values, as families demand continuation of care even if there is no chance of recovery or meaningful survival for the patient.

There is another aspect to the dilemma we now face. We have been given a significant proportion of our society's wealth, enough to build, equip, and staff substantial structures for modern medicine.

Technological advances have made it possible to maintain moribund and comatose patients in a state of suspended animation for prolonged and sometimes indefinite periods. The treatment of such patients by life-support systems cannot strictly be said to be "medically futile" as it maintains vital signs even though it does not restore the patient to consciousness.

There is a great dispute whether a health care system already affected by rapidly increasing costs should force physicians to go against their expert judgement when families insist on maintaining prolonged coma for reasons that are defensible only in emotional terms. Hospitals have the responsibility to promote ethically sound decision-making through well-drafted policies which will inform patients and families regarding the circumstances for withholding or withdrawing futile procedures in the institution. Moves to curtail excesses in health care delivery may now provide financial incentives to limit health care unless it is clearly beneficial. The introduction of economic considerations in individual patient decision-making is clearly perilous but may be necessary as society begins its debate on the most effective use of its limited health resources.

The nature of modern medicine is interventionist. "Aggressive supportive care" for comatose patients has been considered a contradiction in terms on the one hand, but on the other hand La Puma and Schiedermayer in 1989 pointed out why we should talk to comatose patients. Attempts to maintain verbal contact with patients, even when the prognosis for recovery is "hopeless," reinforce the physician's role as a dependable caregiver both for the patient and for those who are able to participate in health care decision-making. Nurses are taught and—in our practice—accompanying persons (family members) are instructed to offer their comatose patients an "environmental enrichment programme." The multimode biofeedback—including verbal stimulation—may help nurses in the difficult task of spending 8 or 12 h giving "total care" and may help the family to become involved in the care.

Physicians may decide to terminate cardiopulmonary resuscitation (CPR) because the patient is not responsive. This demonstrates that withdrawal of care can have the same moral quality or implications as initiating care.

Even though CPR or other life-sustaining manoeuvres may be futile in terms of prolonging life, they can help individual patients and their families if they are of symbolic or psychological value (Crippen, 1992).

Dartmouth Medical School has made an attempt to prepare future doctors for situations likely to be encountered in practice, using "Problem-based Learning of the Social Sciences and Humanities."

This was developed on the premise that doctors should learn to borrow relevant concepts from many humanistic and social disciplines and to integrate them into their daily decision-making process for the benefit of their patients, their communities, and eventually society as whole.

Regarding the future, it may be featured as *chaos making a new science*. By the late 20th century, in ways never before conceivable, images of the incomprehensibly small and the unimaginably large became part of everyone's experience, thanks to microscopes and telescopes.

In the development of a person's mind from childhood, information is clearly not just accumulated but also generated—created from connections that were not there before. The shapes of all natural objects are dynamic processes jelled into physical forms, and particular combinations of order and disorder are typical for them. The paragon of a complex dynamic system is the human body—no object of study available offers such a cacophony of counterrhythmic motion on scales from the macroscopic to the microscopic (James Gleick, 1987).

A new kind of physiology—chaos—is built on the idea that mathematical tools could help scientists understand global complex systems independently of local detail. Researchers have increasingly recognized the body as a place of motion and oscillation and found rhythms that were invisible on frozen microscope slides or daily blood samples. The dynamics are much richer than anybody would guess from reading textbooks.

Pattern born amid formlessness—that is *biology's* and *medicine's* basic beauty and its *basic mystery*.

Chapter 33
Scientists, Doctors and the Nuclear Dilemma

Sir Joseph Rotblat[†], DSc, PhD, KCMG, CBE, FRS

There can be no doubt that the greatest threat to the survival of civilization, perhaps of mankind itself, comes from nuclear arms. At the First Special Session on Disarmament in 1978, the General Assembly of the United Nations was unanimous in declaring that:

> Mankind today is confronted with an unprecedented threat of self-extinction arising from the massive and competitive accumulation of the most destructive weapons ever produced. Existing arsenals of nuclear weapons alone are more than sufficient to destroy all life on earth ... Removing the threat of a world war – a nuclear war – is the most acute and urgent task of the present day. Mankind is confronted with a choice: we must halt the arms race and proceed to disarmament or face annihilation.

In view of this universal condemnation of the nuclear arms race, what is it that keeps it going unabated, indeed accelerating its pace? By its very nature, the nuclear arms race feeds on the continuous input of scientific innovation and technological skill, but many analysts believe that these factors have acquired a momentum of their own, that they have become the masters instead of being the tools. We are frequently told that nowadays technology dictates policy, that new weapons systems emerge not because of any military or security requirements but because of the sheer impetus of the technological process. Lord Zuckerman, for many years scientific adviser to the British Cabinet, had this to say on the subject:

> When it comes to nuclear weapons, the military chiefs of both sides – who by convention are the official advisers on national security – usually serve only a channel through which the men in the laboratories transmit their views. For the man in the laboratory – not the soldier, or sailor, or airman – who at the start proposes that for this or that arcane reason, it would be useful to improve an old or to devise a new nuclear warhead ... It is he who has succeeded over the years in equating, and so confusing, nuclear destructive power with military strength, as though the former were the single and sufficient condition of military success. The men in the nuclear weapons laboratories may never have been in the battle, they may never have experienced the devastation of war; but they know how to devise means of destruction.

This is rather a strong statement. While there can be no doubt that science and technology are vital factors in the nuclear arms race, it seems to me that they are by no means the only factors which contribute to the momentum of the race. Primarily,

---

[†] 1908–2005

the arms race is the product of political forces, and there are many factors, often interacting with each other, which enter into play . . .

But what are the motives of the scientists engaged in these activities? Actually, while we can think of a few scientists who nearly fit the image of the fictional Doctor Strangelove, the great majority of scientists involved in military research do this for other, generally quite prosaic motives.

It is unfortunately a fact that a high proportion of all scientists, variously estimated as between 25 and 40 percent, is occupied on military matters. The proportion of scientists who work in the opposite direction, who give their time, effort and ingenuity to counteract the evils of the arms race, is much, much smaller. But it is about this minority of scientists that I shall be mainly concerned in this paper. Paradoxically, many of the scientists most active in the struggle to stop and reverse the nuclear arms race were the very scientists who were responsible for the development of nuclear weapons in the first instance. The start of the nuclear arms race can be pinpointed to 29 August 1949, when the Russians tested their first atom bomb. But it is not generally realized that preceding that race there was—as many of us thought—another nuclear arms race, between American and British scientists on one side and German scientists on the other side.

This race—to be first to make the atom bomb—was only thought to have existed, because it subsequently turned out that Germans never really entered the race. It also turned out that from the beginning the Soviets were seen as the real adversary.

The work of the scientist is usually unrelated to practical reality. The theoretical ideas, or the experimental data, are initially of a purely academic nature, and it used to take many years before they made an impact on society. The discovery of fission, coming as it did in Nazi Germany in a war atmosphere, changed all this. The release of nuclear energy, talked about for a long time as a theoretical possibility, suddenly became a practical proposition, and many scientists working in this field conceived the idea that the energy could be released in a violent manner, producing an explosion of unprecented destructive power.

But as it was, it posed a frightful dilemma to the scientists. The most outstanding case is that of Albert Einstein. A pacifist from early youth, it is ironical that he should be called "father of the atom bomb".

Other, lesser mortals than Einstein, faced the same dilemma. I can speak of this from first-hand knowledge. Many of us, brought up on humanitarian principles, believed that science should be used in the service of mankind; the idea of utilizing our knowledge to produce an awesome weapon of destruction was abhorrent to us . . . My decision to overcome the moral scruples and initiate and partcipate in the atom bomb project was rationalized on the argument—nowadays very familiar in the arms race vocabulary—namely, deterrence. I argued that the only way to stop the Germans from using the atom bomb against us would be if we too had the bomb and threatened to retaliate: my work on the bomb was therefore solely for the purpose that it should not be used. Looking back with the wisdom of hindsight, I can see the folly of the deterrent argument.

More importantly, once an arms race is started, then sooner or later the arms will be used. As indeed it happened: two bombs were dropped on Japanese cities even though nobody suggested that Japan was thinking of making an atom bomb.

Eight weeks before the atom bomb was dropped scientists working on the Manhattan Project formally voiced their concern about the intended use of the atom bomb and the grave implication of such use. The nuclear age tragically began with the atom bomb that was dropped on Hiroshima on 6 August 1945.

The scientists' plea was ignored. Military and political considerations took precedence over humanitarian appeals, and two Japanese cities were devastated.

Partly as a result of the rift, most academic scientists, in the universities and institutes of technology, removed themselves from military work, and in the course of time became less and less knowledgeable about the detailed technological aspects of nuclear weapons. The work on these is carried out in military establishments and, since the research is classified, the results are not processed by the usual method of refereeing by peers.

The unsoundness of this state of affairs is recognized by the scientific community. It resulted in efforts by independent scientists to spend time on studying the problems involved so that they will be in a position to provide an objective assessment of military projects. The organization which comes nearest to this objective of rousing the conscience of scientists and making an effort to ameliorate the nuclear arms race is the Pugwash Movement, or to give it its full name—Pugwash Conferences on Science and World Affairs.[1]

In recent years the medical profession has become very active on the international arena in the efforts to prevent a nuclear war.

The physicians view a nuclear war as the final epidemic, with the doctors being unable to do anything to ameliorate. Therefore the only remedy they can recommend is prevention of the epidemic; this is the message they endeavour to convey. Unlike the scientists, the image of the physicians has not been tarnished: the average person trusts the doctor, whereas he has good reason to mistrust the scientist. The medical campaign is therefore likely to be more successful in the appeal to the public, but of course the two movements are to a large extent complementary.

The work and conclusions of the World Health Organization are exemplary in this respect.

---

[1] Pugwash and Sir Joseph Rotblat jointly received the Nobel Prize for Peace in 1995.

Chapter 34
Serving the Global Community Through eHealth: The Role of Academia

Kendall Ho, MD, FRCPC

34.1 Introduction

Despite global advances in medical research and sophistication and efficacy in health care management, paradoxically global inequity in health care access continues to persist (WHO, 2006). Underserved populations around the world, in particular, face common challenges in health care access problems including: unclean water and poor sanitation, poverty, geographic isolation, shortage of health professionals and medical supplies, training and supervision of health care workers, and referral systems (Wooton, 2001). These problems reveal that the health of a population or a nation is not only dependent on access to health professionals or treatments, but also governed by societal factors at play in their communities—commonly referred to as social determinants of health (Marmot, 2000).

Recognizing the intricate and undeniable geopolitical and socioeconomic relationships to health statuses of nations, as improving one will certainly influence another, the United Nations Millennium declaration in September 2000 embarked upon "... (setting) time-bound and measurable goals and targets for combating poverty, hunger, disease, illiteracy, environmental degradation and discrimination against women" (United Nations, 2000, 2002). The Millennium Development Goals (MDG), as this initiative has come to be known, and the eight key goals reflecting the essence of social determinants of development, provide a framework for the entire UN system and countries for which to strive with concerted efforts (UNMDG).

In addition to investing global energy in MDG, the chronic global shortage of skilled health professionals also requires strong and simultaneous attention. Dr Lee Jong-wook, the late Director-General of the World Health Organization, stated in the November 2005 high-level forum in Paris, France, that "We have to work together to ensure access to a motivated, skilled, and supported health worker by every person in every village everywhere" (WHO, 2006). It is with the recognition of this global health human resource shortage that the 2006 WHO Report was dedicated to the exploration of global solutions to improve supply of and access to health workers (WHO, 2006).

34.2 Advantage of eHealth

Modern information and communication technologies (ICT), including computers, personal digital assistants, cellular phones, and an ever increasing list of portable communication devices, are making unprecedented and innovative impact on health care service access, delivery, education and research (Ho, 2004a). Some of the clear advantages of ICT for e-health include, but not limited to, anywhere-anytime access to accurate and searchable health information for knowledge and clinical case exchange, large capacity for information storage and organization for health surveillance, and ease of synchronous and asynchronous communication between individuals in different geographic areas for health service delivery (telehealth). As a result, eHealth—the use of ICT in health—is rapidly gaining momentum worldwide as a vital part of the health care system in and amongst nations. For example, National Health Services in the United Kingdom (Department of Health National Programme on IT), in Australia (National e-Health Transition Authority), and Infoway in Canada (Canada Health Infoway) are actively facilitating the establishment of infrastructure and implementation strategies in eHealth to promote its entrenchment in health practices. Collaboration amongst different agencies and organizations is also evident in establishing emerging eHealth networks in other countries such as the African Health Infoway (Africa Health Infoway, 2005).

The flourishing of affordable, interoperable ICTs that can facilitate seamless data communication, as well as increase in both Internet access and usability worldwide, are breaking down geographic barriers. These advances can transform the ways global health access, surveillance, and education will be carried out. Recognizing the potential, the UN General Assembly categorically stated in its Millennium declaration that "... the benefits of new technologies, especially information and communication technologies . . . (should be made) available to all" (United Nations, 2000). Unmistakably, global eHealth can make a substantial and lasting impact in global health access equalization and delivery. It needs champions to lead the cause, research and evaluation to elucidate exemplars and best practices, and education to build capacity for future expansion and entrenchment into the global health system.

34.3 The Socially Responsive Academic Community

While global policy makers such as WHO and UN can steer the direction towards global health improvement and eHealth realization, they would benefit greatly from involvement of other organizations and partners to help implement the vision and achieve the goals. The academy, with its primary mission to achieve excellence in education, research, and exemplary clinical service delivery, can play a unique and effective role in general, and excellent in eHealth delivery in particular.

In 1995, WHO defined the social accountability of medial schools as "the obligation to direct their education, research and service activities towards addressing the priority health concerns of the community, region, and/or nation they have a mandate to serve. The priority health concerns are to be identified jointly by governments, health care organizations, health professionals and the public" (Health Canada). This definition would also be fitting for academia in general, which not only trains medical doctors but also a range of skilled health workers.

While the basic social responsibility of academia is to train and graduate competent skilled health workers, it can contribute significantly more to the well being of the society in many other meaningful ways. For example, in Vietnam, universities work with their governments to provide knowledge and skills to community members to combat poverty through the Canadian International Development Agency's (CIDA) poverty reduction programme (Participatory Poverty Reduction Planning with Ethnic Minorities in Vietnam Workshop Report, 2002). While one institution can address the health concerns of the community in which it is situated, how can likeminded institutions globally find their respective soul mates, and collectively contribute to address the global health concerns and needs? In other words, how can the collective academic body with its many institutions around the world best achieve social accountability in response to a globalized world?

34.4 Academia in Global eHealth

In eHealth, a good example is the ProCOR project (ProCOR), which is committed to excellence in global heart health with a focus on poor countries as its core mission. The site promotes education and international dialogue of knowledge exchange to stimulate formation of global communities to facilitate local engagement and empowerment. The leaders of ProCOR are international academic leaders and researchers stimulating the genesis and propagation of this international network.

Another example is the eHealth initiative of Universitas 21, or U21 for short (Universitas 21). The U21 consortium, consisting of 16 research-intense universities in 8 countries, was established in 1997; all share a joint vision of contributing to the internationalization in knowledge-sharing and service. The U21 e-health steering committee examined how e-health can contribute to global health and respond to the global societal needs (Ho and Sharman, 2005), and identified three pursuits that would bring high impact return: Telehealth for the underserved population (Woolton et al., 2005), Global e-health policy (Scott and Lee, 2005), and Professional portability (Goldberg et al., 2005). This analysis led to U21's collaboration with and provision of assistance to the Swinfen Charitable Trust (Swinfen Charitable Trust), a non-profit organization dedicated to providing telemedicine consultations to underserved countries, through contributions of faculty members and students to build capacity in service delivery and education.

There are many other excellent examples of academia contributing to global health and eHealth through local and international partnerships, fulfilling the social accountability acumen through action. The challenge to the entire academic body is: can we regularize the occurrence of these academic–community partnerships to all corners of our global world? Can we imbue this value universally to all academic institutions? Can academia, through synergistic actions with global policy makers, increase its voice to help introduce positive and cooperative spirit and values through education, service, and research?

34.5 How can Academia Best Contribute?

Studies have illustrated that, for a team to perform, individuals in the team need to deliver their unique contributions in synchrony with the entire team working together to bring cohesive successes, or "collective work products" (Katzenbach and Smith, 2005). Analogously, as a member of a global team of organizations to work together in producing effective collective work products in global eHealth, the academy can make individual and unique contributions in three specific areas:

1. Effective knowledge translation
2. Build capacity in health human resources
3. Innovation and evaluation

34.5.1 Knowledge Translation: From Research to Practice

The Canadian Institutes of Health Research, the leading health research institution in the country, defines knowledge translation (KT) as 'the exchange, synthesis, and ethically-sound application of knowledge - within a complex set of interactions among researchers and users - to accelerate the capture of the benefits of research for Canadians through improved health, more effective services and products, and a strengthened health care system' (CIHR). This definition serves as a lens to characterize an essential process: as health research brings new evidence and knowledge to the fore, what are effective ways to introduce them into routine practice, thereby bringing effective transformation towards evidence-based health care approaches?

Effective and sustainable KT requires synchronized efforts at different levels (Senge, 1990): the *individuals* carrying out the vision towards change, *teams* of individuals working together to drive the culture, and *systems* level transformation to motivate and guide groups to permit certain types of behaviour and encourage the formation of commitment to change. Getting peoples' commitment to change, demonstrating the contributions that they would make, and providing them with appropriate compensation (monetary or otherwise) are powerful driving forces to motivate change on an individual level. Key factors to promote effective change on the teams' level include (Katzenbach and Smith, 2005): jointly owning a shared vision towards an important goal, having effective and distributive leadership for members to effectively contribute, sharing mutual trust and accountability to each other in carrying out the necessary work, having an effective conflict-resolution mechanism to bring differences respectfully to the table for dialogue and resolution, and achieving and celebrating collective work products. Important change management levers such as adjusting the recognition and reward systems, understanding the social and economic impact beyond health care service delivery, the spirit of innovation to generate new evidence and pathways against existing standards, and the promotion of transfer of functions as part of division of labour, and systems' reflection for continuous quality improvement can only be set in motion in the systems' level.

Last but not least, success in sustainable knowledge translation or mobilization requires *harmonization* of motivations at the individual, team, and system's levels. For example, health professional education on global eHealth practices cannot move forward by the academics alone without innovative policy translation by the policy makers, patient, and health consumer demand or preference, or health system redesign and implementation by health administrators. Aligning these different groups to synchronize their respective changes will accelerate KT in causing effective change. Having best practice models and "prototypes" for all individuals involved to visualize how global eHealth can be achieved further to galvanize the resolve of individuals, teams, and systems to effect change. Finally, innovative spirits to adopt best practices from one jurisdiction to their local contexts are needed, as translation of best practices is not a straightforward and mechanical approach, but rather a complex and adaptive process based on solid principles and united steadfastness. Academic institutions are in the best position to coordinate and integrate all these steps to accelerate KT, thereby nurturing the growth of the intrinsic value system and the extrinsic actions of the current and the next generations of health professionals to bias towards global eHealth action.

34.5.2 Health Human Resources Development

Through eHealth, academic institutions can contribute significantly towards HHR planning and implementation in three major directions:

34.5.2.1 Using ICT for eLearning to Promote Innovative Health Professional Learning, Build Capacity, and Promote Quality of Care

Just-in-time e-learning methodologies, such as electronic clinical practice guidelines and drug prescription and interaction databases on handheld computers, are highly effective in assisting health professionals to make sound decisions in their health practices. This approach is increasingly demanded by health professional trainees and new graduates. Evidence is rapidly accumulating that decision support in the form of intelligent electronic health records and clinical decision support systems is closely linked to improved health care and adherence to evidence based health practices (Ho, 2004b; Pusic and Ansermino, 2004). As a result, eLearning enables global health professionals to access high quality continuing health education where they practice and live. In addition, health professionals can carry out knowledge exchange and sharing of clinical practices with their international counterparts, thereby enriching each other's practice approaches. These positive effects can lead directly to increase in capacity of our global health system to train health professionals beyond their regional academic centres, and success in recruitment and retention of health professionals in underserved locations where training actively takes place.

34.5.2.2 Using ICT as an Unprecedented Team Building Medium to Overcome Conventional Practice Boundaries

Many telehealth initiatives have demonstrated success in bringing primary care health professionals from different geographic regions, health jurisdictions, and health disciplines together to improve access to health services and excellence in quality of care to patients. These innovative models need to be promoted, replicated, and entrenched into our regional and global health systems, leading ultimately not only to improved health services to augment existing ones, but also transform our practices towards team-based and patient-centred practices. These exemplars will lead the way towards ground-breaking health care practice models that require physicians, nurses, pharmacists, social workers, and other health professionals to employ team-based skills in addition to their profession-specific training, leading to an increased capacity of the entire health team in managing their patients' health needs and provide timely care to them. This will bring closer the vision that Dr Lee articulated at the WHO high-level forum as quoted earlier in this chapter.

34.5.2.3 Empowering Communities and Citizens to Become Knowledgeable Health Consumers

eHealth can provide health consumers and patients with context-specific health information to help them in appropriate self care. This in turn can assist patients to connect with their health professionals only when appropriate, thereby improving the availability of skilled health workers for needed health interventions. Many call centres deliver this type of telehealth, in addition to many web-based intelligent information systems to facilitate easily negotiable hyperlinked information intended for patients and family members. This approach indirectly yet definitively impacts on HHR through promoting high impact and fitting encounters between patients and health professionals through effective partnership and appropriate self care.

In order for the aforementioned strategies to maximize their effects, an efficiently working eHealth environment needs to be in place as a necessary condition for success. This means that ICT systems need to be operating smoothly and well integrated into health service delivery with adequate technical support to guarantee quality of service (Gagliardi et al., 2003), appropriate policies and legislations to safeguard the practice environment (Dunn, 2004; Major, 2005), regional readiness for eHealth and matching change management strategies for practitioner buy-in and adoption (Jennett et al., 2004; Moehr et al., 2005), and seamless connection between e-learning and eHealth practices to help professionals towards rapid adoption towards habitual workflow. Academic institutions are therefore necessary but insufficient in themselves to bring effective change.

34.5.3 Innovation and Evaluation

Evident from the above discussions, eHealth is introducing many unconventional and transformative ways towards global health practices. Academic institutions can carry out the following activities to help build evidence and illuminate on directions as to how eHealth can make a difference in global health as follows:

- conduction needs assessment of HHR to support both eHealth and community based services (Jennett et al., 2003),
- innovating on health policies to enable eHealth to assist in HHR planning (for example, harmonizing provincial licensing amongst provinces to improve health professional mobility and facilitate inter-jurisdictional practices) (Ho et al., 2006),
- establishing an appropriate evaluation framework to measure eHealth's contribution to HHR and the resultant impact on health service access and outcome (Ho et al., 2004).

34.6 Conclusion

Academic institutions have unique qualities to contribute to global eHealth improvement beyond their regional roles in eHealth implementation and health professional training. At the end of the day, academia not only has the duty to help those who are in need, but also holds a tremendous privilege to contribute. With the academic mission of knowledge translation, evidence generation and evaluation, and cultivation of the next generation of health professionals, academic institutions can be important and pivotal contributing partners to global health and humanitarian need if they so choose.

References

Africa Health Infoway – draft document. November 17, 2005. Accessible at whqlibdoc.who.int/Draft_Afr_h_info.pdf.
Canada Health Infoway web site. Accessible at www.infoway-inforoute.ca.
CIHR. Knowledge translation. www.cihr-irsc.gc.ca/e/24213.html.
Department of Health National Programme on IT, United Kingdom, web site. Accessible at www.dh.gov.uk/PolicyAndGuidance/InformationPolicy/NationalITProgramme/fs/en.
Dunn G.W.: Legal issues confronting 21st century Telehealth. BC Med. J., 46 (6): 290–2, 2004.

Gagliardi A., Smith A., Goel V., DePetrillo D.: Feasibility study of multidisciplinary oncology rounds by videoconference for surgeons in remote locales. BMC Medical Informatics and Decision Making, 3: 1–7, 2003.

Goldberg M.A., Sharman Z., Bell B., Ho K., Patil N.: E-health and the Universitas 21 organization: 4. Professional portability. J. Telemed. Telecare, 11: 230–3, 2005.

Health Canada. Social accountability: A vision for Canadian medical schools, 2001. www.hc-sc.gc.ca/hppb/healthcare/pdf/social_accountability.pdf.

Ho K.: Embedding technologies into health practices, Part I: Technology-enabled health applications (Editorial). BC Med. J., 46: 222–3, 2004a.

Ho K.: Embedding technologies into health practices, Part 2: Decision support on demand – e-health's Killer-app? BC Med. J., 46 (6): 278, 2004b.

Ho K., Sharman Z.: E-health and the Universitas 21 organization: 1. Global e-health through synergy. J. Telemed. Telecare, 11: 218–20, 2005.

Ho K., Bloch R., Gondocz T. et al.: Technology-enabled knowledge translation: frameworks to promote research and practice. J. Contin. Edu. Health Professions, 24 (2): 90–99, 2004.

Ho K., Scott R.E., Novak Lauscher H. et al.: International mobility of skilled health professionals: the impact of Canada's health policy and eHealth. A SSHRC Report. 2006.

Jennett P., Yeo M., Pauls M., Graham J.: Organizational readiness for telemedicine: implications for success and failure. J. Telemed. Telecare, 9 (Suppl 2): 27–30, 2003.

Jennett P., Jackson A., Healy T. et al.: A study of a rural community's readiness for telehealth. J. Telemed. Telecare, 9: 259–63, 2004.

Katzenbach J.R., Smith D.K.: The discipline of teams. Harvard Business Review, 83 (7): 162, 164–71, July–August 2005.

Major J.: Telemedicine and room design. J. Telemed. Telecare, 11: 10–14, 2005.

Marmot M.: Social determinants of health: from observation to policy. Med. J. Aust., 172 (8): 379–82, 2000.

Moehr J.R., Anglin C.R., Schaafsma J.P. et al.: Video conferencing-based telehealth: its implications for health promotion and health care. Meth. Inform. Med., 44: 334–41, 2005.

National e-health Transition Authority, Australia, web site. Accessible at www.nehta.gov.au.

Participatory Poverty Reduction Planning with Ethnic Minorities in Vietnam Workshop Report. December 10–12, 2002. Accessible at www.ngocentre.org.vn/file_lib/ethnicminoritiesworkshop_dec02_eng.pdf.

ProCOR. Accessible at www.procor.org.

Pusic M., Ansermino M.: Clinical decision support systems. BC Med. J., 46 (5): 236–9, 2004.

Scott R.E., Lee A.: E-health and the Universitas 21 Organization: 3. Global policy. J. Telemed. Telecare, 11: 225–9, 2005.

Senge P.M.: The fifth discipline: the art and practice of the learning organization. Currency Doubleday, New York, 1990.

Swinfen Charitable Trust. Accessible at www.uq.edu.au/swinfen/.

United Nations General Assembly. Resolution adopted by the General Assembly. 55/2. United Nations Millennium Declaration. September 18, 2000. Accessible at www.un.org/millennium/declaration/ares552e.pdf.

United Nations. The millennium development goals and the United Nations Role. UN fact sheet. October 2002. Accessible at www.un.org/millenniumgoals/MDGs-FACTSHEET1.pdf.

United Nations Millennium Development Goals (UNMDG). Accessible at www.un.org/millenniumgoals/index.html.

Universitas 21. Accessible at www.universitas21.com.

Wootton R.: Telemedicine and developing countries – successful implementation will require a shared approach. J. Telemed. Telecare, 7 (suppl.1): 1–6, 2001.

Wootton R., Jabamani L.S., Daw S.A.: E-health and the Universitas 21 organization: 2. Telemedicine and underserved populations. J. Telemed. Telecare, 11: 221–4, 2005.

World Health Organization (WHO). World Health Report 2006 – Working Together for Health. Accessible at http://www.who.int/whr/2006/en/index.html.

Part VI
Society, Health and Equity

Chapter 35
The Humanization of Medicine—A Religious Viewpoint

F. Fabò, DD

The subject of the humanization of medicine and health care has been widely discussed for many years. It is a paradox that a matter such as health, which by its very nature is a humanitarian reality, should need to be humanized. But the facts prove the urgent need "to make health realities human, i.e. worthy of man."

Such calls for a "personalization" or "humanization" of medicine reflect an increased critical capacity in the health field, and today the literature often carries references to the topic. When we speak of man or the person, we are referring both to the irreducible identity and interiority that make up each single individual and to his/her fundamental relationship with others that is basic to the human community.

Persons, individual beings, are also social beings. Human beings are truly human insofar as they actualize the essentially social element of their constitution as persons who are members of groups, be they social, religious, civil, professional, or other, who, together, form the surrounding society to which they belong. Although affirming the basically social character of human existence, Christian civilization nonetheless recognizes the absolute value of the person as well as the importance of individual rights and cultural diversity. However, in the created order, there will always be a certain tension between the individual person and the demands of social existence.

"Criticisms of hospitals are these days presented with certain keywords: technology, prohibition, and isolation. Hospitals are seen as total institutions. But patients, even in hospital, continue to be living beings, i.e. people with needs that are not only physical but also social, psychological, and spiritual. The distance between the outside world and the hospital world should be overcome or reduced as much as possible" (Von Engelhardt, 1994).

The problem of the humanization of health also has a clear cultural and social dimension. One need only think of WHO's definition of health. However, the ministers and servants of life all too often today live submerged in a culture of death. To illustrate this aspect, Veronesi (2003) has this to say: "The way a society treats the dying is a photograph of the particular moment in history which that society is going through.". But if health is a value and not a mere biological fact, it becomes a priority to re-establish a proper scale of values in society and to disseminate the culture of life and solidarity (Commissione episcopale per la pastorale dei vescovi spagnoli, 2003).

We have mentioned cultural and social dimensions. We cannot forget the political, juridical, and economic aspects, which turn the subject of medicine, its objectives, and its actual practice into something that is very complex. To put it in a nutshell, it is easy enough to explain these principles but very hard to carry them out in practice.

The explosive increase of scientific knowledge and technological capacity in the modern epoch has brought mankind considerable advantages, but it also poses some difficult challenges. In the light of our knowledge of the immensity and the antiquity of the universe, the position and importance of man within it appear much less weighty and certain. Technological progress has considerably increased our capacity to control and direct the forces of nature, but it has also had the effect of producing an unexpected and possibly uncontrollable impact on our environment and even on humanity itself.

For all these reasons a profession, mission, or vocation such as that of the health worker naturally requires a solid preparation and continuous training in moral matters in general and in bioethical matters in particular. In the presence of cases that have been rendered ever more complex by the possibilities offered by biotechnology, health workers—and in particular doctors—cannot and must not be left alone under the weight of unsustainable responsibilities. This is all the more the case if we consider that many of these possibilities are still in an experimental phase and are of great sociosanitary importance in the field of personal and public health (Bonifacio Honings).

Bioethical profiles are not just one of the many aspects of the matter—they are one of its essential nuclei. For if the doctrine and practice of medicine occupy a central position in the panorama of bioethical studies, the consideration of human conduct in the sector of life sciences and health care is one of its principal objectives (Parere sugli scopi, rischi e limiti della medicina, 2001).

Without a doubt the true humanization of science and medical technology is at stake, that is, also in the field of medicine it is necessary to construct "that civilization of love and life without which the existence of individual persons and of all society loses its most authentically human meaning" (Evangelium Vitae).

The problem of the humanization of medicine is closely related—also chronologically peaking—to the birth of bioethics. Among other things, this was triggered by certain savage forms of medical experimentation on man.

For example, it came to be known that in Willowbrook State Hospital (New York) some 700 retarded children were deliberately infected with the hepatitis virus between 1965 and 1971; and the fact that in 1964, in the Jewish Chronic Disease Hospital (New York), live cancerous cells were inoculated into 22 elderly men and women set up a strong reaction among the population in general and in the world of scientists. And that is not all: from 1932 to 1972, in a town in Alabama, 399 Afro-American farm workers suffering from syphilis were not treated nor even informed of the true nature of their disease (Tuskegee Syphilis Study). Nuremberg was very soon forgotten, too soon.

In the 1960s, in the context of the Cold War, fear about the nuclear threat and for the future of our planet began to spread. Hence the birth of bioethics.

Of all the sciences that study nature, medicine is the only one that should never be entirely thought of as mere technique. For a doctor, technique or "theoretical" knowledge is never enough. There must also be practical know-how.

In people's collective imagination, doctors are people who cure the sick, who look after patients. All their activity involves a holistic activity of the organism, which is a vital activity. Indeed, "the term and the concept of health mean everything related to the prevention, diagnosis, therapy, and rehabilitation for a better equilibrium and physical, psychological, and spiritual welfare of the person." This concept should not be confused with that of the person, who, instead "regards policies, legislation, programming and health facilities" (John Paul II).

The exceptional and rapid progress of medical science gives rise to repeated ethical and deontological questions, and the finding of an adequate response, on the ethical level, ultimately depends on the concept one has of medicine and of man.

> Today the medical profession is at a sort of crossroads: in today's cultural and social context, in which medical science and art run the risk of losing their native ethical dimension, doctors may sometimes be strongly tempted to transform themselves into ministers of the manipulation of life or even into operators of death. In the face of such a temptation their responsibility is today enormously enlarged and finds its deepest inspiration and strongest support precisely in the intrinsic and inalienable ethical dimension of the health profession.
>
> (John Paul II, 2000)

Medical action is—and must be—intrinsically moral because it is intrinsically human. An amoral, neutral medicine that does not wager on behalf of man is inhuman and immoral because it goes against man and because it has failed in what was its basic function: to serve life.

The peculiarity of the art of medicine is the fact that it acts not only on agriculture or on the breeding of animals but also on human beings who have to be treated. This condition defines the sphere of the doctor's scientific competence from a new point of view. It means that the sick, the patients are, above all, people. When this personal condition is neglected, forgotten, or ignored, medicine loses its specificity and becomes a different art, one that is all too often perverse and inhuman.

> Their action [i.e. that of doctors or health workers], as human action, contains in itself a truth that does not depend on them, on their will, or on their feelings. It depends, on the contrary, on the reality of the people to whom they direct their action and whose vital principle is intrinsic, and depends only extrinsically on doctors, in a vicarious or surrogate form, inasmuch as they are capable of eliminating the pathology or accompanying it in its development.
>
> That is how the truth of medical practice should be understood, on which the very goodness of such action depends and in which the very goodness of doctors is at stake, as they establish the right relationship with their patients, in such a way as to treat them with objective reality and to support and promote what is good for them and what they rightly deserve.
>
> (Noriega, 2002)

"The basic evaluation criterion," as Pope John Paul II affirmed, "lies in the defence and promotion of the integral good of human beings, according to their individual dignity. To this regard it is worth remembering that all medical action on a person is subject to limits that are not limited to any technical impossibilities of realization but rather are linked to respect for human nature itself, taken in its fullest meaning: what is technically possible is not for that simple reason morally admissible" (Speech by His Holiness John Paul II, 2000).

We said here at the start that "in the created order there will always be a certain tension between individual people and the demands of social existence." Freedom, responsibility, law, and duty are firm categories of which we speak at length. At this point—almost provocatively—I would like to recall some thoughts expressed by Joseph Ratzinger, published in his book *Truth – Tolerance – Freedom*.

> Freedom is related to a criterion, the criterion of reality – to truth. The freedom to destroy oneself or to destroy another person is not freedom but its diabolical parody. [...] The freedom of man is a shared freedom, freedom in the togetherness of freedoms, which limit each other reciprocally and thus reciprocally support each other: freedom has to measure itself by what I am, by what we are – otherwise it suppresses itself. [...] The law is not a limitation of freedom, it constitutes freedom. The absence of law is the absence of freedom.

What is a law that conforms to freedom? How must a law be structured for it to constitute a right to freedom? For there undoubtedly exists an apparent right, which is a slave's right and therefore not a right but a regulated form of injustice. [...] The criterion for a real law that can authentically define itself as such, and therefore as a right to freedom, can thus only be the good of all, that is, goodness itself. Understanding this, Hans Jonas declared that the concept of responsibility was the central ethical concept. This means that freedom, to be properly understood, must always be considered together with responsibility.

[...] The question of the way in which responsibility and freedom have to be set in their proper relation cannot be decided simply by a calculation of effects. [...] The reality of the individual person, properly comprehended, brings with it a reference to the collectivity, to the other person. We will therefore say: there exists in every one of us the common truth of the unique human essence, which traditionally was called "human nature." [...] Responsibility would therefore mean: to live our lives as an answer to what we really are (Ratzinger).

In the context of the reform of the United Nations, I should like to conclude with the words pronounced by Cardinal Angelo Sodano:

> To the human race, exposed to the pandemics of today and to others that threaten to develop, to the masses of people denied access to basic health, aspirin, and drinking water, we must not offer an ambiguous, oversimplified, or even ideological vision of health. For example, would it not be better to speak clearly of "the health of women and children" instead of using the expression "reproductive health!" Can it be that there is a desire to speak of a right to abortion?
>
> (Sodano, 2006)

Bibliography

Von Engelhardt D.: Cultura e Medicina. In: "Dizionario di Bioetica", 218–9, Leone S., Privitera S. (eds), EDB-ISB, Bologna-Acireale, 1994.
Veronesi U.: Eutanasia ed etica del medico. Bioetica: Rivista Interdisciplinare, 11: 228–9. 2003.
Commissione episcopale per la pastorale dei vescovi spagnoli. Final document of "Chiesa e Salute" National Congress, Bioetica: Rivista Interdisciplinare, 11: 556–64. 2003.

Commissione teologica internazionale, Comunione e servizio, la persona umana creata a imagine Dio, n. 1.

Father Bonifacio Honings, O.C.D.: Consultor of the Congregation for the Doctrine of the Faith and of the Pontifical Council of the Pastoral for Health Workers, citing "The Health Workers' Charter", no. 5.

Parere sugli scopi, rischi e limiti della medicina, Italian National Bioethics Committee, 14 December 2001.

Evangelium Vitae, 27.

Tuskegee Syphilis Study.

John Paul II: To the Plenary Assembly of the Pontifical Council for Health Workers, 9 February 1990. In: Teachings XIII/2, p. 405, n. 4.

John Paul II: "Nothing can justify the elimination of a life which can be a gift of love for a family even in the suffering of the final days". In: Medicina e Morale, 50 (IV): 761. 2000.

Noriega J.: L'azione medica e la sua bontà. La cura del malato in stato vegetativo permanente. In: "Né accanimento né eutanasia", 153–62, Lateran University Press, Rome, 2002.

Speech by His Holiness John Paul II: Eighteenth International Congress of the Transplantation Society, August 2000. Cf. Donum Vitae, no. 4.

Ratzinger J.: "Truth – Tolerance – Freedom", 261–9.

Speech by Cardinal Angelo Sodano: Secretary of State, on 16 September in New York during the Summit Meeting of Heads of State and Government, United Nations Organization. J. Humanitarian Med.,VI (4): October–December, 2006.

Chapter 36
Urban Social Exclusion—The Samusocial Response

Xavier Emmanuelli, MD

36.1 Introduction: A Widespread Social Ill—People in Cities Around the World Face Social Exclusion

The socially disadvantaged desparately need society's attention. The Samusocial concept and operation are one such humanitarian response.

Eighty per cent of Europe's population live in cities. Estimates suggest that in the short term, by 2030, sixty per cent of humanity will live in major urban areas. This development will lead to significant changes in how we live and think, as well as how we behave.

When most people lived in essentially rural, traditional societies, their existence was governed by laws, but also by the rhythm of the seasons, rites and customs. This provided a certain level of social cohesion because people were united, symbolically, by a common purpose. For example, life was marked by ploughing, harvesting and grape picking. Even personal life followed the rhythm of rites familiar to all—the transition to adolescence, the marriage ritual and entrance into the community through baptism. Even the dying were sent to their graves with a ceremony to mark their passing. Night followed day in a cycle of history celebrated by all.

These rites and myths are unnecessary to city life. Work rhythms have assumed a different pattern and the sense of membership of a group has disappeared. Social cohesion has lessened and people have become more isolated. The notion of the larger family, its responsibilities and its limitations has changed radically. The implicit notion of an individual's obligations towards others, both as individuals and collectively, represented a security net that has unravelled. City life is characterized, then, by the absence of symbolic points of reference that used to underpin the notion of community. The most fragile individuals (the physically or emotionally disabled, the homeless, the elderly and the marginalized) no longer receive support from this implicit connection. Societies are now liberated from symbolic representations that no longer need to exist. The community is unaware of the distress these individuals experience because it lacks the codes to recognize them. Thus, the weaker members are left to themselves and to their solitude.

Institutions provide aid but many of these people exist beyond the institutional world's field of vision. This, then, represents urban exclusion. Humanitarian organizations and aid measures have been created in an effort to remedy this exclusion, but such efforts are inadequate in the face of the mechanism that promotes the exclusion of the weakest. Modern society is further characterized by a rural exodus and large-scale migrations that push entire populations to reassemble in megalopolises, creating rejection and alienation.

Samusocial is an aid organization that can respond to large-scale social exclusion.

36.2 Samu Medical and Samusocial: Two Entities Working in Emergency Settings

Samusocial was founded in Paris in November 1993, as a parallel organization to the SAMU (Service d'Aide Médical d'Urgence, the French national Emergency Medical Service). Additional Samusocial organizations have since opened in 70 cities, in partnership with the French Red Cross. The SAMU (from which *Samusocial* takes its name) aids accident victims by dispatching a mobile medical unit to the scene. Victims can then be treated on site before being transported to the appropriate hospital. SAMU emergency services are provided in response to calls to its *toll-free number, 15,* throughout France. The service operates as a "hospital without walls."[1]

Samusocial (*Service d'Aide Mobile d'Urgence Sociale,* the emergency social service) operates similarly. It assists socially isolated persons and those in distress, but who do not have injuries that require emergency medical care. The Samusocial *telephone number is 115.* The Samusocial mobile unit responds by sending out a team composed of a nurse, driver and social worker. Both organizations—medical and social—operate around the clock.

36.3 Samusocial: Tools and Methods

The Samusocial is an emergency response entity that *operates only in cities.* It relies on *seven tools:*

1. Mobile aid teams;
2. A free public telephone number;
3. Emergency housing centres (CHU);
4. Emergency housing centres with nursing care (CHUSI), referred to as LHSS (Lits Halte Soins Santé);
5. A storefront centre that is open during the day (ESI, Espace Solidarité Insertion);
6. A research unit that analyses the data gathered by teams and staff; and
7. A "family shelter" (Maison relais) that offers housing to individuals identified by Samusocial. Following an evaluation of their level of independence, they can live in a facility that provides both autonomy and contact with other residents in common areas. The family shelter is directed by a Housemistress, who acts as a community organizer–manager, not as a social worker.

---

[1] See also the "World Open Hospital" concept elsewhere in this book.

36.3.1 Methods

The Samusocial teams are easily identified by their jackets. The teams circulate in city streets night and day, watching for individuals who are too marginalized to even be able to ask for help, either because:

- they cannot assess their own situation;
- they are resigned to it; or
- they know that "traditional" aid programmes will not help them.

Street people always congregate at the same location. This is their *living space* that, by means of an age-old reflex, involves building a substitute home. They can thus be located and monitored.

The team's tasks include:

- developing a credible and respectful approach to these individuals;
- evaluating the individual's status;
- offering treatment or emergency shelter;
- confirming their physical and emotional status in order to establish a connection and offer appropriate solutions;
- directing or transporting individuals to the most appropriate aid.

Whatever the approach, it involves a lengthy educational process in the street to transmit the "social codes" that will ensure the individual's ultimate re-entry into society.

The *Housing Centres*[2] provide temporary shelter, along with a meal and a shower, as well as services such as a locker and a medical consultation (possibly with a gynaecologist, psychiatrist, dermatologist or other specialist) and social work assistant. Medical and social service files are established. In the *housing centres with nursing care* (CHUSI), individuals may receive short-term treatment, chemotherapy, alcohol treatment, wound care and anticoagulant injections or, simply, a place to rest while they return to an acceptable state of health or until they can be transferred to an appropriate facility, rest home, therapeutic housing or CHRS (Centre d'Hébergement et de réinsertion Sociale, temporary housing placement).

36.4 Samusocial International

Exclusion is a paradoxical result of development and is a universal phenomenon. As cities grow, a certain population category is increasingly marginalized and faces problems including crowding, sanitation, nutrition, exposure to infectious disease, shelter and transportation. This is the corollary of our globalized culture's lifestyle. Megalopolises result in exclusion. The Samusocial approach is one way to provide aid to the most marginalized populations.

---

[2] See below: outreach services and the Housing Centres.

Samusocial agencies have been created in France's large cities. Some have a greater presence than others, but all share the following features:

1. Round-the-clock operations and, in particular, at night,
2. Mobility: Mobile clinics travel throughout the city, particularly to locations where homeless people are known to gather regularly,
3. Shelter, offered by a multidisciplinary team (medical–mental health–social work) and through treatment, a rebuilding of the person and the personality with the ultimate goal of social inclusion.

Samusocial International was founded on this model in 1998. Its goal is to aid the most at-risk populations in distress in large cities around the world. Those populations most often include street children.

A *university diploma programme* has been established in two Paris universities to train Samusocial staff. The programme, "Abord des enfants errants en danger dans les rues des mégalopoles," addresses outreach to street children in major urban areas. Trainers may also go on site to train local staff.

There are *16 Samusocial* organizations in existence or formation around the world: Lima (Peru), Cayenne (Guyana), Fort de France (Martinique), Brussels (Belgium), Paris and 70 cities (France), Moscow (Russia), Budapest (Rumania), Algiers (Algeria), Casablanca (Morocco), Bamako (Mali), Ouagadougou (Burkina Faso), Dakar (Senegal), Pointe Noire (Congo) in start-up, Saigon (Vietnam), Cairo (Egypt) in the planning phase and Athens (Greece).

36.5 Street Children

Urban street children are a phenomenon of the last 30 years. They can be seen on every continent, but this development is more visible and less tolerable in developing countries, which often lack legal tools and protective measures to help the children.

The presence of street children is a late-stage symptom and its causes vary. They may include family breakdown, polygamy, poverty, rural exodus, political or economic migration and cultural aberrations, like the phenomenon of the "talibes," beggar children sent out to the streets by religious leaders. Regardless, all street children adopt the same behaviour:

- They live in groups of varying size and structure;
- Leadership develops, as do relationships of dominance and domination;
- The group members are involved in begging or perform small jobs, carrying out various errands;
- Drug addiction (glue or solvents) is a nearly constant social practice;
- They occupy very well-defined spaces: night-time areas, areas for earning money and so on;
- Adults exploit them (criminality, pedophilia, clandestine labour).

However, the children's activities are characterized by the "game." These playful activities—like hide-and-seek with irritated shopkeepers, the police and others—complicate institutional relationships.

The children often suffer from a range of pathologies, including traumas, skin problems, sexually transmitted diseases and, among girls, prostitution and early pregnancy.

36.6 The Role of Samusocial International

Three principles guide the work of Samusocial: round-the-clock availability, mobility and shelter. They make it possible for the organization to work with these persons day or night, on their territory, after negotiating with their leader, or leaders, and focus initially on the most vulnerable. This intervention is followed up by regular visits so that the children can give up street survival codes and replace them with social codes, including those that involve representation of the body, time and relationships with others.

These children suffer from the syndrome known as *paradoxical overadaptation*. In other words, to survive, they adapt to street life. As time passes, they adapt increasingly—even *overadapt*—to their experience. The more they adapt to that life, the less *adaptable* they are to life in society and to social life.

With the tools at its disposal, Samusocial works on the streets, on a long-term, personal basis with each child, which may involve stays in housing centres. In most cases, the organization manages to help children leave dangerous and precarious situations. Samusocial is an emergency, first-line response. It can function only via a network approach since its strategy is based on three phases: Emergency, Post-emergency, Inclusion. Each requires a specific approach:

- Emergency: initial contact, first aid and orientation;
- Post-emergency: relearning social codes;
- Inclusion: long-term activities including apprenticeship, literacy and so on.

It is thus a "preliminary phase" tool that takes the form of a non-profit group addressing both emergency aid and development needs.

36.7 Outreach Services and Housing Centres

The goal of the Paris Samusocial outreach service is to establish or maintain contact with homeless people. There are not—and will never be—enough emergency housing placements to meet all the needs. The emergency housing centre is, and can only be, a transition "space" that:

1. provides shelter in case of severe weather conditions (extreme cold or heat) and
2. in particular, provides the opportunity to conduct a health and social services evaluation as the first step in a process leading to permanent housing and social inclusion.

As such, the emergency housing centre is a *tool* for following up the treatment and support services provided on arrival at the centre with reasonable and appropriate next steps.

Emergency housing centres must:

- be adequate in number,
- provide dignified accommodation, be well-equipped and function in a professional manner.

Individuals with health problems are housed in emergency housing centres with **nursing care** (LHSS).

Those individuals with social welfare-related concerns will be housed in centres that provide only emergency housing.

The emergency housing centres are among the social supports intended to achieve health and social reintegration.

Individuals will need to participate in a long educational process to acquire, or reacquire, the "codes" required to interact in society and live independently:

- corporal codes: a sense of the physical self, which allows the individual to seek treatment and develop a concern for his/her health,
- temporal codes: a sense of time and the ability to plan for the future (learning about making and keeping appointments),
- code of the "Other:" the ability to create, through one's own action, tools for interpersonal exchange and
- spatial codes: the ability to move from place to place and expand one's environment and sense of living space, broadly defined.

Emergency housing centres are not intended for medium- or long-term stays, but are temporary "treatment sites" that, during outreach missions, can help to:

- strengthen the institutional connection and
- provide a period for rest, recovery and restoration. They complement the lengthy treatment and education conducted in the streets to help individuals change so that they can reintegrate into society.

Chapter 37
Social and Medical Progress Through Patient Education in Chronic Diseases

J. P. Assal, MD, FMH

37.1 Psychosocial and Pedagogic Dimensions of Long-Term Follow-up: Other Roles for the Physician Enlarging his Biotechnical Ability

Because of social progress, improved medication, and increasing life expectancy, chronic diseases—whether among the elderly or the young—are becoming more prevalent, their treatment more demanding, and more important to health care delivery and decision-making. The medical profession and society are being forced to develop new strategies and more imaginative approaches to meet the growing needs.

Long-term education of the chronically ill is proving to be one of the most successful key strategies to meeting the challenge, which is for an extended management system that adds pedagogic, psychological, and sociologic dimensions to traditional responses. It should also expand the role of the physician and health care team beyond the established biomedical approach.

The treatment of diabetes mellitus illustrates remarkably well the evolution of therapeutic strategies and management of chronic patients. In this context it certainly represents a model for the treatment of chronic diseases. Taking the example of insulin-dependent diabetes, four significant phases can be distinguished (Figure 37.1).

37.1.1 First Phase: 1921

The discovery of insulin introduced a radical correction of a metabolic problem that was theretofore fatal.

37.1.2 Second Phase: 1946

The advent of antibiotics, which made it possible to control many infections that caused severe metabolic failure. Many diabetics had to have limb amputation for

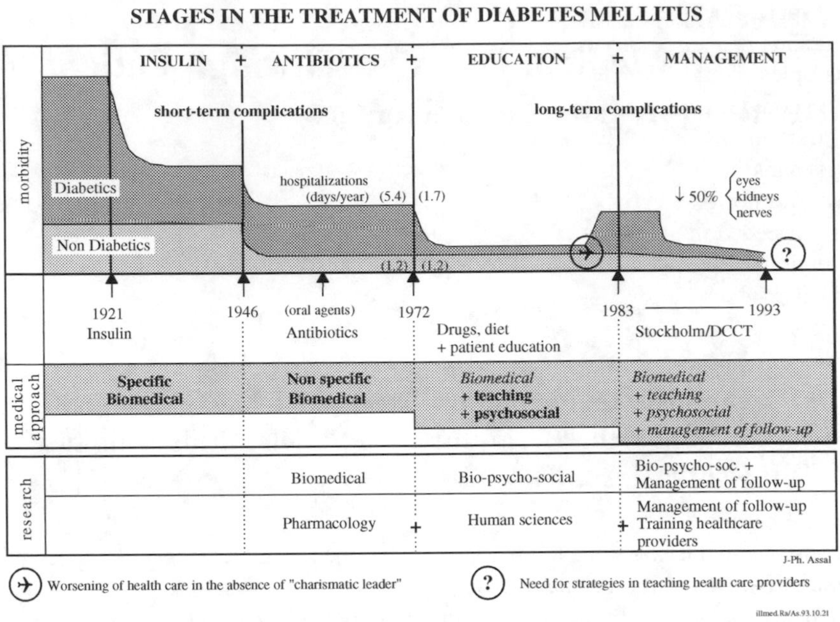

STAGES IN THE TREATMENT OF DIABETES MELLITUS

Fig. 37.1 The four phases in the history of the treatment of diabetes

osteomyelitis secondary to infected neuropathic foot! In these two phases, improvement in the control of diabetes was due to research and treatment in the biomedical field, diabetes-specific for insulin, and non-diabetes-specific for the antibiotics.

37.1.3 Third Phase: 1972

The arrival of pedagogy and patient education in the field of therapeutics, thanks to the work of Leona Miller (Miller and Goldstein, 1972). For instance, among the Mexican-American population of Los Angeles, with an underprivileged patient community, this physician introduced a patient education programme that reduced hospital stay from 5.4 days per year, per patient, to 1.7 days. This statistically shortened period was the same as that for non-diabetic hospital patients, at 1.2 days/year/patient. For the first time in the history of medicine it was proven on a large scale that the patient's education played a therapeutic role of prime importance, even though the medical profession had the advantage of remarkable tools for treatment: highly purified insulin, diabetes auto-control techniques, and a choice of antibiotics that covered most of the microorganisms.

The biomedical dimension of a diabetic's treatment was therefore optimal, but its efficiency could only be manifested through another dimension, that of patient education. The epidemiological proof was thus established: psychosocial and pedagogical approaches came to the rescue of biological therapy.

It must, however, be mentioned that right from the discovery of insulin several clinicians had insisted, in their own centres, on the role of the patient's training. Examples include E. Allen in London (Jackson), E.P. Joslin in Boston, E. Roma in Lisbon, G. Constam in Switzerland, M. Derot and H. Lestradet in France, and J. Pirart in Belgium. The list can be extended for every country. These eminent physicians had shown the path, without, however, quantifying their approaches. They did not describe their technique of patient education. Their experiences had not succeeded in motivating the medical profession at the international level. These exceptional clinicians, charismatic personalities, bound by their daily activities did not have the time to structure and to organize the training of the medical and nursing professions in their therapeutic environment.

Leona Miller's study, published in the New England Journal of Medicine in 1972, on the effects of training 6,000 patients, provided an official approval to this method of treatment. To reinforce the biomedical approach, the treatment of diabetes thus benefited from the human sciences: a new challenge for the medical profession, a new role for the physician—that of integrating pedagogy and psychology into medical practice. The centres that applied this integrated approach for diabetes and patients were able to diminish by about 80 % the cases of failure, of keto-acidotic coma and of hypoglycaemic coma. As for prevention of amputations in high-risk patients, those with loss of pain sensitivity or with arterial deficiency, the rate of amputations fell by about 75 %.

Thanks to technological improvements, auto-control of glycaemia made it possible for patients to manage their diabetes on a day-to-day basis. Results have shown that in the 1970s and 1980s the auto-control of blood sugar was perhaps more useful in the control of acute failures (hypo- or hyperglycaemic comas) than in a permanent improvement of metabolic balance. There is a similar auto-control possibility in other diseases also, such as asthma, with regular assessment of peak flow, or in Parkinson's disease, with a recorded diary of the frequency and length of kinetic crises that helps the patient to adapt the timing of his L-dopa therapy.

37.1.4 Fourth Phase: 1993

The organization of patient follow-up as assurance for long-term metabolic quality control.

The American study of Diabetes Complications Control Trial (DCCT) (Diabetes Control and Complications Trial Research Group, 1993) and six European studies (Reichard et al., 1993; Wang et al., 1993) analysed the effects of diabetes control on the incidence and long-term progress of complications. These investigations have shown similar results: a fall of about 50 % in the incidence of long-term progression of complications involving diabetic retinopathy, kidney disease, and neuropathic deterioration. A study of the activities of all these centres shows that, in addition to patient education, the organization of follow-up of the patients was a determinant factor in long-term metabolic quality control. These centres had structured their follow-up in an optimal fashion, with multidisciplinary teams that included physicians, nurses, dietitians, and psychologists. These investigations, especially DCCT, have shown to the profession the importance of organizing in long-term care, the dynamics of interdisciplinarity within the health care team as well as the regular assessment of the patients' performance.

One example among many is worth citing: in the DCCT investigation, every fortnight the patient had to bring to the physician or the nurse the results of his blood sugar readings and metabolic value controls. He or she also had to show how he or she had modified the treatment according to his findings. Telephone and fax were used regularly; telephone terminals were provided so that the patient could have constant access to information and advice on the management of his treatment programme. Guidance by psychologists was included in these services to reinforce the patients' motivation for treatment. This fourth phase shows that education alone is not enough and that it must be completed by organizing the medical follow-up. The accent is therefore on the medical 'management' of the patient, an aspect that until now depended on the common sense and personal initiative of the health care team, but which had never been thought out within the structure and organization of long-term care. Here is a new field in which expertise must be developed to ensure quality of care.

A diabetes clinic, as in any continuing care of chronically ill patients, can no more be based entirely on biomedical technology or knowledge, however important these may be at the pathophysiological level. Diabetes mellitus, like any other chronic disease, necessitates, therefore, medical training based on follow-up techniques and integration of the patient in a continuous process of care.

Here biotechnical and psychosocial dimensions are fundamentally complementary and can no more be separated or opposed, as is often the case with medicine. It behoves the physician to unite these two sectors, quite a difficult mission even today, as little has been done to close the gap between these dimensions of medicine. The treatment and continuing care of chronic patients offer a unique opportunity to develop such an integrated approach.

Experience shows that health practitioners are not sufficiently conscious of the peculiarities of the kind of medicine they practice; little do they know how much the type of service they provide (e.g. emergency medicine) can complicate and interfere with the transition to another type of care, such as follow-up of chronic illness. Such problems are seen when a hospital-based physician leaves his institutionalized position and goes into private practice.

37.2 Long-Term Follow-up of a Patient

An important part of out-of-hospital activity is the long-term care of patients suffering from chronic illnesses such as cardiovascular diseases (arterial hypertension, anginal claudication, cardiac insufficiency), metabolic and nutritional diseases (diabetes, hyperlipidaemia, high blood urea, overweight), rheumatological conditions (arthritis, backache, rheumatism), neurological diseases (cerebral arteriosclerosis, Alzheimer's disease, epilepsy, Parkinson's disease), pulmonary conditions (chronic bronchitis, obstructive syndromes, bronchial asthma), and gastrointestinal diseases (gastroduodenal ulcer, colonic conditions, cholecystopathies, hepatitis).

Each one of these conditions has probably been seen within the hospital in an acute stage, such as pulmonary oedema, diabetic coma, herniated disc, epileptic attack, acute asthma, gastrointestinal haemorrhage, jaundice, and so on. There the physician will have learned to treat the emergency and to have "cured" it. But he or she will not have learned to treat these illnesses on a long-term basis, most of which cannot be cured but can well be kept under control. Although these diseases are different, they share certain common characteristics:

Chronic illness

- is often incurable.
- is silent outside acute exacerbations.
- if there is pain, it tends to be persistent.
- often there is little relationship between the complaints and biological findings.
- its progress is unpredictable.
- may be related to the patient's lifestyle.

The treatment

- is important for survival and/or daily comfort.
- has variable effects.
- often necessitates the training of the patient to ensure its management.
- implies daily discipline.
- usually takes the patient's time.
- often interferes with social life.

The patient

- may not be cured of the illness, but can control it.
- must manage the treatment according to various factors related to his private life.
- outside acute episodes, his illness is usually silent.
- as soon as surveillance weakens the disease relapses.
- must be trained to act rapidly in case of crisis.
- must accept a certain degree of loss of his integrity.

The physician

- prescribes the treatment but only indirectly controls the illness.
- must train his patient for treatment; must share his medical power.
- must manage the illness often in its silent phase.
- must urgently treat the acute episodes.
- must be vigilant to detect late complications.
- must ensure psychological and social support.
- must be prepared to accept a new medical identity.

The medical identity associated with the treatment of acute illness imprisons the physician often in a stereotyped functional mode and prevents him from being fully effective in his new role for long-term care. He or she is bound by biomedical and pharmacological specificities and finds it difficult to adapt himself or herself to the requirements of long follow-up of these chronic patients.

Several physicians have developed some very effective approaches to these patients, but unfortunately these experiences have rarely been conceptualized, such that the required training, extending from a hospital system to an ambulatory system, remains inadequate.

37.3 The Physician's Training: What Requirements for Long-Term Patient Care?

Centred principally on pathophysiology of disease, on establishing a diagnosis and choosing a treatment, medical studies have not trained the student for long-term patient care. Such training will be provided only if the philosophy of medical education is changed. To the above-mentioned established themes, it is necessary to add training in strategies of treatment management, especially in long-standing illnesses.

In medical studies the student first encounters a cadaver (anatomy and dissection lectures) while his earliest experiences should also have been based on the ordinary patient model. Such training would have allowed him to complete his theoretical knowledge with know-how in treatment and follow-up strategies. In this regard some recommendations can be made for the training of health personnel:

- avoid education based exclusively on factual knowledge: promote a process of understanding by stimulating the problem-solving approach;
- enlarge the notions of pharmacological action and therapeutic indication of drugs with an understanding that promotes treatment management by the patient;
- overcome the temptation of intellectual arrogance and learn to manage ambiguity and uncertainty in diagnosis and therapy;
- be able to pass from the domain of biological thinking to the less precise but real domain of the patient's experiences and beliefs concerning his or her illness, health, and treatment;
- complete the physician's biomedical competence with knowledge acquired in the consulting room from the realities of daily life.

It is difficult to introduce such a change; it requires modifying certain traditions and habits of the medical profession and overcoming certain convictions. In the present context it means providing the physician with a wider education that meets the various needs of the patient, needs that far outweigh the purely biomedical dimension. It is therefore indispensable that any person looking after chronic patients should master certain elements in the following fields: (a) education of the patient, (b) psychology of the patient, and (c) organization and management of long-term follow-up.

Considered together and oriented towards clinical activity, these themes could include the following:

Training in treatment education; helping the patient to manage his treatment.

37.4 Practical Training for the Therapeutic Education of Patients

At the request of WHO–Euro, a group of experts have prepared a special report (Therapeutic patient Education: Continuing Education for Healthcare Providers in the Management of Chronic Diseases) indicating the need of the medical community for more specific training of health care providers in the management and long-term follow-up of chronic diseases (World Health Organization, 1998). One key concept emerged from this expert group: Patient education should be replaced by *therapeutic* patient education (Lacroix and Assal, 2003).

When health care providers teach patients, they tend to spend more time and energy speaking about the disease than providing the patient with the appropriate skills for the daily management of his or her condition. Therapeutic patient education therefore focuses on the skills for effective self-management of the treatment adaptation to a chronic disease and coping processes and skills, while also taking into consideration the cost to the patient and society.

Therapeutic patient education is an essential component for the efficient self-management and quality of care of all long-term diseases and conditions. However, patients with acute diseases should not be excluded from its benefit.

37.5 The Need for Educational Programmes in Therapeutic Patient Education

The World Health Organization has defined therapeutic patient education as follows:

- *Therapeutic Patient Education should enable patients to gain and maintain abilities that allow them an optimal management of life with their disease.*
- *Therapeutic Patient Education is therefore a continuous process, integrated in health care.*
- *It is patient-centred; it includes organized awareness, information, self-care learning, and psychosocial support activities, regarding disease, prescribed treatments, care, hospital, and other health care settings, organizational information, health, and illness behaviour.*
- *Its aim is to help patients and their families to understand the disease and the treatment, cooperate with health care providers, manage their own health and maintain and/or improve their quality of life.*

Description of these various needs is beyond the scope of this article, but the following is a list of topics that are now part of a postgraduate and continuing education curriculum given at the Faculty of Medicine of the University of Geneva. It leads to a diploma in the field of therapeutic education of patients with chronic diseases.

- The characteristics of chronic diseases compared to the acute medical situations (how to adapt the behaviour of physicians to the specificity of chronic diseases).
- Understanding how the patient with a chronic disease functions with regard to his treatment and daily management of the control of his illness.
- Taking into account the patient's coping strategies with the diseases (which counter-attitude do physicians develop in front of a patient who is in revolt or in the bargaining stage with his treatment?).
- Communicating with the patient and mastering the "active listening" technique (which strategies should be used to facilitate the communication?).
- Giving therapeutic instructions to the patient (which approach should help the physician deal with the health beliefs of the patient? How can the physician evaluate if the patient's locus of control is external or internal?).
- Assisting a patient in coping with his illness and its treatment (mastering the various barriers that interfere with the patient's adherence to the treatment, developing specific attitudes that would reinforce the process of coping).
- Integrating the patient's own experience in his therapeutic educational programme (which educational strategies are recommended to help the patient acquire the skills for self-management?).
- Evaluation of a learning process and methods used (methodologies for the evaluation of courses given to patients and the evaluation of the impact of the courses on the patients).
- Long-term follow-up of patients (which strategies are needed to integrate patients' relapse prevention, therapeutic education, and psychosocial support into the biomedical activity of the physician?).

37.6 Conclusions

The physician's identity has been moulded during medical school and years of hospital training into a way of thinking about specific sub-systems dealing with pathology, biochemistry, and organic and laboratory diagnostic procedures—each of these representing a sub-system, a speciality in itself, a rather "closed" entity. Management of chronic diseases forces the physician, whether he or she likes it or not, to face other sub-systems that deal with the entire person, two persons, the family, the community, and society. In this perspective, professional specialities (endocrinology, diabetology, etc.) always fall short of the need to simultaneously handle the various problems and requirements of the patient as the bearer of the disease and his family.

A professional who accepts this inter-relatedness will eventually face an identity crisis, discovering that his sub-speciality is only part of the whole. Although it is not within the scope of this chapter to address the problematic issue of professional identity, it is important here to note, at least, that this broadening of professional orientation is often initially experienced by the physician as a loss of his or her specialized medical power.

Medical training is slowly, but surely, improving. The fact that WHO is now strongly recommending training in therapeutic patient education and that some medical schools already have developed specific training programmes into their medical curricula is a major step forward for the quality of care. This training is also an answer to what patients and patients' associations have asked for, for so many years.

References

1. Miller L.V., Goldstein J.: More efficient care of diabetic patients in a county hospital setting. N. Eng. J. Med., 286: 1388–91, 1972.
2. Diabetes Control and Complications Trial Research Group. The effect of intensive treatment of diabetes on the development and progression of long-term complications in insulin-dependent diabetes mellitus. N. Eng. J. Med., 329 (14): 977–86, 1993.
3. Reichard P., Nilsson B.Y., Rosenqvist U.: The effect of long-term intensified insulin treatment on the development of microvascular complications of diabetes mellitus. N. Eng. J. Med., 329 (5): 304–9, 1993.
4. Wang P.H., Lau J., Chalmers T.C.: Meta analysis of effects of intensive blood-glucose control on late complications of type I diabetes. *The Lancet*, 341: 1306–9, 1993.
5. World Health Organization (WHO). Regional Office for Europe, Copenhagen. Report of a WHO Working Group. Therapeutic Patient Education. Continuing education programmes for healthcare providers in the field of prevention of chronic diseases, 1998.
6. Lacroix A., Assal J-Ph.: L'éducation thérapeutique des patients. Nouvelles approches de la maladie chronique. 2ème édition complétées. Editions Maloine, Paris, 2003.

Chapter 38
An Equitable Society Protects the Health of its Weakest Members: Women and Children

G. Masellis, MD, D. Vezzani, MD and G. Gargano, MD

In our professional activity in the field of women's health, in a well-supplied country where the majority of women who work are educated, and act responsibly in the management of their lives, certain conditions of social equity and stability are an expected part of our daily work and are indeed taken for granted. In other parts of the world, however, where the social scene presents different requirements, the health of women and children is also different, being affected by variables that from our point of view would be considered to be extraneous to a physician's daily task.

We would like to consider here the particular features of the health of women and children. Women's health is often identified with their reproductive capacity, while in fact this represents only one aspect of female health. In general, female reproductive health is looked upon as an asset in all cultures and in all conditions, but there is no such universal appreciation of the efforts that a society should make—even a small society like the family—in order to keep women "healthy." The safeguard of the central role of female welfare as a requisite for the welfare of both family and children is common to all points of view. This means that women, their families, and social groups can everywhere share the value of programmes for the defence of women's health.

In the Beijing Declaration in 1995 the governments participating in the Fourth World Conference on Women declared the intention to ensure the application of the human rights of women and girls as an integral and indivisible part of human rights and of basic freedoms.

This affirmation of principles led to a platform outlining strategic objectives and possible action to achieve them in a number of fields: poverty, education, health, violence against women, the economy, access to decision-making levels, and many others. In particular, in *actions for women and health*, it is stated that "women have the right to have the highest attainable level of physical and mental health" and that "the achievement of this right is fundamental to their life, their well-being, and their possibility of full participation in family and public life". In national and international forums women have regularly pointed out that for the achievement of these health standards three conditions are necessary: peace, development, and equity in family and social responsibilities.

The achievement of good health standards is obstructed by barriers related to various differences: not only of gender (male/female) but also of geographical, social, and ethnic differences. Women do not have the same access to health resources, and in conditions of poverty and conflict this difference increases. A further discrimination occurs in childhood because girls are discriminated from boys as regards access to play, food, and health services. The limited decision-making capacity allowed to many women regarding, in particular, their sexual and reproductive life is a widespread reality that has a negative impact on women's health. This disparity is further aggravated by the greater presence among women of poverty, economic dependence, experiences of violence, and discrimination.

Women's and children's health is also negatively affected by the unequal distribution of food in the family for women and girls and by the lack of adequate hygienic and housing conditions, especially in rural areas and poor city quarters. The enjoyment of good health is a *sine qua non* for the successful performance of all the tasks involved in caring for a family and participation in productive social activity at all levels.

After this preamble we should agree with the World Health Organization (WHO) that reproductive health is a state of physical, psychic, and social well-being, in all its various aspects, related to the reproductive system and its functions and processes, a state of well-being in which people must be able to enjoy a satisfactory and safe sexual life and to have the opportunity to reproduce, as well as freedom to decide if, when, and how to do so.

Reproductive health is negatively affected in the world by:

- inadequate knowledge of human sexuality;
- prevalence of risky sexual behaviour patterns;
- poor quality or inappropriateness of available services and information;
- discriminatory social practices, such as strict segregation of the sexes even between those caring for others and those being cared for;
- limited decisional power of many women and girls on their own lives.

All these factors lead to diseases related to pregnancy, abortion performed in unsafe conditions, and the spread of sexually transmitted diseases and AIDS, often as a consequence of sexual violence on younger women and of commerce in women for sexual exploitation.

Sexual or gender violence in its various forms, violence in the home, psychological abuse, and exploitation for sexual purposes are all factors that place women and girls at high physical and mental risk, exposed to illness and unwanted pregnancies. When health problems originate from such conditions, a feeling of shame will often deter women from approaching their family or health services. The disparity is further aggravated by the greater prevalence among women of poverty, economic dependence, and experiences of violence and discrimination.

Reproductive health assistance thus becomes the sum total of all the methods, techniques, and services that by promoting cultural and social development, prevention, and adequate health assistance contribute to health and reproductive well-being.

   Reproductive health is in fact related to a series of determinant factors that can directly provide protection from diseases or, on the contrary, cause them, since health touches on matters related to lifestyle, the environment, the population, employment, economic considerations, information, education, and health service organization.

   The World Health Organization has proposed 17 indicators for the monitoring of reproductive health that can be applied in all conditions of economic development. The actions necessary for the improvement of these indicators should constitute a privileged basis for collaboration between the highly developed countries and the developing ones. These indicators are commented upon in the *Report on the Monitoring of the World Population in 2002* by the United Nations, devoted to reproductive rights and health.

   We present in Table 38.1 some of the proposed indicators:

Table 38.1 Overall indicators of reproductive health

Overall fertility rate		Objectives proposed in the International Conference on Population and Development
Number of children per woman		Although the Programme of actions does not quantify the objective for the increase in population and its distribution, it points out that a stabilization of the world population would contribute to the achievement of the objectives of sustainable development.
– Italy	1.2	
– EU	1.5	
– USA	2.1	
– Developing countries	4.6	

   The fertility rate has dropped everywhere. One cause of this, that is amply documented, is the decisive role played by the improvement in women's education and the reduction in the number of pregnancies per woman.

   Reproductive behaviour has been affected everywhere by women's increased decisional capacity and their greater autonomy, which have led to better capacity in women to control their fertility.

   School attendance affects two main aspects of fertility: age at first marriage and the use of contraceptives. Even a limited number of years of school attendance makes a difference: women who complete an elementary school education have fewer children than women who are illiterate.

   The use of contraception has considerably increased all over the world (Table 38.2). It is estimated that 60 % of couples in developing countries now use contraceptives, compared with 10 % in the 1960s. Developed regions and developing areas present certain differences as regards the type of contraception employed. In developed regions contraception is usually by reversible, short-duration methods

Table 38.2 Prevalence of contraception

Percentage of women of reproductive age who use (or their partner uses) contraceptive methods	By the year 2005, 60% of family planning services should offer as wide a range as possible of safe and effective contraceptive methods.

(pill, condom, traditional methods), while, on the contrary, in developing countries long-duration and highly effective methods are used (sterilization, intra-uterine device) which often put a permanent end to the capacity for reproduction.

38.1 Maternal Deaths

Every year 515,000 women die owing to pregnancy-related complications. There are five main causes of death due to obstetric complications: haemorrhage (25%), sepsis (15%), eclampsia/hypertension (13%), dystocia (7%), and abortion in unsafe conditions (13%) (Table 38.3).

Table 38.3 Maternal death rate

Number of mothers deceased per 100,000 live births		National states should do everything in their power to achieve a significant reduction in maternal mortality and morbidity by the year 2015: a reduction to one-half that of 2000.
– Africa	1000	
– Asia	280	
– Europe	28	
– North America	11	

38.2 Obstetric Assistance

Many obstetric complications can be avoided by simple interventions performed by trained health personnel, especially during labour and the actual delivery. But in developing countries only 35 % to 53 % of births are attended by trained personnel (in Italy the percentage is 98 %) (Table 38.4).

Action to reduce maternal mortality depends on the availability of easily accessible services to assist the pregnancy and delivery and to prevent unwanted pregnancies, especially in cases of poor maternal health.

Table 38.4 Percentage of births attended by trained health personnel

Percentage of births attended by health personnel	Every birth should be attended by trained personnel. By the year 2005, 80% of births should be attended by trained personnel, 85% in 2010, and 90% by 2015.
Developing countries *35-50%*	
Developed countries *98-100%*	
Availability of basic obstetric assistance *Number of services for basic obstetric assistance (including antibiotic parenteral therapy, oxytocics, sedatives for eclampsia, manual assistance and removal of placental residue) per 500,000 inhabitants. This refers to the technical capacity to provide vaginal operative deliveries, treatment of eclampsia and severe infections, repair of lacerations, manual intervention*	Promote availability of obstetric services capable of assisting births and coping with obstetric emergencies.
Availability of overall obstetric assistance *Number of services for essential obstetric assistance per 500,000 inhabitants, including surgery, anaesthesia and possibility of transfusions, capable of offering not only the services defined immediately above but also obstetric surgery (Caesarian section), anaesthesia, and transfusions*	By the year 2005, 60% of primary and family planning services should offer obstetric assistance directly or by transfer to another facility.

Poverty and limited access to economic and educational resources reduce women's capacity to decide matters related to their own health and nutrition. A poor diet and overwork are major negative factors affecting maternal health. Women are often unable to decide autonomously when they have to seek help—they have to wait for the opinion of their husbands or mothers-in-law (Table 38.5).

It is not only back-street procured abortion that has negative effects on female health, there is also the lack of adequate care following spontaneous miscarriage.

In North Africa, where abortion is illegal, it is estimated that one obstetric hospitalization in five is due to the effects of procured abortion or spontaneous miscarriage. Some studies have estimated the abortion rate in countries where it is in fact illegal: in Bangladesh the estimated annual rate is 750,000, that is 28 per 1000, a rate similar to that in Nigeria and the Philippines.

Table 38.5 Percentage of hospitalizations due to abortion

Percentage of hospitalizations due to complications of abortion (spontaneous or procured): every year 78,000 maternal deaths following abortion	Women must have access to quality services for treatment of the complications of abortion.

After an illegal abortion only 10–50% of women seek assistance. Every year 78,000 maternal deaths occur due to complications of abortion procured in unsafe conditions, that is one maternal death in eight. The number of permanent lesions is incalculable. In countries where the risk of illegal abortion is higher, services for contraception are inadequate or non-existent (e.g. they are provided only to married couples or are not available as basic services).

38.3 Sexually Transmitted Disease

To protect women's health and dignity there is one type of legal restriction that should be enforced: that of the selective abortion of female foetuses. This type of restriction, however, introduced by the Indian government in 1994, has encountered great difficulty for its acceptance (Table 38.6).

Sexually transmitted disease (STD) is the cause of acute illness and long-term morbidity for both men and women, but women suffer the greater social and

Table 38.6 Sexually transmitted disease rate in pregnant women

Percentage of pregnant women aged 15-24 yr attending prevention and treatment services	By the year 2005, 60% of primary and family planning services must provide prevention and treatment for genital infections, including sexually transmitted diseases, in addition to spreading information about barrier methods for the prevention of infection.
HIV-positive rate among women *Percentage of pregnant women (aged 15-24 yr) presenting to prenatal services found to be HIV-positive*	The HIV-positive rate in persons aged 15-24 yr must be reduced by 25% in highly endemic countries by the year 2005. Globally, it must be reduced by 25% by 2010.

economic consequences. The commonest form of female neoplasia in the developing countries, that is cancer of the uterine cervix, is related to STD. The consequences of STD also affect pregnancy: low birth weight, premature birth, morphological damage, and blindness due to untreated eye infections. In countries where AIDS is endemic, the infection rate is five times as high in females as in males of the same age. The reasons for this are both biological (greater sensitivity to infection) and social. The network of these girls' sexual partners often consists of adult males who have many partners and a high probability of being HIV-positive. Young women have fewer opportunities and possibilities of negotiating the use of condoms and their partner's fidelity. Also, with regard to young women, sexual coercion is very frequent (e.g. sex acts in exchange for food and lodging).

Services for reproductive health are often directed at pregnant married women, such that adolescents are excluded, also for reasons of natural reserve.

Primary prevention is directed at every aspect that prevents contracting the disease: health education, information on safe sex, use of condoms (not only with prostitutes), and lowering of the age when sexual activity initiates. This prevention is equally effective for HIV and other STDs (Table 38.7).

Secondary prevention is the treatment of infection, to interrupt the chain of transmission. As regards HIV/AIDS, interruption of the chain of transmission involves education of the patient: treatment slows down transmission by reducing the patient's infectiousness. The condom, which provides effective and cheap protection against further spread of infection, is used by adult males in their relations with prostitutes, but is little used in married couples' sex. A married adolescent female runs a very low risk of contracting such diseases.

It is easy to understand how the growing co-operation between the north and south of the world increases the risk of triggering social conflict in the field of sexual health. If this co-operation fails to respect basic rights and cultural differences, the defence of reproductive health can clash with common concepts of male/female relationships and of religious/non-religious law in various countries.

Common to all concepts is the safeguard of female well-being as a prerequisite for the well-being of the family and of children. This means that everywhere women, their families, social groups, and co-operation programmes are favourable to the defence of women's health.

Table 38.7 Prevalence of low birth weight

Prevalence of low birth weight *Percentage of babies with birth weight under 2500 g*	Improving women's state of nutrition, particularly if pregnant, and children. Action to reduce the low birth weight rate includes improvement of maternal nutrition and increasing the time interval between births.
Developing countries 18.6% *Developed countries 7%* *World 15.5%*	

38.4 Children

Infantile mortality is especially serious in African countries because of poor sanitary and social conditions, while in the more advanced countries the rate is fairly stable at values of less than 10 per 1000. With regard to children's health problems, there are three main scenarios where there appear to be close links between maternal health, human rights, economic development, and infantile health that affect infantile mortality.

First, the problem of low birth weight is closely related to the mother's health conditions. Second, the question of respiratory infections, among other things, stresses the need to promote combined action for the instruction of families with regard to the most appropriate methods of care for sick children. The third problem is AIDS, which poses the most dramatic health emergency at the start of this new century.

38.4.1 Low Birth Weight

Children undernourished in utero are more likely to die in the early years of life. They have lower immune defences and are therefore more subject to disease and more exposed to later pathologies of adult life, such as diabetes and cardiac diseases, and they are more likely to develop intellectual deficits that reduce future professional opportunities (Table 38.7).

In developing countries, low birth weight is mainly due to poor conditions of maternal health and nutrition. Inadequate maternal nutrition before and during pregnancy accounts for a large proportion of deficits of foetal growth. Also, diseases during pregnancy such as diarrhoea and malaria can further reduce the mother's energy reserves. Among the causes of low neonatal weight, pregnancy in adolescent females who have not yet completed their physical growth is a problem common to both industrialized and developing countries. The main studies monitoring the evolution of this indicator have not demonstrated any substantial modification in the situation in the past few years.

38.4.2 Respiratory Infections

Acute respiratory infections are the leading cause of mortality in children aged less than 5 years. In 2000 they caused the death of two million children in developing countries. Sixty per cent of these deaths could have been avoided by the selective use of antibiotics. To prevent death from respiratory infection it is crucial that the signs of the illness (coughing and variations in the breathing rate) should be recognized by the family and that the children should be taken to the appropriate medical facilities where the necessary drugs are available. The object of the promotion of health in

Table 38.8 Prevalence of acute respiratory in-fections

In 2000, two million children in developing countries died of acute respiratory infections.	Improve parents' information, the availability and accessibility of services, and the availability of drugs.

this case is to improve the knowledge of the parents and of all caretakers of such children. In developing countries, only 50% of children with respiratory symptoms receive adequate care. This means that if we are going to have any incisive effect on the problem our action must extend in four directions: improvement of the families' knowledge, availability and accessibility of services, availability of drugs, and improvement of the social environment (Table 38.8).

38.4.3 HIV/AIDS

Since its first appearance, the AIDS epidemic has spread to all four corners of the world and in many countries is reversing the economic and social improvements achieved in recent years, destroying resources and human lives, and extending the gap between rich countries and poor. In the world today, of the 36 million persons suffering from HIV, 45 % are women and 1.4 million are babies and children aged less than 15 years. Transmission from mother to foetus is responsible for 90 % of infections in children. In areas where the disease is most prevalent infantile mortality is expected to double in the next few years. With regard to HIV-positive breast-fed children, 20 % of them contract the infection during the mother's pregnancy, 50 % during the birth process, and 30 % during feeding. Breastfeeding increases the child's risk of infection by 20%, but many infected mothers do not have access to the clean water and hygienic conditions necessary for the preparation of artificial milk. Recent studies have also shown that mixed feeding is riskier than breastfeeding alone in mother-to-child transmission (Table 38.9).

Table 38.9 Prevalence of HIV-positivity among children

Prevalence of HIV-positivity among children *1.4 million babies and children < 15 yr HIV-positive*	Improve pharmacological prophylaxis and safe procedures for feeding of children, and promote awareness on the part of the mother of mother-to-child transmission.

Transmission of the virus from mother to child must in all cases be fully understood if effective prevention is to be achieved. The means available are: pharmacological prophylaxis (at sustainable costs, doses, and social impact), safe procedures for feeding children, and awareness on the part of women. As things stand today, in countries where AIDS is highly endemic, 50 % of women do not know that the virus can be transmitted from mother to child.

38.5 Discussion and Conclusions

As health professionals we might be tempted to stand aside from the disparity between advanced and developing countries, which is a matter of the availability of health resources, in the name of the presumed superiority of the medical profession. However, we no longer have the right to consider ourselves *super partes*, inasmuch as the taking of a neutral stance endorses injustices and social inequalities.

We have to realize that with the appropriate health practices we can contribute to the wider diffusion of concepts: that of the rights of the person, an economic model, a model of society (e.g. the relationship between the value of the individual and that of the family or social group of origin), and an interpretation of the relationship between human beings and the forces of nature (i.e. the concept that illness can be overcome by organization and knowledge rather than magic or religion).

Caring for people involves much else besides—it produces a cascade of other effects besides the mere treatment of a disease. All of us carry within us a set of values in whatever acts of care that we perform: some people will limit themselves to carrying out surgical operations, others will discuss ideas, yet others will exchange life experiences, while others again will seek points in common between different worlds and different cultures.

One question is whether the offer of a model of high-cost medicine to a limited number of persons, in communities that require low-cost medical action over a wide range, might not be contradictory. Or whether one might not give an equivalent impulse by improving the lives of individuals and families by tackling high-tech treatment in rich countries, and thereby liberating resources in developing countries that could be devoted to basic treatment.

Another question concerns the matter of supplying some of our resources and facilities to treat persons coming from less affluent countries. It is good to host a certain number of patients and to involve doctors and those responsible for managing resources, our hospital corporations, and regional administrations. Basically, we would be continuing to do what we already know. It is more difficult to create initiatives to be applied in the developing countries and to request that essential drugs be reasonably priced and that opportunities for the health of women and children be related to programmes that come into force prior to the, destruction of local systems, rather than in the aftermath of an emergency. Not all of us have the necessary courage or determination to go out and practise medicine in the less developed countries, but we can all act to affirm the ethics of rights and knowledge, which offer to all individuals the awareness that would change the quality of life of disadvantaged women and children. This is where the World Open Hospital (WOH) of the International Association for Humanitarian Medicine (IAHM) can play a most useful role. It is not simple to co-operate for health in the world, as multicultural health requires the recognition of equal dignity between different cultures and genders.

The difficulty of working for health in the world is often related to the fact that the confrontation of different systems prevails over the confrontation between individuals—which means that we can have a direct experience of the relationship between the North and South when we have had first-hand direct experience of suffering and disease.

We discover in such moments that people the world over suffer and rejoice for the same reasons, while if we compare the complexities of different systems (cultural, religion, political, race, wealth, poverty), walls and defences build gradually set up that accentuate the differences.

All this underlines the profound inequalities that exist in the world, inequalities that are the result of an "inconsiderate egoism" that does not take into account among us the weakest or the future generations, rich or poor as they may be; it is not difficult to imagine that this sort of egoism may drag the entire human race to the brink of catastrophe (Erice Declaration, March 2001, on the Quality and Right of Health).

We would like to make an appeal to an "intelligent egoism" that takes into account the principles of sustainability, that practises generous and constructive forms of international solidarity, guarantees everyone access and availability of health and education services, and that opposes all forms of discrimination. It is difficult to speak of humanitarian medicine at a time when national states are unable to settle their problems peacefully, and when thousands of deaths of women and children occur. However, if it is declared by the governments that health is a universal human right, this right must be defended and asserted even under most difficult conditions. This assertion is the testing ground of our own humanity.

In the exercise of our profession we have to learn to safeguard the dignity of the human person, respect for life, and equity, and we have to realize that there is a right to being different that merits protection and recognition. We have to learn to provide health in a context where several moral concepts exist side by side and we also have to realize that the moral authority to impose a concept on others, without their consent, is only a limited authority. If we recognize the right to differences we also recognize a parity between cultures, which in turn means respect for collective cultural rights: in this way we can make a positive contribution to peace.

Technicosanitary co-operation also entails the promotion of better living conditions—otherwise such co-operation soon becomes ineffective. Medical action has to be accompanied by the promotion of society: that is by access to education, to micro-credit, to equality, to social justice—in a nutshell, to projects for life.

Bibliography

WHO Reproductive Health Indicators for Global Monitoring. Report of the Second Intera-
    gency Meeting 2001. *http://www.who.int/reproductive-health publications/RHR 01 19/RHR01
    19/RHR 01 19 content.en.html*
Gill Z.: Implementing emergency obstetric care in developing countries. Workshop Report, 2001.
Reproductive Health in Refugee Situations. An Interagency Field Manual. United Nations
    High Commissioner for Refugees 1999. *http://www.who.int./reproductive-health/publications/
    interagency manual on RH in refugee situations/index.en.htm*
Link to UNICEF STATISTICS site. *http://www.safemotherhood.org/resources/pubs/actionagenda
    pdfs.html*
International Journal of Gynecology and Obstetrics: AMDD papers
    http://www.womenshealth-elsevier.com/doc/journal/ijgo amdd.html
Masellis M., Gunn S.W.A.: Humanitarian medicine: A vision and action. J. Humanitarian Med., 2:
    33–9, 2002.
Gunn S.W.A.: The right to health through international cooperation. J. Humanitarian Med., 1:
    1–3, 2000.
Gunn S.W.A.: Commentary on female genital mutilation. World J. Surgery, 23: 1087, 1999.

Chapter 39
The Humanitarian Force of the UN Millennium Development Goals

Hanifa Mezoui, PhD

39.1 Summary

As the United Nations celebrates its 60th anniversary, it is time for renewal, a time to commit again to Security for All, a time for development.

Development had been placed prominently as one of the four overarching subjects to be considered at the 2005 World Summit and by the 60th General Assembly. Not only these bodies considered the future of world development, but they also reflected on the progress made since the Millennium Summit five years ago. Primarily, the Millennium Development Goals (MDGs), as derived from the Millennium Declaration, will be the guidelines used to assess the progress made with respect to the past and the future.

Concurrently, the World Summit and the General Assemblies (GA) will speak to issues regarding humanitarianism, its changing role in an evermore interconnected world, and nations' changing abilities to address humanitarian concerns.

While both issues are prominently being discussed throughout the United Nations, an important connection can be described linking the two issues and showing that the implementation of one can have significant benefits for the other. The relationship between the MDGs and humanitarian concerns is complex and cooperative. There is no simple cause and effect relationship. To add to the complexity, the MDGs are multifaceted. They have exceptional relevance to a number of GA agenda items. Humanitarian concerns are just one of the many issues that relate and benefit from MDG progress. It is their simplicity that drives the allure of nations to the MDGs and provides the ability to encompass a number of issues. The MDGs are not policy or even recommendations; they are simply a means of measure and a springboard for the development agenda. Humanitarian concerns, just one of these issues that relate to the MDGs, benefit significantly from their implementation.

Today, the challenge is for governments and leaders of the UN to recognize that humanitarian concerns will benefit from the implementation of the MDGs as well as work to understand the degree of their effect and contemplate what could be done to expand their effect. Promoting the MDGs, which many nations at least claim to be doing wholeheartedly, could be equally as great for the overall promotion of humanitarian affairs as it is for the development agenda itself. With an understanding of their relationship, it becomes clear that it is time to develop the humanitarian approach to development and recognize the positive contributions of the MDGs to humanitarian concerns.

39.2 Humanitarian Issues

Of the issues addressed in the MDGs therein lie humanitarian issues that simultaneously benefit from the effort put forth to achieve the eight goals. While this is not a comprehensive list of humanitarian issues, it is intended to encompass the greatest range. These issues that will be addressed further in this chapter are:

- Principles: humanity, independence, neutrality, and impartiality;
- Protection and promotion of human rights through the protection of the vulnerable and the establishment of the rule of law;
- Effectiveness of emergency aid;
- Response to natural disaster;
- Response to disasters of war and instability;
- Response to internal and external displacement;
- Preventing and responding to health issues, specifically HIV/AIDS;
- Allowing humanitarian actors safe and unimpeded access to vulnerable populations.

39.3 Humanitarian Issues and the MDGs

The MDGs were created to focus on eight different points of development including: the eradication of extreme poverty, achievement of universal primary education, promotion of gender equality, the reduction of child mortality, the improvement of maternal health, improving the international condition of health crisis (like HIV/AIDS), ensuring environmental stability, and the creation of a global partnership for development. While none of these goals specifically addresses any of the humanitarian issues listed above, the analysis in this section will show that success in completing any of these goals will have a transitory effect on the improvement of the humanitarian issues.

It is important to note before comparing humanitarian concerns with the MDGs that the goals stand solely as a point of measure and not as a means of development. Humanitarian concerns and humanitarian progress rest more on the goals' means of implementation and the end result than on the goals themselves. For this reason drawing a connection between humanitarian concerns and the MDGs will often require a second step regarding potential means of implementation of the goals.

Additionally, it must be understood that the goals were written to be succinct and relate to specific issues regarding development that can be calculated. The humanitarian issues that are related are derivative and are not easily calculable.

39.3.1 Promotion of the Principles: Humanity, Independence, Neutrality and Impartiality

Of all the humanitarian concerns addressed in this chapter, the promotion of humanitarian principles is by far gaining the greatest support from the MDGs. This is simply due to the humanitarian nature of the MDGs and their intrinsic mission for the improvement of the world's societies. Humanitarianism and its principles of humanity and independence are based on individuals and nations of the world providing and supporting others. Similarly, it is the MDGs, goals to provide and support for the world's nations. While the MDGs do not say that any nation is required to help any other nation to any degree, the intent is clear that a great deal of the support that is spoken about in the MDGs is contingent on aid, debt forgiveness, and an overall adjustment to the world's financial system (mainly discussed in Goal 8.) With the MDGs and their implementation comes a change in attention focusing the world more on development and humanitarian goals than other issues. There are a number of examples, but the recent discussion and recommitment to the 0.7 % of GDP aid contributions that many member nations of the UN are bringing before the table of the summit and the GA is an exceptional display of recommitment to the humanitarian charge. This change in international focus displays clearly, through the call for additional aid, as an effect of the MDGs and the humanitarian policies that are hidden within them.

Goal 1 plays a primary role, as it is the basis for many humanitarian projects. Simply stated, it is the goal to end poverty. It is clear that the principles of humanity and independence are directly linked to the ability to provide one's self and one's family with food, water, and shelter. The eradication of poverty and hunger is significant to allowing individuals throughout the world the basic ability to fulfil basic needs.

Fighting poverty and hunger, however, are not new endeavours for the UN. But with the implementation of the MDGs there is potential to elevate the assistance given from simply aid to a greater importation of knowledge and technology that will distribute the means for individuals to provide for themselves. With a productive capacity individuals can produce more than their own share of food, a basic start to the long process of structural development and capital accumulation necessary for economic growth. As individuals and nations become more self-reliant, productive, and wealthy, their need for humanitarian assistance will decline. Basic standards of human living can be upheld and those that begin the process of development will also be more capable of helping others needing assistance. Further, independence is closely tied to an individual's freedom to produce and provide for himself. Lack of dependence in parts of the world will allow humanitarian assistance to be more concentrated and effective in other locations. Of course, the MDGs are universal and should have positive effects in all locations if properly applied, but their implementation and overall completion will surely take place at different rates in different areas.

Neutrality and impartiality are dependent on the individual's ability to make his own decisions in an educated and informed way. Education and equality amongst sexes are representative of the complete fulfillment of this issue as well (These issues represent goals 2 and 3). Health too, without progress, limits one's ability to travel, to work, and to enjoy one's experience. Without health improvements humanitarian efforts are often lost to the overwhelming preconditions of a nation suffering from epidemics. Further, nations that are bordering other nations, upon improvement of health and education, will be more capable of supplying aid to their neighbours in case of emergency. This displays the main contribution the MDGs have on humanitarian affairs. Humanitarian concerns will greatly benefit from the creation of more nations capable of looking to their neighbours to distribute aid as those nations who used to be importers of aid begin the process of development which leads to their ability to contribute.

39.3.2 Protection and Promotion of Human Rights Through the Protection of the Vulnerable and the Establishment of the Rule of Law

The MDGs play a fundamental role in the protection and promotion of human rights. Human rights are contingent on the stability of a nation through economic development, social tranquility, and effective representative government. As the MDGs become implemented their contribution to stability will be clear and profound. Education, lack of poverty, and reduction of epidemics will all contribute to overall stability as well as allow the individual's attention to be drawn to human rights abuses rather than simply be focused on surviving.

Further, the international community's attention being directed to the poorest and the most ill of the world will also draw more attention to the gravest abusers of human rights. Many governments will be incapable of neglecting at least basic human rights without also breaking many of the MDGs. The parallel attention will be symbiotically beneficial. The MDGs, in this circumstance, can be used as a humanitarian tool to address many issues of human rights abuse. This will become even more effective as more and more nations fulfil the goals.

Indeed, human rights are contingent on the protection of the rule of law and the promotion of democracy. Their interlinked structure mutually reinforces a universal and indivisible core of values and principles of the United Nations. The Universal Declaration of Human Rights and other human rights institutions are supported by and provide support for the MDGs. Benefiting both, the Goals and human rights need each other for long-term success. The MDGs tack eight of the most ingrained hindrances to the ability to experience and enjoy the rights and fundamental freedoms of all persons; upon their achievement the MDGs will allow greater access to human rights to all persons. It is often the goals of humanitarian organizations to re-establish human rights to persons of a derelict country. The MDGs will complete that goal in many situations by simple economic stability, health, and development.

Gender rights are also closely linked to human rights and often represent the need to protect the vulnerable (Goals 3 and 6 speak directly to this linkage). It is also important to mention Goal 7, the improved environmental regulations and policies. A clean and controlled environment is a human right and a necessity for stability. The environment, while not commonly considered a humanitarian concern, will become more prevalent in the near future as abusers neglect and pollute the public good, the environment. The MDGs' attention to the changes and their call for positive improvement are deeply rooted in issues such as human rights.

39.3.3 Effectiveness of Emergency Aid

Today, more than ever before, we live in a global, interdependent world. No State can stand wholly alone. Akin to this, humanitarian issues of concern are interlinked and require nations to be equally prepared and capable to respond. It is the MDGs' purpose to standardize each nation's ability to address the issues of humanitarian concern.

Often emergency aid is necessary in nations in which poverty and hunger are the worst. If the MDGs can effectively spur the management of poverty this statistic would quickly become obsolete.

The key point is that the MDGs make nations more capable of helping themselves get out of emergency situations, and more importantly, make all nations more capable of helping their neighbour in times of need and distress. Development coalitions (Goal 8) and intercommunication will only further the capabilities of emergency aid networks. Further, progress made by the MDGs will inherently reduce the necessity or the amount of emergency aid simply by removing the demand for it. When there is a reduction in demand, those that do demand aid will receive more direct and more comprehensive assistance.

39.3.4 Response to Natural Disasters

Natural disaster response is always a difficult activity. In some circumstances, such as the events in Southeast Asia during December of 2004, humanitarian response is often perceived as good, while in other circumstances, such as the State of Louisiana in August of 2005, it is perceived as bad. However, in both cases it can be seen that the international response was both positive and effective. The latter circumstance only shows that even the most economically and militarily powerful nation in the world can be devastated by a natural disaster.

Whether the response was good or not does not really matter. In fact, it is clear that whatever the response, it could always have been better. The MDGs can play an important contributing factor in improving response to natural disasters. First, as discussed in the above issue, an economically developed neighbour will be more capable of providing aid and response in emergency situations. Second, development, particularly the goal of eradicating poverty and the goal of reducing the global spread of disease, inherently prevents natural disasters from exacerbating already disastrous situations. When people are not hungry and are not ill they are more capable of surviving, coping with disasters, and helping.

39.3.5 Response to Disasters of War and Instability

Specific issues of development and response to disasters of war have been recently addressed in the preparatory paperwork for the World Summit. *In Larger Freedom*, written by Kofi Annan, speaks to the facilitation of more rapid humanitarian response by improving timeliness of aid and greater funding.

Speed of aid is contingent on the amount that can be given from the reserves of one nation to another. Certainly, as nations work to accomplish the MDGs, there will be an increase in the overall ability of nations to aid each other. Former Least Developing Countries (LDCs) will have the capability of contributing to aid their neighbours. Further, an individual country's capability to control its citizens will improve with development as poverty reduction, education, and health services promote stability and reduce the likelihood of civil strife.

39.3.6 Response to Internal and External Displacements

There is a clear need to strengthen the inter-agency and country-level responses to the needs of internally and externally displaced persons. There are already international standards for the minimum level of support for those persons, but commitment to refugee protection plans and holding higher standards of support would be more beneficial.

Clearly, development, as described in the MDGs, would allow for citizens of one nation to be more capable of hosting refugees from another, or even within one nation. As seen by the internally displaced in America in the aftermath of Hurricane Katrina, developed nations are more capable of boarding and supporting their own citizens. In locations with large numbers of refugees, namely Africa, development in one nation, through the elimination of poverty and the eradication of epidemic illnesses, would be exceptionally beneficial to those displaced to that location.

39.3.7 Preventing and Responding to Health Issues, Specifically HIV/AIDS

Clearly, this humanitarian issue has the most in common with any one of the MDGs. Goal 6 is exactly this: come to a global conclusion and then act to eradicate global health issues such as HIV/AIDS, malaria, and others. Success in performing this goal is contingent on a great humanitarian effort to share technologies and medications and support a global exchange of ideas on how to combat these horrific illnesses.

Further, as stated above, limiting horrific health crises will be beneficial to humanitarian emergency aid efforts because the populations receiving help will not have their problems exacerbated by disease. Also, there will be a greater number of humanitarian workers and supplies to be redirected to other emergency situations.

39.3.8 Allowing Humanitarian Actors Safe and Unimpeded Access to Vulnerable Populations

The MDGs call for the implementation of development policies. While they do not enumerate those policies, or even make recommendations, they are supportive of whatever policies might be necessary to generate development. Clearly, humanitarian efforts will become easier as development occurs. Illness will decline as health issues are addressed, and disruption and war will decline as stability is created by a reduction of poverty. Further, with global attention drawn to the MDGs, nations will be less likely to inhibit humanitarian projects.

39.4 Conclusion

The humanitarian issues, ranging from responsiveness to natural disasters to protection and promotion of human rights, are mutually reinforcing and cannot be enjoyed without each other. Thus, it is necessary to recognize the importance of the MDGs to humanitarian issues and bring forward questions on how to further the MDGs, speed their progress, and increase their effectiveness so that the humanitarian benefits that have been discussed in this report can benefit further by the quick implementation of the goals.

Many nations are promoting the MDGs, especially those in need of development. In Africa, knowledge of the MDGs is almost universal among government officials and civil society organizations. It is important that, if the external benefits of the MDGs are to be realized, the goals are implemented and enacted by all nations. It is clear that it is time to develop a humanitarian approach to development and recognize the positive contributions of the MDGs to humanitarian progress.

WHO on Poverty and Health

The World Health Organization is committed to promote the highest attainable level of health for every human being, as of right. Poverty is one of the principal impediments to health and must be overcome in every way.

The following two chapters from WHO highlight the nefarious effects of poverty on health and the ways to control them.

Chapter 40
Science and the Health of the Poor

Jong-Wook Lee[†] MD

During the last half of the 20th century we saw examples of dramatic progress in health: sharply reduced infant mortality rates and longer average lifespan in many countries; the eradication of smallpox and highly effective vaccination programs against other illnesses; and new technologies for controlling both communicable and noncommunicable diseases. Yet the fruits of progress in health have been unevenly distributed, and for hundreds of millions of people the possibility of a healthier and safer life for themselves and their families remains a promise unfulfilled.

The directions taken by the World Health Organization in this first decade of a new millennium will have far-reaching implications. They will affect public health globally, and will inevitably change the organization itself. Most importantly, our policies will have consequences for communities and individuals—especially the poor. It is time for WHO to reassert the global vision of health that excludes no one. Our Constitution demands exactly this in stating as our objective "the attainment by all peoples of the highest possible level of health."

Rigorous science is the basis of our credibility and of our capacity to get results. In recent months, the fight against SARS has confirmed WHO's scientific leadership in the global struggle against disease. Yet solid science is only the beginning. Scientifically excellent public health guidelines and other reliable information sit inert in journals and databases unless there is political commitment—on the part of governments, communities, and individuals—to turning knowledge into action that will get results on the ground. In this WHO's political role of leadership, partnership building is essential. Both technical excellence and political commitment have no value, however, unless they have an ethically sound purpose. For us now the objective is to correct a dangerous and unacceptable imbalance: the majority of the world's population are still exposed to severe and fatal diseases which are in most cases preventable and curable.

Scientific and political conditions are the variables in our work, requiring a new response as the significance of each new piece of evidence becomes clear. But there is also this constant, which is the value of human health itself, and everyone's need for it, and society's obligation to meet that need. National health authorities exist to uphold the value of health as a matter not only of self-interest but of principle. Global interdependence makes an international health authority necessary for the same reason: to defend this principle regardless of the state of play between nations.

Recognizing health as an absolute human need, and thus an absolute obligation for society to provide for all its members as best it can, is one argument for putting the poor first, but it is by no means the only one. Some emphasize instead the utilitarian view that investing in the health of the disadvantaged will strengthen the global economy and bring greater prosperity and safety to all. Others see international health work as part of a wider effort to build a global society that maximizes the freedom of all to develop their own capabilities and live lives they consider to be valuable. These and other such arguments come from different political horizons but they converge in supporting urgent action in favor of those most in need. WHO's task is to lead this global action.

In the coming years it is results in countries that will be the measure of our success. More specifically, we must support countries in building up health systems that can meet the needs of everyone through the reliable provision of basic care. Global targets in nutrition, maternal and child health, access to essential medicines, and the control of specific diseases will contribute to an across-the-board strengthening of health systems, with a focus on primary health care. We will advance a major, new initiative to build country-level capacity in health surveillance and measurement. Meanwhile, we must ensure that the communities most directly concerned have an active say in setting health agendas. People's participation in making decisions that affect their lives is fundamental to a just and sustainable global order.

In no area is the union of science, moral vision, and political courage more urgent than in the treatment of HIV/AIDS. I have pledged to attack the AIDS crisis with new determination, and strongly support the "3 × 5" goal: three million people in developing countries on antiretroviral combination therapy by the end of 2005. Work toward "3 × 5" will be a testing ground for new ways of working within WHO. Responsibility will be delegated, administrative and financial transparency increased. Thinking and action will be less hierarchical and more flexible. Civil society groups representing grassroots communities will be key partners. Our constant focus will be on outcomes on the ground. To get results on the scale required, we must innovate. Creative input must come from all points in the network, not just the top. Collaborative work patterns can be greatly enhanced by information technology. But beyond new tools we need a more humane organizational culture, based on openness and mutual respect. The spirit of cooperation begins at home. Changes of this kind will enable the organization to make more effective use of its greatest resource—its people.

In our work, the hard sciences are entwined with economic social, political, and cultural determinants of health that often cannot easily be quantified. Attention to all these issues and their interconnections is vital for responsible scientific practice in the contemporary world. This is where the *Bulletin of the World Health Organization* will continue to make a very important contribution, as an independent voice within WHO, and a model of the open debate I will seek to nurture throughout this Organization.

Enormous challenges lie before the public health community. They will engage all WHO's capacities—scientific, political, and ethical. Yet the present situation also presents us with an opportunity to make bold progress. Global health issues are high on the international agenda. Many of the tasks before us are already well defined. Now is the time to "make it happen where it matters," by turning scientific knowledge into effective action for people's health.

Courtesy, Bulletin of the World Health Organization 81 (7): 473, 2003.

Chapter 41
Poverty and Disease—Health and Prosperity*

Report from WHO and UN agencies shows that the main diseases that cause and perpetuate poverty can be successfully controlled

Joint WHO and UN Report

A report jointly issued by six United Nations agencies claims that worsening AIDS, TB, and malaria epidemics are not inevitable, as shown by the many successful strategies to turn back these diseases and prevent the deaths they cause, deployed by several developing countries. The targets for reducing the toll of these illnesses, set by the world's leaders at successive summits over the years, are feasible. What is needed are the funds and systems that will enable widespread implementation of actions that have shown to be effective, the report says.

In a joint report—"Health, a Key to Prosperity: Success Stories in Developing Countries"—the World Health Organization (WHO), the United Nations Children's Fund (UNICEF), the United Nations Educational, Scientific and Cultural Organization (UNESCO), the Joint United Nations Programme on HIV/AIDS (UNAIDS), the United Nations Population Fund (UNFPA), and the World Bank outline key factors for combating AIDS, tuberculosis, malaria, childhood diseases, and maternal and perinatal conditions, even in resource-poor settings.

"The prospects of intervening to prevent death in developing countries have never been better," said Dr Gro Harlem Brundtland, former Director-General of WHO. "The evidence refutes those who doubt that the world's poorest communities can be protected from AIDS, tuberculosis (TB), malaria, childhood diseases, and maternal mortality. With a concerted effort from the international community we can turn the promise of these success stories into a reality in the coming years."

The publication of the Report came shortly after a meeting where representatives from the "Group of Eight" countries agreed to significantly scale up its global work to fight diseases in the world's poorest countries.

The Report contains success stories from 20 different countries, encompassing the widest variety of economic, social, and geographic conditions. It shows, for example, how countries such as Senegal, Uganda, and Thailand have developed strategies that successfully can reduce HIV infection rates, how Azerbaijan and Viet

---

* WHO Press WHO/78.

Nam have cut in half the number of deaths from malaria, how China, India, and Peru have cut TB deaths by half, and how Sri Lanka has drastically reduced maternal mortality.

"The success stories described in these pages demonstrate how far many nations have come in defining viable strategies to attack these public health threats and in scaling up for a national impact," said Mr James Wolfensohn, President of the World Bank.

> The stories illustrate many lessons. They demonstrate that success is possible even when resources are scarce. They show that inputs such as drugs or vaccines, as important as they are to improving health, are not enough. Political commitment, capacity-building, human resources, education and communication, local adaptation, and community involvement are critical. They also signal that strengthening and increased financing of underlying health systems and social services is key to ensuring a large-scale and more sustainable response.

The Report identifies six important characteristics of programs that have succeeded in controlling diseases of poverty:

- *political commitment* at the highest level is key to achieving results and sustaining programs.
- successful disease and mortality prevention has often involved new ways of working, for example, entering into *partnerships* with the private sector, nongovernmental organizations, and UN agencies.
- *innovation*, born out of a pragmatic approach to achieving results, has made all the difference in some countries.
- promoting the *home as the first hospital* helps reduce child deaths. In particular, the training and education of mothers has been a key to success.
- widespread *availability of supplies*, medicines, and other low-cost tools at community level is essential.
- *measuring results* is key to planning control measures.

Yet UNICEF Executive Director Carol Bellamy said many of these success stories remain invisible to a largely pessimistic world. "There's widespread scepticism about controlling disease in the developing world. In light of this report, such fatalism is simply unacceptable," said Ms Bellamy. "Given what we know, over the next decade it will be possible to make huge gains worldwide. But if we don't make a concerted effort now, we are, in essence, condemning millions of people to death, especially young children."

The Report is broken down into five sections: tuberculosis, malaria, AIDS, childhood disease, and maternal and perinatal conditions. Among its highlights are:

41.1 Tuberculosis

Almost two million people die from TB every year—98% in poor developing countries. And yet anti-TB medicines are 95% effective in curing TB and cost as little as US$ 10 for a six-month course of treatment.

In Peru, for example, high-level political commitment has produced one of the most successful TB-control programs in the world. On current trends, the number of new TB cases could be halved every 10 years. Diagnosis and treatment are provided free of charge, and low-income families receive food packages to encourage compliance with treatment.

In general, elements of successful TB control using WHO's DOTS (Directly Observed Treatment Short-course) strategy include:

- government commitment to sustained TB control,
- detection of TB cases through sputum smear microscopy among symptomatic people,
- regular and uninterrupted supply of high-quality anti-TB drugs,
- 6–8 months of regularly supervised treatment,
- reporting systems to monitor treatment progress and program performance.

41.2 Malaria

Malaria kills over one million people per year, mostly in Africa, and most of them children. And women are especially vulnerable to malaria during pregnancy, when the disease can lead to life-threatening anemia, miscarriages, and the birth of premature, low birth-weight babies.

More rapid and effective treatment of malaria with antimalarial drugs could prevent malaria deaths. Antimalarial drugs cost as little as US$ 0.12 per treatment. Meanwhile, many child deaths from malaria can be prevented through the widespread use of low-cost, insecticide-treated bednets. But, so far, only an estimated 1% of African children today sleep under a bednet, due to poverty.

The main prongs of the Roll Back Malaria partnership's strategy to reduce the ill health and poverty which malaria induces include:

- access to rapid diagnosis and treatment at village/community level,
- preventive treatment for pregnant women,
- multiple measures to prevent mosquito bites,
- a focus on mothers and children—the highest risk groups,
- better use of existing malaria control tools,
- research to develop new medicines, vaccines, and other tools,
- improved surveillance to improve epidemic forecasting and response.

Azerbaijan, Ethiopia, Kenya, and Viet Nam have all shown success in rolling back malaria. In Viet Nam, for example, government commitment, largely in the form of the supplying of free insecticide-treated bednets and the use of locally produced, high-quality antimalarial drugs, reduced the malaria death toll by 97% in a 5-year timespan. The concerted drive against the disease involved a major investment in training and disease reporting systems, the use of mobile teams to supervise health workers, and the mobilization of volunteer health workers. And in Kenya, an innovative scheme involving a community bednet-sewing industry, workplace promotion of bednets, and employer-sponsored payroll purchasing schemes has helped reduce malaria cases, slash overall healthcare cost, reduce absenteeism, decrease poverty, and increase productivity among the workers involved.

41.3 AIDS

While figures show that HIV/AIDS killed an estimated three million people in 2000, the United Nations argues against accepting a worsening AIDS pandemic as inevitable. Although there is no AIDS vaccine and antiretroviral therapy is still unaffordable for most poor, developing countries, experience in countries such as Senegal, Thailand, and Uganda has shown that reduction in infection rates is possible. Effective prevention measures include:

- access to condoms,
- prophylaxis and treatment of opportunistic infections including STIs and TB,
- sex education at school and beyond,
- access to voluntary counseling and testing,
- counseling and support for pregnant women and efforts to prevent mother-to-child transmission of HIV,
- promotion of safe injection practices and blood safety,
- access to safe drug-injecting equipment.

The example of Thailand, for instance, shows how government determination to promote 100% condom use in brothels and to ensure wide access to HIV-prevention campaigns through schools, the mass media, and the workplace has been a key factor in lowering HIV infection rates; the Report notes that by 1997, for example, HIV infection rates among 21-year-old military conscripts had fallen to 1.5%, from a peak of 4% in 1993.

The Report also notes that a year's supply of condoms costs only US$ 14.

"Twenty years of experience of the epidemic have demonstrated some key components of an effective response: strong leadership, partnerships, overcoming stigma, addressing social vulnerability, linking prevention to care, focusing on young people, and encouraging community involvement in the response," explained Dr Peter Piot, Executive Director of UNAIDS.

The UN agencies emphasize in the Report that even the Thai approach may not be sustainable if the program focuses just on heterosexuals, and if there is not continuous adequate funding.

"Girls and women are most vulnerable to HIV infection, given the social and economic disadvantages they face in their day-today lives," added Dr Nafis Sadik, Executive Director of UNFPA. "The burden of caring for entire families falls increasingly on the shoulders of women as AIDS continues to devastate families and communities. Further efforts must be made to empower women and girls and create a space for female decision-making in private as well as public life. The success stories included in this report serve as an important reminder of the power of committed and focused multilateral partnerships."

"The AIDS epidemic is eroding the educational systems of many countries, especially in sub-Saharan Africa," added Mr Koichiro Matsuura, Director-General of UNESCO.

An alarming percentage of teachers are affected by HIV, and millions of children and adolescents are no longer able to go to school. There is no infrastructure to deal with the crisis, which is undermining these countries' economic, social, and human development. It is imperative that the international community rallies to the rescue of these teachers and students. Equally indispensable is the need for extensive AIDS-prevention educational programs, which, to be effective, must be respectful of the cultural context of the populations they target.

41.4 Childhood Diseases

In developing countries, 70% of childhood deaths—over 8 million—are caused by no more than five conditions: pneumonia, diarrhea, malaria, measles, and malnutrition. Three out of every four children who seek healthcare are suffering from one or more of these conditions. Yet low-cost interventions are available to prevent or treat them. These are diseases of poverty.

In Mexico, for example, determined efforts by the government to promote the use of oral rehydration therapy (which costs as little as US$ 0.33), to immunize children against measles, and to improve access to safe water and sanitation have succeeded in reducing childhood deaths from diarrheal diseases by 60% in less than a decade. Other key factors in this success have included an increase in education levels among women, investment of adequate resources, and the widespread use of case management guidelines.

41.5 Maternal and Perinatal Conditions

Every year, more than half a million women worldwide die from complications of pregnancy and childbirth—mainly severe bleeding, infections, unsafe abortions, hypertension, and obstructed labour. Almost 90% of these deaths occur in Asia and poor sub-Saharan Africa. And most of them could be prevented at low cost. WHO's Mother–Baby package, for example, costs no more than US$ 3 in low-income countries. The strategy involves ensuring access to:

- antenatal care,
- normal delivery care assisted by a skilled birth attendant,
- treatment for complications of pregnancy,
- neonatal care,
- family planning advice,
- management of STIs.

Sri Lanka, for example, is a major success story. In that country, where a third of the population is estimated to live below the poverty line, maternal mortality rates are among the lowest in the developing world. Most deliveries take place in a health facility, with the support of a skilled birth attendant. This achievement is the result of government's commitment to improving education and health in Sri Lanka, the relatively high status of women, and high female literacy rates.

The Editors

S. William A. Gunn, MD, MS, FRCSC, FRCSI(Hon), DSc(Hon), Dr h c, is a surgeon and senior international health official involved in humanitarian medicine and disaster management. Formerly Head of the WHO Emergency Humanitarian Operations, he has conducted numerous field missions, advised governments and organized programmes for complex emergencies, services recognized by Honorary Doctorates and other distinctions. Founding President of the WHO Medical Society and the International Association for Humanitarian Medicine, he is editor of the Journal of Humanitarian Medicine and author of eleven books, including the classic Dictionary of Disaster Medicine and International Relief, translated into several languages. Fellow of the Royal College of Surgeons of Canada, with several university affiliations, he is interested in the interactions between health, human rights, basic surgical needs and sustainable development particularly in emerging societies. He is the principal editor of this book.

Michele Masellis, MD, is an Italian surgeon with extensive activities in burn therapy, reconstructive surgery and international health. Formerly Professor of Plastic and Reconstructive Surgery at the Universities of Padua and Palermo, he co-founded and is now President of the Mediterranean Council on Burns and Fire Disasters. Among a rich contribution to surgical literature, he is co-editor of three books and of the periodicals Annals of Burns and Fire Disasters and Journal of Humanitarian Medicine. Member and Honorary Member of several professional associations, he has been awarded the Spanish Red Cross Silver Medal and the Italian President's Gold Medal for Public Health. He is currently the Director of the International Association for Humanitarian Medicine, and co-editor of this book.

Index